Teen Health Series

Pregnancy and Birth
SOURCEBOOK

Third Edition

Third Edition

Pregnancy and Birth

SOURCEBOOK

Basic Consumer Health Information about Pregnancy and Fetal Development, Including Facts about Fertility and Conception, Physical and Emotional Changes during Pregnancy, Prenatal Care and Diagnostic Tests, High-Risk Pregnancies and Complications, Labor, Delivery, and the Postpartum Period

Along with Tips on Maintaining Health and Wellness during Pregnancy and Caring for Newborn Infants, a Glossary of Related Terms, and a Directory of Resources for Additional Help and Information

Edited by
Amy L. Sutton

Omnigraphics

P.O. Box 31-1640, Detroit, MI 48231

Bibliographic Note
Because this page cannot legibly accommodate all the copyright notices, the Bibliographic Note portion of the Preface constitutes an extension of the copyright notice.

Edited by Amy L. Sutton

Health Reference Series
Karen Bellenir, *Managing Editor*
David A. Cooke, MD, FACP, *Medical Consultant*
Elizabeth Collins, *Research and Permissions Coordinator*
Cherry Edwards, *Permissions Assistant*
EdIndex, Services for Publishers, *Indexers*

* * *

Omnigraphics, Inc.
Matthew P. Barbour, *Senior Vice President*
Kevin M. Hayes, *Operations Manager*

* * *

Peter E. Ruffner, *Publisher*

Copyright © 2009 Omnigraphics, Inc.
ISBN 978-0-7808-1074-7

Library of Congress Cataloging-in-Publication Data

Pregnancy and birth sourcebook : basic consumer health information about pregnancy and fetal development ... / edited by Amy L. Sutton. -- 3rd ed.
   p. cm.
   Summary: "Provides basic consumer health information about the reproductive process from preconception through the postpartum period, with facts about fertility, maintaining health during pregnancy, coping with high risk pregnancies and complications, and newborn care. Includes index, glossary of related terms and directory of resources"--Provided by publisher.
   Includes bibliographical references and index.
   ISBN 978-0-7808-1074-7 (hardcover : alk. paper) 1. Pregnancy--Popular works. 2. Childbirth--Popular works. 3. Pregnancy--Complications--Popular works. I. Sutton, Amy L.
   RG525.P676 2009
   618.2--dc22
                                                                    2009029246

∞

This book is printed on acid-free paper meeting the ANSI Z39.48 Standard. The infinity symbol that appears above indicates that the paper in this book meets that standard.

Printed in the United States

Table of Contents

Visit www.healthreferenceseries.com to view *A Contents Guide to the Health Reference Series*, a listing of more than 15,000 topics and the volumes in which they are covered.

Part II: Understanding Pregnancy-Related Changes and Fetal Development

Part V: Pregnancy Complications

Part VIII: Additional Help and Information

Preface

About This Book

Although the months of anticipation before a woman becomes a parent can be joyous and fulfilling, they can also mark a time filled with uncertainty and worry over potential birth defects, pregnancy complications, and chronic health conditions. These worries are not unfounded. Recent statistics show increases in preterm deliveries, low birthweight babies, and the incidence of cesarean sections among U.S. births. Fortunately, maternal and fetal monitoring, prenatal care, and healthy habits can reduce the risk of complications and make labor, delivery, and the postpartum period less stressful.

Pregnancy and Birth Sourcebook, Third Edition provides health information about the reproductive process—from preconception through the postpartum period. It provides information about fertility, infertility, and pregnancy prevention. The book's chapters explain the physical and emotional changes that occur during pregnancy, and they discuss topics related to staying healthy during pregnancy, including eating nutritiously, exercising regularly, obtaining prenatal care, and avoiding harmful substances. Facts about high risk pregnancies—such as those in women with chronic medical conditions, advanced maternal age, or weight concerns—are included. Finally, the book answers common questions about labor and delivery, postpartum recovery, newborn screening, and infant care. A glossary of terms and a directory of resources for information and support are also provided.

How to Use This Book

This book is divided into parts and chapters. Parts focus on broad areas of interest. Chapters are devoted to single topics within a part.

Part I: Preconception Health: Preparing for Pregnancy provides information about health habits, screenings, and interventions women may need prior to conception. This part also addresses factors that influence fertility (such as age and stress), details common causes of infertility, and identifies methods of preventing unintended pregnancies.

Part II: Understanding Pregnancy-Related Changes and Fetal Development provides trimester-by-trimester details about physical changes in the fetus. The part also identifies early signs of pregnancy, suggests strategies for determining conception and due dates, and discusses emotional concerns and physical changes that may occur during pregnancy, including depression, back pain, pelvic floor and bladder problems, and vision and oral changes.

Part III: Staying Healthy during Pregnancy highlights strategies women can undertake to help promote a healthy pregnancy. These include getting prenatal care and related medical tests, using medication safely, eating nutritiously, exercising, preventing excessive weight gain, and avoiding toxic substances and other harmful exposures. This part also offers advice on how pregnant women can stay safe at work or during travel.

Part IV: High-Risk Pregnancies discusses pregnancies at high risk due to maternal age, multiple fetuses, or chronic health conditions, including allergies, asthma, cancer, diabetes, epilepsy, lupus, sickle cell disease, thyroid disease, eating disorders, and obesity.

Part V: Pregnancy Complications describes diseases and disorders that may influence a pregnancy's outcome, such as amniotic fluid abnormalities, birth defects, bleeding, blood clots, gestational diabetes, hypertension, severe nausea and vomiting, placental complications, Rh incompatibility, umbilical cord abnormalities, and sexually transmitted diseases and other infections. This part also offers information about preterm labor and pregnancy loss, including ectopic pregnancy, miscarriage, and stillbirth.

Part VI: Labor and Delivery includes information about planning for labor and delivery by choosing a birthing center or hospital, selecting a birth partner or doula, and preparing a birth plan. This part also provides details on the stages of labor, pain relief during labor, vaginal and cesarean births, and emergency situations that may occur during childbirth.

Part VII: Postpartum and Newborn Care discusses common postpartum concerns, including recovery expectations for new mothers, newborn care and screening tests, breastfeeding and formula-feeding tips, strategies for bonding with a new baby, and considerations for working after a child's birth.

Part VIII: Additional Help and Information includes a glossary of important terms and a directory of organizations that provide help, information, and assistance to low-income pregnant women and their partners.

Bibliographic Note

This volume contains documents and excerpts from publications issued by the following U.S. government agencies: Agency for Healthcare Research and Quality (AHRQ); AIDSinfo; Center for Devices and Radiological Health (CDRH); Center for the Evaluation of Risks to Human Reproduction (CERHR); Centers for Disease Control and Prevention (CDC); Environmental Protection Agency (EPA); National Cancer Institute (NCI); National Heart, Lung, and Blood Institute (NHLBI); National Human Genome Research Institute (NHGRI); National Institute of Arthritis and Musculoskeletal and Skin Diseases (NIAMS); National Institute of Child Health and Human Development (NICHD); National Institute of Diabetes and Digestive and Kidney Diseases (NIDDK); National Institute of Environmental Health Sciences (NIEHS); National Institute of Mental Health (NIMH); National Institute of Neurological Disorders and Stroke (NINDS); National Institute on Alcohol Abuse and Alcoholism (NIAAA); National Institutes of Health (NIH); Office of Women's Health; U.S. Department of Health and Human Services (HHS); U.S. Department of Labor (DOL); and the U.S. Food and Drug Administration (FDA).

In addition, this volume contains copyrighted documents from the following organizations: Academy of General Dentistry; A.D.A.M., Inc.; American Academy of Family Physicians; American College of Allergy, Asthma and Immunology; American College of Nurse-Midwives; American Pregnancy Association; American Society for Reproductive Medicine; American Society of Anesthesiologists; BabyCenter LLC; Childbirth Connection; Children's Hospital of Pittsburgh; DONA

International; Hepatitis B Foundation; Hyperemesis Education and Research Foundation; Institute for Women's Policy Research; Henry J. Kaiser Family Foundation; Lamaze International; March of Dimes Birth Defects Foundation; National Campaign to Prevent Teen and Unplanned Pregnancy; National Network for Immunization Information; The Nemours Foundation; Obesity Action Coalition; Organization of Teratology Information Services (OTIS); Prevent Blindness America; and the University of Pittsburgh Medical Center.

Full citation information is provided on the first page of each chapter or section. Every effort has been made to secure all necessary rights to reprint the copyrighted material. If any omissions have been made, please contact Omnigraphics to make corrections for future editions.

Acknowledgements

Thanks go to the many organizations, agencies, and individuals who have contributed materials for this *Sourcebook* and to medical consultant Dr. David Cooke and document engineer Bruce Bellenir. Special thanks go to managing editor Karen Bellenir and research and permissions coordinator Liz Collins for their help and support.

About the Health Reference Series

The *Health Reference Series* is designed to provide basic medical information for patients, families, caregivers, and the general public. Each volume takes a particular topic and provides comprehensive coverage. This is especially important for people who may be dealing with a newly diagnosed disease or a chronic disorder in themselves or in a family member. People looking for preventive guidance, information about disease warning signs, medical statistics, and risk factors for health problems will also find answers to their questions in the *Health Reference Series*. The *Series*, however, is not intended to serve as a tool for diagnosing illness, in prescribing treatments, or as a substitute for the physician/patient relationship. All people concerned about medical symptoms or the possibility of disease are encouraged to seek professional care from an appropriate health care provider.

A Note about Spelling and Style

Health Reference Series editors use *Stedman's Medical Dictionary* as an authority for questions related to the spelling of medical terms and the *Chicago Manual of Style* for questions related to grammatical structures, punctuation, and other editorial concerns. Consistent adherence is not always possible, however, because the individual volumes within the *Series* include many documents from a wide variety of different producers and copyright holders, and the editor's primary goal is to present material from each source as accurately as is possible following the terms specified by each document's producer. This sometimes means that information in different chapters or sections may follow other guidelines and alternate spelling authorities. For example, occasionally a copyright holder may require that eponymous terms be shown in possessive forms (Crohn's disease *vs.* Crohn disease) or that British spelling norms be retained (leukaemia *vs.* leukemia).

Locating Information within the Health Reference Series

The *Health Reference Series* contains a wealth of information about a wide variety of medical topics. Ensuring easy access to all the fact sheets, research reports, in-depth discussions, and other material contained within the individual books of the *Series* remains one of our highest priorities. As the *Series* continues to grow in size and scope, however, locating the precise information needed by a reader may become more challenging.

A Contents Guide to the Health Reference Series was developed to direct readers to the specific volumes that address their concerns. It presents an extensive list of diseases, treatments, and other topics of general interest compiled from the Tables of Contents and major index headings. To access *A Contents Guide to the Health Reference Series*, visit www.healthreferenceseries.com.

Medical Consultant

Medical consultation services are provided to the *Health Reference Series* editors by David A. Cooke, MD, FACP. Dr. Cooke is a graduate of Brandeis University, and he received his M.D. degree from the University of Michigan. He completed residency training at the University of Wisconsin Hospital and Clinics. He is board-certified in Internal Medicine. Dr. Cooke currently works as part of the University of Michigan Health System and practices in Ann Arbor, MI. In his free time, he enjoys writing, science fiction, and spending time with his family.

Our Advisory Board

Health Reference Series *Update Policy*

The inaugural book in the *Health Reference Series* was the first edition of *Cancer Sourcebook* published in 1989. Since then, the *Series* has been enthusiastically received by librarians and in the medical community. In order to maintain the standard of providing high-quality health information for the layperson the editorial staff at Omnigraphics felt it was necessary to implement a policy of updating volumes when warranted.

Medical researchers have been making tremendous strides, and it is the purpose of the *Health Reference Series* to stay current with the most recent advances. Each decision to update a volume is made on an individual basis. Some of the considerations include how much new information is available and the feedback we receive from people who use the books. If there is a topic you would like to see added to the update list, or an area of medical concern you feel has not been adequately addressed, please write to:

Editor
Health Reference Series
Omnigraphics, Inc.
P.O. Box 31-1640
Detroit, MI 48231
E-mail: editorial@omnigraphics.com

Part One

Preconception Health: Preparing for Pregnancy

Chapter 1

Overview of Reproductive Health

What is reproductive health?

Reproductive health includes a variety of topics, such as:

- menstruation and menopause;
- pregnancy and preconception care;
- fertility/infertility;
- contraception;
- sexually transmitted diseases and AIDS/HIV [acquired immunodeficiency syndrome/human immunodeficiency syndrome]; and
- health and function of the male and female reproductive systems.

What is the menstrual cycle?

The menstrual cycle is the process by which a woman's body gets ready for the chance of a pregnancy each month. The average menstrual cycle is 28 days from the start of one to the start of the next, but it can range from 21 days to 35 days.

From "Reproductive Health," by the National Institute of Child Health and Human Development (NICHD, www.nichd.nih.gov), part of the National Institutes of Health, February 5, 2008.

Most menstrual periods last from three to five days. In the United States, most girls start menstruating at age 12, but girls can start menstruating between the ages of 8 and 16.

What is pregnancy?

Pregnancy is the term used to describe when a woman has a growing fetus inside of her. In most cases, the fetus grows in the uterus.

Human pregnancy lasts about 40 weeks, or just more than 9 months, from the start of the last menstrual period to childbirth.

What are prenatal and preconception care and why are they important?

Prenatal care is the care woman gets during a pregnancy. Getting early and regular prenatal care is important for the health of both mother and the developing baby.

In addition, health care providers are now recommending a woman see a health care provider for preconception care, even before she considers becoming pregnant or in between pregnancies.

Both preconception care and prenatal care help to promote the best health outcomes for mother and baby.

What is infertility?

Infertility is the term health care providers use for women who are unable to get pregnant, and for men who are unable to impregnate a woman, after at least one year of trying.

In women, the term is used to describe those who are of normal childbearing age, not those who can't get pregnant because they are near or past menopause. Women who are able to get pregnant but who cannot carry a pregnancy to term (birth) may also be considered infertile.

Infertility is a complex problem—it does not have a single cause because getting pregnant is a multi-step chain of events. The cause of infertility can rest in the women or the man, or can be from unknown factors or a combination of factors.

What is contraception?

Contraception, also known as birth control, is designed to prevent pregnancy. Some types of birth control include (but are not limited to):

- Barrier methods, such as condoms, the diaphragm, and the cervical cap, are designed to prevent the sperm from reaching the egg for fertilization.

- Intrauterine device, or IUD, is a small device that is inserted into the uterus by a health care provider. The IUD prevents a fertilized egg from implanting in the uterus. An IUD can stay in the uterus for up to 10 years until it is removed by a health care provider.

- Hormonal birth control, such as birth control pills, injections, skin patches, and vaginal rings, release hormones into a woman's body that interfere with fertility by preventing ovulation, fertilization, or implantation.

- Sterilization is a method that permanently prevents a woman from getting pregnant or a man from being able to get a woman pregnant. Sterilization involves surgical procedures that must be done by a health care provider and usually cannot be reversed.

The choice of birth control depends on factors such as a person's overall health, age, frequency of sexual activity, number of sexual partners, desire to have children in the future, and family history of certain diseases. A woman should talk to her health care provider about her choice of birth control method.

It is important to remember that even though birth control methods can prevent pregnancy, they do not all protect against sexually transmitted diseases or HIV.

Chapter 2

Preconception Considerations

Chapter Contents

Section 2.1

What to Do before You Conceive

From "Healthy Pregnancy: Before You Start Trying," by the Office of
Women's Health (www.womenshealth.gov), part of the U.S. Department
of Health and Human Services, March 2007.

Some foods, habits, and medicines can harm your baby—even before he is conceived. Find out what to do and what to avoid when you're
trying to get pregnant.

Before Pregnancy

If you're thinking about getting pregnant, or are already pregnant,
taking care of your health is more important than ever. Follow these
tips for a healthy pregnancy:

- **Get 400 micrograms (or 0.4 mg) of folic acid daily.** Eat
  foods fortified with folic acid, take a multivitamin, or take a
  folic acid pill to get your daily dose. Taking folic acid in a pill is
  the best way to be sure you're getting enough. Including 0.4 mg
  of folic acid (or folate) in your diet before you get pregnant and
  in the first three months of pregnancy can help prevent some
  birth defects. If you don't get enough folic acid, your baby's spine
  may not form right. This is called spina bifida. Also, your baby
  needs folic acid to develop a healthy brain. Many doctors will
  prescribe a vitamin with folic acid. But you also can buy vitamins or folic acid pills at drug and grocery stores. Some foods
  rich in folate include: leafy green vegetables, kidney beans, orange juice and other citrus fruits, peanuts, broccoli, asparagus,
  peas, lentils, and whole-grain products. Folic acid is also added
  to some foods like enriched breads, pastas, rice, and cereals.

- **Start watching what you eat.** Load up on fruits, vegetables,
  and whole-grains (such as whole-wheat breads or crackers).
  Eat plenty of calcium-rich foods such as non-fat or low-fat yogurt, milk, and broccoli. Your baby needs calcium for strong
  bones and teeth. When fruits and vegetables aren't in season,

frozen vegetables are a good option. Avoid eating a lot of fatty foods (such as butter and fatty meats). Choose leaner foods when you can (such as skim milk, chicken and turkey without the skin, and fish).

- **Tell your doctor if you smoke or use alcohol or drugs.** Quitting is hard, but you can do it. Ask your doctor for help.

- **Get enough sleep.** Try to get seven to nine hours every night. Take steps to control the stress in your life. When it comes to work and family, figure out what you can and can not do. Set limits with yourself and others. Don't be afraid to say no to requests for your time and energy.

- **Move your body.** Once you get pregnant, you can't increase your exercise routine by much. So it's best to start before the baby is on the way.

- **Get any health problems under control.** Talk to your doctor about how your health problems might affect you and your baby. If you have diabetes, monitor your blood sugar levels. If you have high blood pressure, monitor these levels as well. If you are overweight, talk to your doctor about how to reach a healthy weight.

- **Ask your mother, aunts, grandmother or sisters about their pregnancies.** Did they have morning sickness? Problems with labor? How did they cope?

- **Find out what health problems run in your family.** Tell these to your doctor. You can get tested for health problems that run in families before getting pregnant (genetic testing).

- **Make sure you have had all of your immunizations (shots), especially for rubella (German measles).** If you haven't had chickenpox or rubella, get the shots at least three months before getting pregnant.

- **Get checked for hepatitis B and C, sexually transmitted diseases (STDs), and HIV [human immunodeficiency virus].** These infections can harm you and your baby. Tell your doctor if you or your sex partners have ever had an STD or HIV.

- **Go over all of the medicines you take (prescription, over-the-counter, and herbals) with your doctor.** Make sure they are safe to take while you're trying to get pregnant or are pregnant.

Planning Conception

While trying to conceive, you can use natural planning methods such as the ovulation method (have intercourse just before or after ovulation) or the symptothermal method (evaluating fertility based on your daily temperature). Remember: women are more likely to become pregnant if intercourse takes place just before or just after ovulation. This is because the unfertilized egg can live for only 12–24 hours in your body. If you've been trying for a few months with no results, don't get discouraged. Only 20% of women trying to get pregnant are successful on the first attempt. So don't lose hope or assume something is wrong.

Adoption and Foster Care

If you are having fertility problems, you and your partner might want to explore other ways to raise a child. Find out more about adoption and foster care. Adopting or becoming a foster parent could be one of the most rewarding experiences of your life.

Section 2.2

Understanding Genetic Counseling and Evaluation: Is It Right for You?

From "Frequently Asked Questions About Genetic Counseling," by the National Human Genome Research Institute (NHGRI, www.genome.gov), March 28, 2008.

What are genetic professionals and what do they do?

Genetics professionals arc health care professionals with specialized degrees and experience in medical genetics and counseling. Genetics professionals include geneticists, genetic counselors, and genetics nurses.

What is genetic counseling and evaluation?

Genetic professionals work as members of health care teams providing information and support to individuals or families who have genetic disorders or may be at risk for inherited conditions. Genetic professionals:

- assess the risk of a genetic disorder by researching a family's history and evaluating medical records;
- weigh the medical, social, and ethical decisions surrounding genetic testing;
- provide support and information to help a person make a decision about testing;
- interpret the results of genetic tests and medical data;
- provide counseling or refer individuals and families to support services;
- serve as patient advocates;
- explain possible treatments or preventive measures; and
- discuss reproductive options.

11

How do I find a genetic professional?

Your health care provider may refer you to a genetic professional. Universities and medical centers also often have affiliated genetic professionals or can provide referrals to a genetic professional or genetics clinic.

As more has been learned about genetics, genetic professionals have grown more specialized. For example, they may specialize in a particular disease (such as cancer genetics), an age group (such as adolescents), or a type of counseling (such as prenatal).

How do I decide whether I need to see a geneticist or other specialist?

Your health care provider may refer you to a geneticist—a medical doctor or medical researcher—who specializes in your disease or disorder. A medical geneticist has completed a fellowship or has other advanced training in medical genetics. While a genetic counselor or genetic nurse may help you with testing decisions and support issues, a medical geneticist will make the actual diagnosis of a disease or condition. Many genetic diseases are so rare that only a geneticist can provide the most complete and current information about your condition.

Along with a medical geneticist, you may also be referred to a physician who is a specialist in the type of disorder you have. For example, if a genetic test is positive for colon cancer, you might be referred to an oncologist. For a diagnosis of Huntington disease, you may be referred to a neurologist.

Chapter 3

Questions and Answers about Preconception Care

What is preconception health?

Preconception health is a woman's health before she becomes pregnant. It focuses on the conditions and risk factors that could affect a woman if she becomes pregnant. Preconception health applies to women who have never been pregnant, and also to women who could become pregnant again. Preconception health looks at factors that can affect a fetus or infant. These include factors such as taking prescription drugs or drinking alcohol. The key to promoting preconception health is to combine the best medical care, healthy behaviors, strong support, and safe environments at home and at work.

What is preconception health care?

Preconception health care is care given to a woman before pregnancy to manage conditions and behaviors which could be a risk to her or her baby. There are many topics covered under preconception care, including:

- folic acid supplements to prevent neural tube defects;
- rubella vaccinations to prevent congenital rubella syndrome;

Excerpted from "Preconception Care Questions and Answers," by the Centers for Disease Control and Prevention, National Center on Birth Defects and Developmental Disabilities (NCBDDD, http://www.cdc.gov/ncbddd), April 12, 2006.

- detecting and treating existing health conditions to prevent complications in the mother, and reduce the risk of birth defects. Complications include:

  - diabetes;

  - hypothyroidism;

  - HIV/AIDS [human immunodeficiency virus/acquired immunodeficiency syndrome];

  - hepatitis B;

  - PKU [phenylketonuria];

  - hypertension;

  - blood diseases; and

  - eating disorders;

- reviewing medications that can affect the fetus or the mother, such as epilepsy medicine, blood thinners, and some medicines used to treat acne, such as Accutane;

- reviewing a woman's pregnancy history;

- stopping smoking to reduce the risk of low birth weight;

- eliminating alcohol consumption to prevent fetal alcohol syndrome, and other complications;

- family planning counseling to avoid unplanned pregnancies; and

- counseling to promote healthy behaviors such as appropriate weight, nutrition, exercise, oral health. Counseling can help a woman avoid substance abuse and toxic substances. It can help women and couples understand genetic risks, mental health issues (such as depression), and intimate partner domestic violence.

Good preconception health care is about managing current health conditions. By taking action on health issues before pregnancy, future problems for the mother and baby can be prevented. Preconception health care must be tailored to each individual woman. It means helping women and their partners reduce risks and get ongoing care. Men and other family members are also very important in supporting the goals of preconception health.

14

Does preconception health apply to women who do not plan to get pregnant?

Absolutely. Every woman should be thinking about her health and whether or not she wants to get pregnant. Some of the basic recommendations for preconception health include healthy weight and nutrition and identifying and managing existing conditions and infections. All women should quit smoking and avoid other harmful substances. These are important health goals for everyone, not just women planning to get pregnant.

Since over half of all pregnancies in the United States are unplanned, women who might be sexually active with male partners should consider their health. As they might not know they are pregnant, women need to avoid risks, such as using medications that could harm a fetus, whenever possible.

CDC recommends that men and women think about a reproductive life plan. This means deciding the ideal time and conditions for having children and learning how to achieve these goals. This can include effective contraception. Women's lives are rich and complex, and the possibility of pregnancy is only one factor affecting women's health choices. The more that women know about the health care relevant to their own circumstances, the more empowered they are to make the right choices for their lives.

How long before becoming pregnant should a woman start preparing for pregnancy? What are the five most important things she should do before pregnancy for her and her baby's health?

Every man and woman should prepare for pregnancy before becoming sexually active, or at least three months before conception. Women should begin some of the recommendations even sooner—such as quitting smoking, reaching healthy weight, and adjusting medications. Planning for pregnancy is also a good time to talk about other concerns. Issues such as intimate partner domestic violence, mental health, and previous pregnancy problems need to be discussed. Although men and women can do much on their own, a health care provider is necessary for finding and treating existing health problems. They can also help a woman improve her health before pregnancy.

The five most important things a woman can do for preconception health are:

1. Take 400 mcg of folic acid a day for at least 3 months before becoming pregnant to reduce the risk of birth defects.

2. Stop smoking and drinking alcohol.

3. If you currently have a medical condition, be sure these conditions are under control. Conditions include but are not limited to asthma, diabetes, oral health, obesity, or epilepsy. Be sure that your vaccinations are up to date.

4. Talk to your doctor and pharmacist about any over-the-counter and prescription medicines you are taking, including vitamins and dietary or herbal supplements.

5. Avoid exposures to toxic substances or potentially infectious materials at work or at home, such as chemicals or cat and rodent feces.

The new recommendations say that everyone should have a reproductive life plan. What does this really mean?

A reproductive life plan is a set of personal goals about having (or not having) children. It also states how to achieve those goals. Everyone needs to make a reproductive plan based on personal values and resources. Here are some examples:

- "I'm not ready to have children now. I'll make sure I don't get pregnant. Either I won't have heterosexual sex, or I'll correctly use effective contraception."

- "I'll want to have children when my relationship feels secure and I've saved enough money. I won't become pregnant until then. After that, I'll visit my doctor to discuss preconception health. I'll try to get pregnant when I'm in good health."

- "I'd like to be a father after I finish school and have a job to support a family. While I work toward those goals, I'll talk to my wife about her goals for starting a family. I'll make sure we correctly use an effective method of contraception every time we have sex until we're ready to have a baby."

- "I'd like to have two children, and space my pregnancies by at least two years. I'll visit my certified nurse midwife to discuss preconception health now. I'll start trying to get pregnant as soon as I'm healthy. Once I have a baby, I'll get advice from a

16

health professional on birth control. I don't want to have a second baby before I'm ready."

- "I will let pregnancy happen whenever it happens. Because I don't know when that will be, I'll make sure I'm in optimal health for pregnancy at all times."

There are many kinds of reproductive life plans. What's important is that you think about when and under what conditions you want to become pregnant. Then make sure your actions support these goals. Health care providers and counselors can help you understand the clinical and lifestyle options that are best for you.

What can men do to support the preconception health of their female partners and their future babies?

Men can make a big difference in promoting good preconception health. As boyfriends, husbands, fathers-to-be, partners, and family members, they can learn how their loved ones can achieve optimal preconception health. They can encourage and support women in every aspect of preparing for pregnancy.

There are other ways men can help. Men who work with chemicals or other toxins need to be careful that they don't expose women to them. For example, men who use fertilizers or pesticides in agricultural jobs should change out of dirty work clothes before coming near their female partners. They should handle and wash soiled clothes separately.

The family health histories of men are also important when planning a pregnancy. Understanding genetic risks from both sides enables providers to give more accurate advice. Screening for and treating STIs (sexually transmitted infections) in men can help make sure that the infections are not passed to female partners. Men can improve their own reproductive health by reducing stress, eating right, avoiding excessive alcohol use, not smoking, and talking to their health care providers about their own medications. It is also important for men who smoke to stop smoking around their partners to avoid the harmful effects of secondhand smoke.

What should my health care provider be doing about preconception care at my regular visits?

Health care providers have a lot to cover during an appointment, so it's always a good idea to make a list and bring up any issues on your mind. Do this even if the health care provider doesn't ask about them. The first thing to discuss is your plan for pregnancy. If you tell your provider that you might become pregnant in the near future, there will be a number of things to discuss. You may need to schedule another visit to make sure everything gets covered.

Your health care provider should:

- review your family's medical history. This includes your previous experiences with pregnancy, fertility, birth, and use of birth control methods.

- ask about your lifestyle, behaviors, and social support concerns that affect your health. Do you smoke, drink alcohol, use drugs, or have psychological problems, including depression? Do you have nutrition and diet issues? Concerns about health conditions in your or your partner's family? Are there issues around intimate partner domestic violence? What are the medications you are taking? Are there chemicals, solvents, radiation, or other potential risks at your workplace or home that could harm you or your baby?

- schedule health screening tests—Pap smear, urinalysis, blood tests. Your provider needs to know your blood type, Rh factor, and whether you have diabetes, hypertension, sexually transmitted infections, or other conditions.

- review your immunization status and update them if needed.

- perform a physical exam, including a pelvic exam and a blood pressure check.

Based on your individual health, your health care provider will suggest a course of treatment or follow up care as needed.

Chapter 4

Factors That Affect Fertility

Chapter Contents

Section 4.1

Age and Fertility

From "Maternal Age," *Child Health USA 2007*, U.S. Department of Health and Human Services, Health Resources and Services Administration, Maternal and Child Health Bureau, 2008.

In 2005, the general fertility rate rose slightly to 66.7 births per 1,000 women aged 15–44 years. The birth rate among teenagers aged 15–19 years continued to decline, reaching another record low (40.5 births per 1,000 women aged 15–19).

This rate was 35 percent lower than the most recent peak reported in 1991 (61.8 births per 1,000). The highest birth rate was among women aged 25–29 (115.5 per 1,000), followed by women aged 20–24 years (102.2 per 1,000). There was a 2.0 percent increase in birth rates among women aged 35–39 years and 40–44 years, since 2004, to 46.3 and 9.1 per 1,000, respectively.

In 2005, 10.2 percent of births were to women aged 19 years and younger, and 52.5 percent of births were to women in their twenties; more than one-third of births were to women in their thirties, and 2.7 percent were to women aged 40–54 years. The average age at first birth was 25.2 years; this is an increase of almost 4 years since 1970.

Among non-Hispanic Black and Hispanic women, more than 56 percent of births were to women in their twenties, while just over half of births to non-Hispanic White women occurred in the same age group. The proportion of births to teenagers was higher among non-Hispanic Black and Hispanic women (17.0 and 14.1 percent, respectively) than to non-Hispanic White women (7.3 percent). Non-Hispanic White women giving birth were more likely to be in the 30- to 54-year-old age range than were either non-Hispanic Black or Hispanic women.

Section 4.2

Stress and Fertility

Stress can come from just about anything that you feel is threatening or harmful. A single event (or your worry about it) can produce stress. So can the little things that worry you all day long.

Acute stress, caused by a single event (or your fear of it), makes your heart beat faster and your blood pressure go up. You breathe harder, your hands get sweaty, and your skin feels cool and clammy. Chronic stress, which is when you are always stressed, can cause depression and changes in your sleep habits. It can also decrease your chances of fighting off common illnesses.

Stress makes many body organs work harder than normal and increases the production of some important chemicals in your body, including hormones.

Is stress causing my infertility?

Probably not. Even though infertility is very stressful, there isn't any proof that stress causes infertility. In an occasional woman, having too much stress can change her hormone levels and therefore cause the time when she releases an egg to become delayed or not take place at all.

Is infertility causing my stress?

Maybe. Many women who are being treated for infertility have as much stress as women who have cancer or heart disease. Infertile couples experience stress each month: first they hope that the woman is pregnant; and if she is not, the couple has to deal with their disappointment.

21

Why is infertility stressful?

Most couples are used to planning their lives. They may believe that if they work hard at something, they can achieve it. So when it's hard to get pregnant, they feel as if they don't have control of their bodies or of their goal of becoming parents. With infertility, no matter how hard you work, it may not be possible to have a baby.

Infertility tests and treatments can be physically, emotionally, and financially stressful. Infertility can cause a couple to grow apart, which increases stress levels. Couples may have many doctor appointments for infertility treatment, which can cause them to miss work or other activities.

What can I do to reduce my stress?

- Talk to your partner.

- Realize you're not alone. Talk to other people who have infertility, through individual or couple counseling, or support groups.

- Read books on infertility, which will show you that your feelings are normal and can help you deal with them.

- Learn stress reduction techniques such as meditation, yoga, or acupuncture.

- Avoid taking too much caffeine or other stimulants.

- Exercise regularly to release physical and emotional tension.

- Have a medical treatment plan with which both you and your partner are comfortable.

- Learn as much as you can about the cause of your infertility and the treatment options available.

- Find out as much as you can about your insurance coverage and make financial plans regarding your fertility treatments.

Who can help us?

RESOLVE is a national support organization for couples with infertility. For information on local chapters, you can reach them at 1310 Broadway, Somerville, Massachusetts 02144; (617) 623- 0744. Also, support information and weekly Internet chat sessions can be found through the American Fertility Association at www.afafamilymatters .com.

Section 4.3

Sperm Shape: Does It Affect Fertility?

How do doctors decide if a man might have a fertility problem? For many years, experts have focused on semen analysis, but research studies show that the number of sperm (count) and the movement of sperm (motility) do not always predict fertility very well by themselves. It may also be useful to look at the shape of the sperm (morphology), which is also one of the important parts of the semen evaluation.

An updated way of determining sperm shape is called the Kruger's strict morphology method. Kruger morphology is a useful system that helps doctors determine if a sperm is normally shaped or not. It was originally used to predict the success of in vitro fertilization (IVF), a fertility treatment in which the sperm are mixed with the woman's egg in a laboratory. More recently, it has been used to tell if intracytoplasmic sperm injection (ICSI) is a necessary treatment. ICSI is a procedure that helps a sperm fertilize an egg by injecting a single sperm directly into the center of the egg.

Even though it is used for these purposes, not all physicians and scientists are sure that strict morphology method alone predicts success with IVF or whether it indicates the need for ICSI.

Characteristics of normal sperm. A normal sperm has:

- a smooth, oval shaped head that is 5–6 micrometers long and 2.5–3.5 micrometers around (less than the size of a needle point);

- a well defined cap (acrosome) that covers 40% to 70% of the sperm head;

- no visible defect of neck, midpiece, or tail;

23

- no fluid droplets in the sperm head that are bigger than one-half of the sperm head size.

Intercourse versus artificial insemination. For patients with fertility problems, sperm morphology may have an effect on your ability to achieve a pregnancy. If the strict sperm morphology is more than 4%, there may be little difference in success whether timed intercourse or artificial insemination is utilized.

In vitro fertilization. A successful pregnancy using IVF depends on many of factors: how many eggs are fertilized, whether the fertilized eggs grow into embryos, and whether the embryo implants in the woman's uterus. When strict morphology is 4% or less, eggs may have a better chance of fertilization with the use of ICSI.

Frequently Asked Questions

If an abnormally shaped sperm fertilizes the egg, does that mean that my child will have genetic abnormalities?

There's no scientific link between the shape of a sperm and its chromosomal content. Once the sperm penetrates the egg, fertilization has a good chance of taking place. However, there may be some male offspring who will inherit the same type of morphology abnormalities. Whether routine investigation of Y-chromosome abnormalities should be initiated when low morphology is noted is controversial.

Are there any substances that I can reduce or eliminate exposure to (e.g., alcohol, tobacco, caffeine) in order to improve the shape of my sperm?

Studies haven't shown a clear link between abnormal sperm shape and these factors, but it's a good idea to try to eliminate use of tobacco and recreational drugs and limit your consumption of alcohol. These substances reduce sperm production and function in several ways. They may hurt sperm DNA (material that carries your genes) quality. Studies have not shown a clear link between caffeine consumption and changes in sperm shape.

Are there any dietary supplements or vitamins that I can take to improve morphology?

Dietary supplements or vitamins have not been clearly shown to improve sperm morphology. Some specialists do recommend that you take a daily multivitamin to improve a number of body functions, including reproductive health.

Section 4.4

Paternal Exposures to Toxins

"Paternal Exposures and Pregnancy," © 2002 Organization of Teratology Information Services (OTIS). Reprinted with permission. Member programs of OTIS are located throughout the U.S. and Canada. To find the Teratogen Information Service in your area, call OTIS toll-free at 866-626-OTIS (866-626-6847), or visit www.otispregnancy.org. Reviewed by David A. Cooke, MD, FACP, April 29, 2009.

This text talks about the risks that paternal exposures can have during pregnancy. With each pregnancy, all women have a 3% to 5% chance of having a baby with a birth defect. This information should not take the place of medical care and advice from your health care provider.

What is a paternal exposure?

A paternal exposure is anything the father of the baby is exposed to before conception or during his partner's pregnancy. Examples include recreational drugs, alcohol, cigarette smoking, chemotherapy or radiation treatments, environmental or occupational exposures, and prescription or over-the-counter medications.

Do paternal exposures cause any problems related to pregnancy?

Yes. Certain exposures may affect a man's ability to father a child by changing the production, size, shape, or performance of sperm. Such changes may cause infertility, delay in getting his partner pregnant, or early pregnancy loss. Data from animal and human studies suggest that paternal exposures may cause genetic changes in sperm which may cause an embryo to fail to develop or cause an increased risk for childhood cancers in an exposed man's children.

Do paternal exposures cause birth defects?

Agents that may cause birth defects do not reach the developing fetus through the father as they do from the pregnant woman. Substances that a father is exposed to may be found in small amounts in the semen, but there is no evidence that these small amounts interfere with normal fetal development. Currently, there is no evidence that paternal exposures increase the risk of birth defects. However, further study is needed in this area.

Can recreational drugs, if used by the father, affect my pregnancy?

These substances may be found in the semen. Recreational drug use may affect sperm quality or provide limited direct exposure to the developing fetus. However, there is no clear evidence that birth defects may result from the use of these substances by the father.

Can alcohol use by the father affect my chances of getting pregnant or affect the baby during pregnancy?

Heavy alcohol use in males may affect sperm formation and function, or may cause impotence. Whether a father's alcohol use increases the risks for birth defects is still being investigated. A recent study suggested that paternal alcohol use may be associated with an increased risk for certain rare heart defects in newborns. More information is needed in this area before a conclusion can be made.

What if the father of the baby smokes cigarettes?

Paternal smoking has been associated with small reductions in sperm quality, but there have been no reports of reduced fertility due to smoking in men. A small association between adverse pregnancy effects and paternal smoking, and a slight increase in certain types of cancer in offspring of smoking fathers has been seen. One study on a small number of babies born with rare heart defects found an association with paternal smoking. Additional studies on the effects of paternal smoking on pregnancy outcome are needed.

Can chemotherapy or radiation for cancer treatments given to the father affect my pregnancy?

Sperm production is frequently affected during cancer treatment. Sometimes, sperm production may return to normal after certain chemotherapy or radiation treatments, but it is not guaranteed.

Men who are facing cancer treatment may wish to consider sperm banking prior to starting treatment. It is recommended that men undergoing chemotherapy wait for at least three months after the end of treatment before attempting to father a child. Certain chemotherapy treatments have been shown to increase the chance of having a fetus with more or less than the normal number of chromosomes.

Damage to the structure of chromosomes in sperm of cancer patients may also occur. It is believed that most of the damage is not permanent, but some studies have detected higher than normal levels of abnormal sperm years after the end of chemotherapy. At this time, there are no data demonstrating an increase in birth defects in the children of cancer patients.

Can the father's workplace exposures affect my pregnancy?

According to the National Institute of Occupational Safety and Health (NIOSH), a number of workplace substances including lead, organic solvents, pesticides, and radiation have been identified as reproductive hazards to men. Some studies in humans suggest that such exposures may be associated with decreased sperm production, increased sperm abnormalities, decreased fertility, and an increased risk of miscarriage in the wives of these workers.

In addition, men exposed to heavy metals, pesticides, and other chemicals in the workplace may carry very small amounts of these agents on their clothes and shoes into the home. This may cause direct exposure of their partner prior to conception or during pregnancy. However, no data are available at this time regarding any increases in birth defects due to such exposures. Further studies are needed in these areas.

Can prescription or over-the-counter medications taken by the father affect my pregnancy?

Paternal exposure to medications prescribed for conditions like high blood pressure or high cholesterol have not been associated with an increased risk of birth defects in the developing fetus. Likewise, over-the-counter medications to treat other conditions have not been associated with an increased risk of birth defects. However, it is important to discuss any concerns you may have with your physician.

References

Brent R, et al. 1993. Ionizing and nonionizing radiations. In: *Occupational and Environmental Reproductive Hazards: A Guide for Clinicians,* Ed.: Maureen Paul, Williams, and Wilkin. Baltimore, MD.

Cohen FL. 1986. Paternal contribution to birth defects. *Nurs Clin North Amer* 21:49–64.

Colie CF 1993. Male mediated teratogenesis. *Reprod Toxicol* 7:3–9.

Correa-Villasenor A, et al. 1993. Paternal exposures and cardiovascular malformations. The Baltimore-Washington Infant Study Group. *J Expo Anal Environ Epidemiol Suppl* 1:173–185.

Generoso WM, et al. 1990. Concentration-response curves for ethylene oxide-induced heritable translocations and dominant lethal mutations. *Environ Mol Mutagen* 16:126–131.

Generoso WM, et al. 1995. Dominant lethal and heritable translocation tests with chlorambucil and melphalan in male mice. *Mutat Res* 345:167–180.

Generoso WM, et al. 1975. 6-Mercaptopurine: an inducer of cytogenetic and dominant lethal effects in premeiotic and early meiotic germ cells of male mice. *Mutat Res* 28:437–447.

Hunt PA. 1987. Ethanol-induced aneuploidy in male germ cells of the mouse. *Cytogenet Cell Genet* 44(1):7–10.

Jensen BK, e al. 1991. The negligible availability of retinoids with multiple and excessive topical application of isotretinoin 0.05% gel (Isotrex) in patients with acne vulgaris. *J Am Acad Dermatol* 24:425–428.

Ji BT, Shu XO, Linet MS, Zheng W, Wacholder S, Gao YT, Ying DM, Jin F (1997) Paternal cigarette smoking and the risk of childhood cancer among offspring of nonsmoking mothers. *J Natl Cancer Inst* 89:238–244.

Obe G and Anderson D. 1987. International Commission for Protection against Environmental Mutagens and Carcinogens. ICPEMC Working Paper No. 15/1. Genetic effects of ethanol. *Mutat Res* 186(3): 177–200.

Pearn JH. 1983. Teratogens and the male. *Med J of Austr* 2:16–20.

Sallmen M, et al. 1998, Time to pregnancy among the wives of men exposed to organic solvents. *Occup Environ Med* 55:24–30.

Sallmen M, et al. 2000 Paternal exposure to lead and infertility. *Epidemiol* 11(2):148–152.

Sallmen M, et al. 1998. Time to pregnancy among the wives of men exposed to organic solvents. *Occup Environ Med.* 55(1):24–30.

Savitz DA, et al. 1991. Influence of paternal age, smoking, and alcohol consumption on congenital anomalies. *Teratology* 44:429–440.

Shelby MD, et al. 1986. Dominant lethal effects of acrylamide in male mice. *Mutat Res* 173:35–40.

Steinberger EK, et al. 2002. Infants with single ventricle: a population based epidemiological study. *Teratology* 65(3):106–115.

Taskinen H, et. al. 1989. Spontaneous abortions and congenital malformations among the wives of men occupationally exposed to organic solvents. *Scand J Work Environ Health* 15:345–52.

Tielemans E, et. al. 1999. Occupationally related exposures and reduced semen quality: a case-control study. *Fert Steril* 71:690–696.

Trasler JM and Doerksen T. 1999. Teratogen update: Paternal exposures reproductive risks. *Teratology* 60(3):161–72.

Vine MF. 1996. Smoking and male reproduction: a review. *Int J Androl* 10(6):323–337.

Chapter 5

Trying to Conceive

Chapter Contents

Section 5.1

Tips for Trying to Conceive

From "Trying to Conceive," by the Office of Women's Health
(www.womenshealth.gov), part of the U.S. Department of Health and
Human Services, April 2006.

Fertility Awareness

The Menstrual Cycle

Being aware of your menstrual cycle and the changes in your
body that happen during this time can be key to helping you plan a
pregnancy, or avoid pregnancy. During the menstrual cycle (a total
average of 28 days), there are two parts: before ovulation and after
ovulation.

- Day 1 starts with the first day of your period.

- Usually by Day 7, a woman's eggs start to prepare to be fertilized by sperm.

- Between Day 7 and 11, the lining of the uterus (womb) starts to
  thicken, waiting for a fertilized egg to implant there.

- Around Day 14 (in a 28-day cycle), hormones cause the egg that
  is most ripe to be released, a process called ovulation. The egg
  travels down the fallopian tube towards the uterus. If a sperm
  unites with the egg here, the egg will attach to the lining of the
  uterus, and pregnancy occurs.

- If the egg is not fertilized, it will break apart.

- Around Day 25 when hormone levels drop, it will be shed from
  the body with the lining of the uterus as a menstrual period.

The first part of the menstrual cycle is different in every woman,
and even can be different from month-to-month in the same woman,
varying from 13 to 20 days long. This is the most important part of
the cycle to learn about, since this is when ovulation and pregnancy

can occur. After ovulation, every woman (unless she has a health problem that affects her periods) will have a period within 14 to 16 days.

Charting Your Fertility Pattern

Knowing when you're most fertile will help you plan or prevent pregnancy. There are three ways you can keep track of your fertile times. They are:

Basal body temperature method: Basal body temperature is your temperature at rest as soon as you awake in the morning. A woman's basal body temperature rises slightly with ovulation. So by recording this temperature daily for several months you'll be able to predict your most fertile days.

Basal body temperature differs slightly from woman to woman. Anywhere from 96 to 98 degrees orally is average before ovulation. After ovulation most women have an oral temperature between 97 and 99 degrees. The rise in temperature can be a sudden jump or a gradual climb over a few days.

Usually a woman's basal body temperature rises by only 0.4 to 0.8 degrees Fahrenheit. To detect this tiny change, women must use a basal body thermometer. These thermometers are very sensitive. Most pharmacies sell them for around $10. You then record your temperature on a special chart.

The rise in temperature doesn't show exactly when the egg is released. But almost all women have ovulated within three days after their temperatures spike. Body temperature stays at the higher level until your period starts.

You are most fertile and most likely to get pregnant:

- two to three days before your temperature hits the highest point (ovulation), and
- 12 to 24 hours after ovulation.

A man's sperm can live for up to three days in a woman's body. The sperm can fertilize an egg at any point during that time. So if you have unprotected sex a few days before ovulation there is a chance of becoming pregnant.

Many things can affect basal body temperature. To get the most useful chart you should take your temperature every morning at about the same time. Things that can alter your temperature include:

- drinking alcohol the night before;

- smoking cigarettes the night before;
- getting a poor night's sleep;
- having a fever;
- doing anything in the morning before you take your temperature—including going to the bathroom and talking on the phone.

Calendar method: This involves keeping a written record of each menstrual cycle on a calendar. The first day of your period is Day 1. Circle Day 1 on the calendar. Do this for eight to 12 months so you know how many days are in your cycle. The length of your cycle may vary from month to month. So write down the total number of days it lasts each time. To find out the first day when you are most fertile, check your list for the cycle with the fewest days. Then subtract 18 from that number. Take this new number and count ahead that many days on the calendar. Draw an X through this date. The X marks the first day you're likely to be fertile. To find out the last day when you are fertile, subtract 11 days from your longest cycle and draw an X through this date. This method always should be used with other fertility awareness methods, especially if your cycles are not always the same lengths.

Cervical mucus method (also known as the ovulation method): This involves being aware of the changes in your cervical mucus throughout the month. The hormones that control the menstrual cycle also change the kind and amount of mucus you have before and during ovulation. Right after your period, there are usually few days when there is no mucus present or "dry days." As the egg starts to mature, mucus increases in the vagina, appears at the vaginal opening, and is white or yellow and cloudy and sticky. The greatest amount of mucus appears just before ovulation. During these "wet days" it becomes clear and slippery, like raw egg whites. Sometimes it can be stretched apart. This is when you are most fertile. About four days after the wet days begin the mucus changes again. There will be much less and it becomes sticky and cloudy. You might have a few more dry days before your period returns. Describe changes in your mucus on a calendar. Label the days, "Sticky," "Dry," or "Wet." You are most fertile at the first sign of wetness after your period or a day or two before wetness begins. This method is less reliable for some women. Women who are breastfeeding, taking hormonal contraceptives (like the pill), using feminine hygiene products, have vaginitis or sexually transmitted diseases (STDs), or have had surgery on the cervix should not rely on this method.

To most accurately track your fertility, use a combination of all three methods. This is called the symptothermal method.

Infertility

It is not uncommon to have trouble becoming pregnant or to experience infertility. Infertility is defined as not being able to become pregnant, despite trying for one year, in women under age 35, or after six months in women 35 and over. Pregnancy is the result of a chain of events. As described in the Fertility Awareness section, a woman must release an egg from one of her ovaries (ovulation). The egg must travel through a fallopian tube toward her uterus. A man's sperm must join with (fertilize) the egg along the way. The fertilized egg must then become attached to the inside of the uterus. While this may seem simple, in fact many things can happen to prevent pregnancy.

Reasons for Infertility

Age

There are many different reasons why a couple might have infertility. One is age-related. Women today are often delaying having children until later in life, when they are in their 30s and 40s. A couple of things add to this trend. Birth control is easy to obtain and use, more women are in the work force, women are marrying at an older age, the divorce rate remains high, and married couples are delaying pregnancy until they are more financially secure. But the older you are, the harder it is to become pregnant. Women generally have some decrease in fertility starting in their early 30s. And while many women in their 30s and 40s have no problems getting pregnant, fertility especially declines after age 35.

As a woman ages, there are normal changes that occur in her ovaries and eggs. All women are born with over a million eggs in their ovaries (all the eggs that they will ever have), but only have about 300,000 left by puberty. Then of these, only about 300 eggs will be ovulated during the reproductive years. Even though menstrual cycles continue to be regular in a woman's 30s and 40s, the eggs that ovulate each month are of poorer quality than those from her 20s. It is harder to get pregnant when the eggs are poorer in quality.

Ovarian reserve is the number and quality of eggs in your ovaries and how well the ovarian follicles respond to hormones in your body. As you approach menopause, your ovaries don't respond as well to your hormones, and in time they may not release an egg each month. A reduced ovarian reserve is natural as a woman ages, but young women might have reduced ovarian reserves due to smoking, a prior surgery on their ovaries, or a family history of early menopause. Also, as a woman and her eggs age, if she becomes pregnant, there is a greater chance of having genetic problems, such as having a baby with Down syndrome. Embryos formed from eggs in older women also are less likely to fully develop, a main reason for miscarriage (early pregnancy loss).

Health Problems

Couples also can have fertility problems because of health problems, in either the woman or the man. Common problems with a woman's reproductive organs, like uterine fibroids, endometriosis, and pelvic inflammatory disease can worsen with age and also affect fertility. These conditions might cause the fallopian tubes to be blocked, so the egg can't travel through the tubes into the uterus.

Some people also have diseases or conditions that affect their hormone levels, which can cause infertility in women and impotence and infertility in men. Polycystic ovarian syndrome (PCOS) is one such hormonal condition that affects many women, and is the most common cause of anovulation, or when a woman rarely or never ovulates. Another hormonal condition that is a common cause of infertility is when a woman has a luteal phase defect (LPD). A luteal phase is the time in the menstrual cycle between ovulation and the start of the next menstrual period. LPD is a failure of the uterine lining to be fully prepared for a fertilized egg to implant there. This happens either because a woman's body is not producing enough progesterone, or the uterine lining isn't responding to progesterone levels at some point in the menstrual cycle. Since pregnancy depends on a fertilized egg implanting in the uterine lining, LPD can interfere with a woman getting pregnant and with carrying a pregnancy successfully.

Certain lifestyle choices also can have a negative effect on a woman's fertility, such as smoking, alcohol use, weighing much more or much less than an ideal body weight, a lot of strenuous exercise, and having an eating disorder.

Unlike women, some men remain fertile into their 60s and 70s. But as men age, they might begin to have problems with the shape and movement of their sperm, and have a slightly higher risk of sperm gene defects. They also might produce no sperm, or too few sperm. Lifestyle choices also can affect the number and quality of a man's sperm. Alcohol and drugs can temporarily reduce sperm quality. And researchers are looking at whether environmental toxins, such as pesticides and lead, also may be to blame for some cases of infertility. Men also can have health problems that affect their sexual and reproductive function. These can include sexually transmitted diseases (STDs), diabetes, surgery on the prostate gland, or a severe testicle injury or problem.

If you or your partner has a problem with sexual function or libido, don't delay seeing your doctor for help.

Treating Infertility

You should talk to your doctor about your fertility if you:

- are under age 35 and, after a year of frequent sex without birth control, you are having problems getting pregnant; or

- are age 35 or over and, after six months of frequent sex without birth control, you are having problems getting pregnant; or

- believe you or your partner might have fertility problems in the future (even before you begin trying to get pregnant).

Your doctor can refer you to a fertility specialist, a doctor who focuses in treating infertility. This doctor can recommend treatments such as drugs, surgery, or assisted reproductive technology. Don't delay seeing your doctor because age also affects the success rates of these treatments.

There are many ways to treat infertility.

Tests

The first step to treat infertility is to see a doctor for a fertility evaluation. He or she will test both the woman and the man to find out where the problem is. Testing on the man focuses on the number and health of his sperm. The lab will look at a sample of his sperm under a microscope to check sperm number, shape, and movement. Blood tests also can be done to check hormone levels. More tests might be needed to look for infection or problems with hormones. These tests can include:

- an x-ray (to look at his reproductive organs);

- a mucus penetrance test (to see if sperm can swim through mucus); or

- a hamster-egg penetrance assay (to see if sperm can go through hamster egg cells, somewhat showing their power to fertilize human eggs).

Testing for the woman first looks at whether she is ovulating each month. This can be done by having her chart changes in her morning body temperature, by using an FDA [U.S. Food and Drug Administration]-approved home ovulation test kit (which she can buy at a drug store), or by looking at her cervical mucus, which changes throughout her menstrual cycle. Ovulation also can be checked in her doctor's office with an ultrasound test of the ovaries, or simple blood tests that check hormone levels, like the follicle-stimulating hormone (FSH) test. FSH is produced by the pituitary gland. In women, it helps control the menstrual cycle and the production of eggs by the ovaries. The amount of FSH varies throughout the menstrual cycle and is highest just before an egg is released. The amounts of FSH and other hormones (luteinizing hormone, estrogen, and progesterone) are measured in both a man and a woman to determine why the couple cannot achieve pregnancy. If the woman is ovulating, more testing will need to be done. These tests can include:

- a hysterosalpingogram (an x-ray to check if the fallopian tubes are open and to show the shape of the uterus);

- a laparoscopy (an exam of the tubes and other female organs for disease); and

- an endometrial biopsy (an exam of a small shred of the uterine lining to see if monthly changes in it are normal).

Other tests can be done to show whether the sperm and mucus are interacting in the right way, or if the man or woman is forming antibodies that are attacking the sperm and stopping them from getting to the egg.

Drugs and Surgery

Different treatments for infertility are recommended depending on what the problem is. About 90 percent of cases are treated with drugs or surgery. Various fertility drugs may be used for women with ovulation problems. It is important to talk with your doctor about the drug to be used. You should understand the drug's benefits and side effects. Depending on the type of fertility drug and the dosage of the drug used, multiple births (such as twins) can occur in some women. If needed, surgery can be done to repair damage to a woman's ovaries, fallopian tubes, or uterus. Sometimes a man has an infertility problem that can be corrected by surgery.

Assisted Reproductive Technology (ART)

Assisted reproductive technology (ART) uses special methods to help infertile couples, and involves handling both the woman's eggs and the man's sperm. Success rates vary and depend on many factors. But ART has made it possible for many couples to have children that otherwise would not have been conceived. ART can be expensive and time-consuming. Many health insurance companies do not provide coverage for infertility or provide only limited coverage. Check your health insurance contract carefully to learn about what is covered. Also, some states have laws for infertility insurance coverage. Some of those include Arkansas, California, Connecticut, Hawaii, Illinois, Maryland, Massachusetts, Rhode Island, Texas, and West Virginia.

In vitro fertilization (IVF) is a type of ART that is often used when a woman's fallopian tubes are blocked or when a man has low sperm counts. A drug is used to stimulate the ovaries to produce multiple eggs. Once mature, the eggs are removed and placed in a culture dish with the man's sperm for fertilization. After about 40 hours, the eggs are examined to see if they have become fertilized by the sperm and are dividing into cells. These fertilized eggs (embryos) are then placed in the woman's uterus, thus bypassing the fallopian tubes. Gamete intrafallopian transfer (GIFT) is similar to IVF, but used when the woman has at least one normal fallopian tube. Three to five eggs are placed in the fallopian tube, along with the man's sperm, for fertilization inside the woman's body. Zygote intrafallopian transfer (ZIFT), also called tubal embryo transfer, combines IVF and GIFT. The eggs retrieved from the woman's ovaries are fertilized in the lab and placed in the fallopian tubes rather than the uterus.

ART sometimes involves the use of donor eggs (eggs from another woman) or previously frozen embryos. Donor eggs may be used if a woman has impaired ovaries or has a genetic disease that could be passed on to her baby. And if a woman does not have any eggs, or her eggs are not of a good enough quality to produce a pregnancy, she and her partner might want to consider surrogacy. A surrogate is a woman who agrees to become pregnant using the man's sperm and her own egg. The child will be genetically related to the surrogate and the male partner, but the surrogate will give the baby to the couple at birth.

A gestational carrier might be an option for women who do not have a uterus, from having had a hysterectomy, but still have their ovaries, or for women who shouldn't become pregnant because of a serious health problem. In this case, the woman's eggs are fertilized by the man's sperm and the embryo is placed inside the carrier's uterus. In this case, the carrier will not be related to the baby, and will give the baby to the parents at birth.

Counseling and Support Groups

If you've been having problems getting pregnant, you know how frustrating it can feel. Not being able to get pregnant can be one of the most stressful experiences a couple has. Both counseling and support groups can help you and your partner talk about your feelings, and to help you meet other couples like you in the same situation. You will learn that anger, grief, blame, guilt, and depression are all normal. Couples do survive infertility, and can become closer and stronger in the process. Ask your doctor for the names of counselors or therapists with an interest in fertility.

Section 5.2

Do Sexual Positions Affect Conception?

Are some sexual positions better than others for conceiving?

There's no evidence that any particular sexual position is more likely to lead to conception. You may have heard that positions that deposit the sperm closest to the cervix—such as the missionary position (man on top)—are more promising than other positions. But there are no studies to back this up.

Proper timing, on the other hand, is a crucial factor. To make conception more likely, have sex a day or two before you expect to ovulate and then again on the day of ovulation.

Will having an orgasm help my chances of conceiving?

Some people believe that a woman who climaxes after her partner ejaculates is more likely to get pregnant, but there's no evidence to support this notion either.

The female orgasm isn't a necessary component of conception, but it is possible that uterine contractions help sperm move toward the fallopian tubes. (Such painless contractions happen involuntarily even when you're not having sex, particularly around the time of ovulation.)

Should I stay lying down afterward?

There's no evidence that it makes a difference, but it can't hurt. Remaining horizontal for 15 minutes or so after intercourse allows more semen to remain in your vagina. Of course, with millions of sperm in every ejaculation, there should be plenty of sperm in your vagina even if you get up right away.

Note: If you've been trying to conceive for a year or more without success (or three to six months if you're 35 or older), or your periods are irregular, your best bet is to see a fertility specialist.

Section 5.3

Using Ovulation Predictor Kits

From "Home-Use Tests: Ovulation (Urine Test)," from the Center for Devices and Radiological Health (www.fda.gov/cdrh), part of the U.S. Food and Drug Administration, February 1, 2003. Reviewed by David A. Cooke, MD, FACP, March 31, 2009.

What does this test do?

This is a home-use test kit to measure luteinizing hormone (LH) in your urine. This helps detect the LH surge that happens in the middle of your menstrual cycle, about 1 to 1½ days before ovulation. Some tests also measure another hormone—estrone-3-glucuronide (E3G).

What is LH?

Luteinizing hormone (LH) is a hormone produced by your pituitary gland. Your body always makes a small amount of LH, but just before you ovulate, you make much more LH. This test can detect this LH surge, which usually happens 1 to 1½ days before you ovulate.

What is E3G?

E3G is produced when estrogen breaks down in your body. It accumulates in your urine around the time of ovulation and causes your cervical mucus to become thin and slippery. Sperm may swim more easily in your thin and slippery cervical mucus, increasing your chances of getting pregnant.

What type of test is this?

This is a qualitative test—you find out whether or not you have elevated LH or E3G levels, not if you will definitely become pregnant.

Why should you do this test?

You should do this test if you want to know when you expect to ovulate and be in the most fertile part of your menstrual cycle. This test can be used to help you plan to become pregnant. You should not use this test to help prevent pregnancy, because it is not reliable for that purpose.

How accurate is this test?

How well this test will predict your fertile period depends on how well you follow the instructions. These tests can detect LH and E3G reliably about nine times out of 10, but you must do the test carefully.

How do you do this test?

You add a few drops of your urine to the test, hold the tip of the test in your urine stream, or dip the test in a cup of your urine. You either read the test by looking for colored lines on the test or you put the test device into a monitor. You can get results in about 5 minutes. The details of what the color looks like, or how to use the monitor varies among the different brands.

Most kits come with multiple tests to allow you to take measurements over several days. This can help you find your most fertile period, the time during your cycle when you can expect to ovulate based on your hormone levels. Follow the instructions carefully to get good results. You will need to start your testing at the proper time during your cycle, otherwise the test will be unreliable, and you will not find your hormonal surges or your fertile period.

Is this test similar to the one my doctor uses?

The fertility tests your doctor uses are automated, and they may give more consistent results. Your doctor may use other tests that are not yet available for home use (i.e., blood and urine laboratory tests) and information about your history to get a better view of your fertility status.

Chapter 6

Frequently Asked Questions about Infertility

What is infertility?

Most experts define infertility as not being able to get pregnant after at least one year of trying. Women who are able to get pregnant but then have repeat miscarriages are also said to be infertile.

Pregnancy is the result of a complex chain of events. In order to get pregnant:

- a woman must release an egg from one of her ovaries (ovulation);

- the egg must go through a fallopian tube toward the uterus (womb);

- a man's sperm must join with (fertilize) the egg along the way;

- the fertilized egg must attach to the inside of the uterus (implantation).

Infertility can result from problems that interfere with any of these steps.

Excerpted from "Infertility: Frequently Asked Questions," Office of Women's Health (www.womenshealth.gov), part of the U.S. Department of Health and Human Services, May 1, 2006.

Is infertility a common problem?

About 12 percent of women (7.3 million) in the United States aged 15 to 44 had difficulty getting pregnant or carrying a baby to term in 2002, according to the National Center for Health Statistics of the Centers for Disease Control and Prevention.

Is infertility just a woman's problem?

No, infertility is not always a woman's problem. In only about one-third of cases is infertility due to the woman (female factors). In another one third of cases, infertility is due to the man (male factors). The remaining cases are caused by a mixture of male and female factors or by unknown factors.

What causes infertility in men?

Infertility in men is most often caused by:

- problems making sperm—producing too few sperm or none at all; or
- problems with the sperm's ability to reach the egg and fertilize it—abnormal sperm shape or structure prevent it from moving correctly.

Sometimes a man is born with the problems that affect his sperm. Other times problems start later in life due to illness or injury. For example, cystic fibrosis often causes infertility in men.

What increases a man's risk of infertility?

The number and quality of a man's sperm can be affected by his overall health and lifestyle. Some things that may reduce sperm number and/or quality include:

- alcohol;
- drugs;
- environmental toxins, including pesticides and lead;
- smoking cigarettes;
- health problems;
- medicines;

- radiation treatment and chemotherapy for cancer; and
- age.

What causes infertility in women?

Problems with ovulation account for most cases of infertility in women. Without ovulation, there are no eggs to be fertilized. Some signs that a woman is not ovulating normally include irregular or absent menstrual periods.

Less common causes of fertility problems in women include:

- blocked fallopian tubes due to pelvic inflammatory disease, endometriosis, or surgery for an ectopic pregnancy;
- physical problems with the uterus; and
- uterine fibroids.

What things increase a woman's risk of infertility?

Many things can affect a woman's ability to have a baby. These include:

- age;
- stress;
- poor diet;
- athletic training;
- being overweight or underweight;
- tobacco smoking;
- alcohol;
- sexually transmitted diseases (STDs); and
- health problems that cause hormonal changes.

How long should women try to get pregnant before calling their doctors?

Most healthy women under the age of 30 shouldn't worry about infertility unless they've been trying to get pregnant for at least a year. At this point, women should talk to their doctors about a fertility evaluation. Men should also talk to their doctors if this much time has passed.

In some cases, women should talk to their doctors sooner. Women in their 30s who've been trying to get pregnant for 6 months should speak to their doctors as soon as possible. A woman's chances of having a baby decrease rapidly every year after the age of 30. So getting a complete and timely fertility evaluation is especially important.

Some health issues also increase the risk of fertility problems. So women with the following issues should speak to their doctors as soon as possible:

- irregular periods or no menstrual periods;
- very painful periods;
- endometriosis;
- pelvic inflammatory disease; and
- more than one miscarriage.

No matter how old you are, it's always a good idea to talk to a doctor before you start trying to get pregnant. Doctors can help you prepare your body for a healthy baby. They can also answer questions on fertility and give tips on conceiving.

Chapter 7

Preventing Unintended Pregnancies

Chapter Contents

Section 7.1

Contraception (Birth Control)

Excerpted from "Birth Control Methods: Frequently Asked Questions,"
by the Office of Women's Health, March 19, 2009.

What Is the Best Method of Birth Control (or Contraception)?

There is no best method of birth control. Each method has its pros and cons.

All women and men can have control over when, and if, they become parents. Making choices about birth control, or contraception, isn't easy. There are many things to think about. To get started, learn about birth control methods you or your partner can use to prevent pregnancy. You can also talk with your doctor about the choices.

Before choosing a birth control method, think about:

- your overall health;
- how often you have sex;
- the number of sex partners you have;
- if you want to have children someday;
- how well each method works to prevent pregnancy;
- possible side effects; and
- your comfort level with using the method.

Keep in mind, even the most effective birth control methods can fail. But your chances of getting pregnant are lowest if the method you choose always is used correctly and every time you have sex.

What Are the Different Types of Birth Control?

You can choose from many methods of birth control. Talk with your doctor if you have questions about any of the choices.

Continuous Abstinence

This means not having sex (vaginal, anal, or oral) at any time. It is the only sure way to prevent pregnancy and protect against sexually transmitted infections (STIs), including HIV [human immunodeficiency virus].

Natural Family Planning/Rhythm Method

This method is when you do not have sex or use a barrier method on the days you are most fertile (most likely to become pregnant).

A woman who has a regular menstrual cycle has about nine or more days each month when she is able to get pregnant. These fertile days are about five days before and three days after ovulation, as well as the day of ovulation.

To have success with this method, you need to learn about your menstrual cycle. Then you can learn to predict which days you are fertile or "unsafe." To learn about your cycle, keep a written record of:

- when you get your period;
- what it is like (heavy or light blood flow); and
- how you feel (sore breasts, cramps).

This method also involves checking your cervical mucus and recording your body temperature each day. Cervical mucus is the discharge from your vagina. You are most fertile when it is clear and slippery like raw egg whites. Use a basal thermometer to take your temperature and record it in a chart. Your temperature will rise 0.4 to 0.8 degrees Fahrenheit on the first day of ovulation. You can talk with your doctor or a natural family planning instructor to learn how to record and understand this information.

Contraceptive Sponge

This barrier method is a soft, disk-shaped device with a loop for taking it out. It is made out of polyurethane foam and contains the spermicide nonoxynol-9. Spermicide kills sperm.

Before having sex, you wet the sponge and place it, loop side down, inside your vagina to cover the cervix. The sponge is effective for more than one act of intercourse for up to 24 hours. It needs to be left in for at least 6 hours after having sex to prevent pregnancy. It must then be taken out within 30 hours after it is inserted.

51

Only one kind of contraceptive sponge is sold in the United States. It is called the Today Sponge. Women who are sensitive to the spermicide nonoxynol-9 should not use the sponge.

Diaphragm, Cervical Cap, and Cervical Shield

These barrier methods block the sperm from entering the cervix (the opening to your womb) and reaching the egg.

- The diaphragm is a shallow latex cup.

- The cervical cap is a thimble-shaped latex cup. It often is called by its brand name, FemCap.

- The cervical shield is a silicone cup that has a one-way valve that creates suction and helps it fit against the cervix. It often is called by its brand name, Lea's Shield.

The diaphragm and cervical cap come in different sizes, and you need a doctor to "fit" you for one. The cervical shield comes in one size, and you will not need a fitting.

Before having sex, add spermicide (to block or kill sperm) to the devices. Then place them inside your vagina to cover your cervix. You can buy spermicide gel or foam at a drug store.

All three of these barrier methods must be left in place for 6 to 8 hours after having sex to prevent pregnancy. The diaphragm should be taken out within 24 hours. The cap and shield should be taken out within 48 hours.

Female Condom

This condom is worn by the woman inside her vagina. It keeps sperm from getting into her body. It is made of polyurethane and is packaged with a lubricant. It can be inserted up to 8 hours before having sex. Use a new condom each time you have intercourse. And don't use it and a male condom at the same time.

Male Condom

Male condoms are a thin sheath placed over an erect penis to keep sperm from entering a woman's body. Condoms can be made of latex, polyurethane, or natural/lambskin. The natural kind do not protect against STIs. Condoms work best when used with a vaginal spermicide, which kills the sperm. And you need to use a new condom with each sex act.

Condoms are either:

- lubricated, which can make sexual intercourse more comfortable; or

- non-lubricated, which can also be used for oral sex. It is best to add lubrication to non-lubricated condoms if you use them for vaginal or anal sex. You can use a water-based lubricant, such as K-Y jelly. You can buy them at the drug store. Oil-based lubricants like massage oils, baby oil, lotions, or petroleum jelly will weaken the condom, causing it to tear or break.

Keep condoms in a cool, dry place. If you keep them in a hot place (like a wallet or glove compartment), the latex breaks down. Then the condom can tear or break.

Oral Contraceptives—Combined Pill (The Pill)

The pill contains the hormones estrogen and progestin. It is taken daily to keep the ovaries from releasing an egg. The pill also causes changes in the lining of the uterus and the cervical mucus to keep the sperm from joining the egg.

Some women prefer the "extended cycle" pills. These have 12 weeks of pills that contain hormones (active) and 1 week of pills that don't contain hormones (inactive). While taking extended cycle pills, women only have their period three to four times a year.

Many types of oral contraceptives are available. Talk with your doctor about which is best for you. Your doctor may advise you not to take the pill if you:

- are older than 35 and smoke;

- have a history of blood clots;

- have a history of breast, liver, or endometrial cancer.

Antibiotics may reduce how well the pill works in some women. Talk to your doctor about a backup method of birth control if you need to take antibiotics.

Oral Contraceptives—Progestin-Only Pill (Mini-Pill)

Unlike "the pill," the mini-pill only has one hormone—progestin. Taken daily, the mini-pill thickens cervical mucus, which keeps the sperm from joining the egg. Less often, it stops the ovaries from releasing an egg.

Mothers who breastfeed can use the mini-pill. It won't affect their milk supply. The mini-pill is a good option for women who:

- can't take estrogen;
- are older than 35;
- have a risk of blood clots.

The mini-pill must be taken at the same time each day. A backup method of birth control is needed if you take the pill more than 3 hours late. Antibiotics may reduce how well the pill works in some women. Talk to your doctor about a backup method of birth control if you need to take antibiotics.

The Patch

Also called by its brand name, Ortho Evra, this skin patch is worn on the lower abdomen, buttocks, outer arm, or upper body.

It releases the hormones progestin and estrogen into the bloodstream to stop the ovaries from releasing eggs in most women. It also thickens the cervical mucus, which keeps the sperm from joining with the egg. You put on a new patch once a week for 3 weeks. You don't use a patch the fourth week in order to have a period.

Shot/Injection

The birth control shot often is called by its brand name Depo-Provera. With this method you get injections, or shots, of the hormone progestin in the buttocks or arm every 3 months. A new type is injected under the skin. The birth control shot stops the ovaries from releasing an egg in most women. It also causes changes in the cervix that keep the sperm from joining with the egg.

The shot should not be used more than 2 years in a row because it can cause a temporary loss of bone density. The loss increases the longer this method is used. The bone does start to grow after this method is stopped. But it may increase the risk of fracture and osteoporosis if used for a long time.

Vaginal Ring

This is a thin, flexible ring that releases the hormones progestin and estrogen. It works by stopping the ovaries from releasing eggs. It also thickens the cervical mucus, which keeps the sperm from joining the egg.

It is commonly called NuvaRing, its brand name. You squeeze the ring between your thumb and index finger and insert it into your vagina. You wear the ring for 3 weeks, take it out for the week that you have your period, and then put in a new ring.

Implantable Rod

This is a matchstick-size, flexible rod that is put under the skin of the upper arm. It is often called by its brand name, Implanon. The rod releases a progestin, which causes changes in the lining of the uterus and the cervical mucus to keep the sperm from joining an egg. Less often, it stops the ovaries from releasing eggs. It is effective for up to 5 years.

Intrauterine Devices or IUDs

An IUD is a small device shaped like a "T" that goes in your uterus. There are two types:

* **Copper IUD:** The copper IUD goes by the brand name ParaGard. It releases a small amount of copper into the uterus, which prevents the sperm from reaching and fertilizing the egg. It fertilization does occur, the IUD keeps the fertilized egg from implanting in the lining of the uterus. A doctor needs to put in your copper IUD. It can stay in your uterus for 5 to 10 years.

* **Hormonal IUD:** The hormonal IUD goes by the brand name Mirena. It is sometimes called an intrauterine system, or IUS. It releases progestin into the uterus, which keeps the ovaries from releasing an egg and causes the cervical mucus to thicken so sperm can't reach the egg. It also affects the ability of a fertilized egg to successfully implant in the uterus. A doctor needs to put in a hormonal IUD. It can stay in your uterus for up to 5 years.

Sterilization Implant (Essure)

Essure is the first non-surgical method of sterilizing women. A thin tube is used to thread a tiny spring-like device through the vagina and uterus into each fallopian tube. The device works by causing scar tissue to form around the coil. This blocks the fallopian tubes and stops the egg and sperm from joining.

It can take about 3 months for the scar tissue to grow, so it's important to use another form of birth control during this time. Then you will have to return to your doctor for a test to see if scar tissue has fully blocked your tubes.

Surgical Sterilization

For women, surgical sterilization closes the fallopian tubes by being cut, tied, or sealed. This stops the eggs from going down to the uterus where they can be fertilized. The surgery can be done a number of ways. Sometimes, a woman having cesarean birth has the procedure done at the same time, so as to avoid having additional surgery later.

For men, having a vasectomy keeps sperm from going to his penis, so his ejaculate never has any sperm in it. Sperm stays in the system after surgery for about 3 months. During that time, use a backup form of birth control to prevent pregnancy. A simple test can be done to check if all the sperm is gone; it is called a semen analysis.

Emergency Contraception (Plan B, Also Called Morning-After Pill)

Emergency birth control is used to keep a woman from getting pregnant when she has had unprotected vaginal intercourse. "Unprotected" can mean that no method of birth control was used. It can also mean that a birth control method was used but did not work—like a condom breaking. Or, a woman may have forgotten to take her birth control pills, or may have been abused or forced to have sex.

Emergency contraception consists of taking two doses of hormonal pills 12 hours apart. They work by stopping the ovaries from releasing an egg or keeping the sperm from joining with the egg. For the best chances for it to work, start the pills as soon as possible after unprotected sex. It should be started within 72 hours after having unprotected sex. Starting emergency contraception within 5 days after having unprotected sex might lower your risk of getting pregnant.

Where Can I Get Birth Control? Do I Need to Visit a Doctor?

Where you get birth control depends on what method you choose. You can buy these forms over the counter:

- male condoms
- female condoms

- sponges
- spermicides
- emergency contraception pills (girls younger than 17 need a prescription)

You need a prescription for these forms:

- oral contraceptives, such as the pill and the mini-pill
- skin patch
- vaginal ring
- diaphragm (your doctor needs to fit one to your shape)
- cervical cap
- cervical shield
- shot/injection (you get the shot at your doctor's office)
- IUD (inserted by a doctor)
- implantable rod (inserted by a doctor)

You will need surgery or a medical procedure for male and female sterilization.

Section 7.2

Mifepristone (The Morning-After Pill)

Excerpted from "Mifeprex (mifepristone)," by the U.S. Food
and Drug Administration (FDA, www.fda.gov), August 29, 2007.

Mifeprex is used, together with another medication called misoprostol, to end an early pregnancy (within 49 days of the start of a woman's last menstrual period). Since its approval in September 2000, the Food and Drug Administration has received reports of serious adverse events, including several deaths, in the United States following medical abortion with mifepristone and misoprostol. Each time FDA receives a report of a serious adverse event or death after medical abortion with these drugs, the agency carefully analyzes the available scientific information to determine whether or not the serious adverse event or death is related to the use of the drugs.

As previously reported by the agency, several of the women who died in the United States died from sepsis (severe illness caused by infection of the bloodstream) after medical abortion with mifepristone and misoprostol. Sepsis is a known risk related to any type of abortion. Most of these women were infected with the same type of bacteria, known as *Clostridium sordellii*. The symptoms in these cases of infection were not the usual symptoms of sepsis. We do not know whether using mifepristone and misoprostol caused these deaths.

Patients should contact a healthcare practitioner right away if they have taken these medications for medical abortion and develop stomach pain or discomfort, or have weakness, nausea, vomiting or diarrhea with or without fever, more than 24 hours after taking the misoprostol. These symptoms, even without a fever, may indicate sepsis. Patients should make sure their healthcare practitioner knows they are undergoing a medical abortion.

All providers of medical abortion and emergency room healthcare practitioners should investigate the possibility of sepsis in women who are undergoing medical abortion and present with nausea, vomiting, or diarrhea and weakness with or without abdominal pain. These symptoms even without a fever may indicate a hidden infection. Strong consideration should be given to obtaining a complete blood count in these patients. Significant leukocytosis with a marked left shift and hemoconcentration may be indicative of sepsis.

FDA recommends that healthcare practitioners have a high index of suspicion for serious infection and sepsis in patients with this presentation and consider immediately initiating treatment with antibiotics that includes coverage of anaerobic bacteria such as *Clostridium sordellii.*

FDA does not have sufficient information to recommend the use of prophylactic antibiotics for women having a medical abortion. Reports of fatal sepsis in women undergoing medical abortion are very rare (approximately 1 in 100,000). Prophylactic antibiotic use carries its own risk of serious adverse events such as severe or fatal allergic reactions. Also, prophylactic use of antibiotics can stimulate the growth of "superbugs," bacteria resistant to everyday antibiotics. Finally, it is not known which antibiotic and regimen (what dose and for how long) will be effective in cases such as the ones that have occurred.

These recommendations are consistent with warnings in the Prescribing Information and information for the patient in the Medication Guide for Mifeprex.

The approved Mifeprex regimen for a medical abortion through 49 day's pregnancy is:

- Day One: Mifeprex Administration: 3 tablets of 200 mg of Mifeprex orally at once.

- Day Three: Misoprostol Administration: 2 tablets of 200 mcg of misoprostol orally at once.

- Day 14: Post-Treatment: The patient must return to confirm that a complete termination has occurred. If not, surgical termination is recommended to manage medical abortion treatment failures.

The safety and effectiveness of other Mifeprex dosing regimens, including use of oral misoprostol tablets intravaginally, has not been established by the FDA.

Do not buy Mifeprex over the Internet. You should not buy Mifeprex over the Internet because you will bypass important safeguards designed to protect your health (and the health of others). Mifeprex has special safety restrictions on how it is distributed to the public. Also, drugs purchased from foreign Internet sources are not the FDA-approved versions of the drugs, and they are not subject to FDA-regulated manufacturing controls or FDA inspection of manufacturing facilities.

Section 7.3

Facts about Abortion in the United States

"Abortion in the U.S.: Utilization, Financing and Access," (#3269-02) The Henry J. Kaiser Family Foundation, June 2008. This information was reprinted with permission from the Henry J. Kaiser Family Foundation. The Kaiser Family Foundation is a non-profit private operating foundation, based in Menlo Park, California, dedicated to producing and communicating the best possible information, research and analysis on health issues.

Approximately one-fifth (19%) of the 6.4 million pregnancies occurring annually in the United States end in induced abortion.[1] While abortion is one of the most common medical procedures for women,[2] access and availability of services has been subject to ethical and political debates. Federal and state policies have a substantial impact on women's access to abortion services. This information provides an overview of the use of abortion services in the United States and reviews state and federal policies that affect women's access.

Incidence and Trends

- In 2005, 1.21 million abortions were performed in the United States, down from 1.61 million (the all-time high) in 1990.[3]

- 49% of pregnancies were unintended in the United States, and of these, 42% resulted in abortions in 2001 (the most recent data available).[4]

- The abortion rate (the number of abortions per 1,000 women aged 15–44) was 19.4 in 2005, a 9% drop since 2000.[5]

- 89% of abortions were performed in the first 12 weeks of pregnancy in 2004, with about 63% in the first eight weeks and 1% of abortions at 21 weeks or later.[6]

- About 19% of women having abortions in the United States are teens; 33% are between the ages of 20 and 24; and 48% are ages

25 and older.[7] Two-thirds (67%) of women have never been married and about 61% of women have given birth before.[8]

- Abortion rates for black women (49 per 1,000 women), Hispanic women (33 per 1,000) and Asian women (31 per 1,000) are higher than those of white women (13 per 1,000).[9]

- Abortion rates are higher among low-income women. The abortion rate for poor women has been increasing since 1994, so that the procedure is becoming increasingly concentrated among poor women, including those on Medicaid.[10]

Methods

- Two general types of abortion are available to women in the United States: surgical and medical (non-surgical) abortions.

- Surgical abortions account for the majority (87%) of abortions performed in the United States.[11] The most common surgical methods include vacuum aspiration, dilation and curettage (D&C), and dilation and evacuation (D&E). Surgical abortion is generally not performed until the sixth week of gestation.

- In September 2000, the U.S. Food and Drug Administration approved mifepristone (also known as "RU-486"), the first drug specifically designed for use as a method of medical abortion. This drug, in conjunction with misoprostol, is the most commonly used method of medical abortion.[12] Methotrexate, usually followed by misoprostol, is also used for medical abortion. Medical abortion can be initiated as soon as a pregnancy is confirmed.

- In 2005, medical abortions accounted for approximately 13% of all abortions (compared to 6% in 2001) and 22% of abortions before nine weeks' gestation.[13]

- Since the 1990s, 31 states have enacted bans on procedures called "partial-birth" abortions, with 14 state laws (GA, IN, KS, LA, MS, MT, NM, ND, OH, OK, SC, SD, TN, UT) in effect. All include an exception to the ban: four states (GA, KS, NM, OH) include a health exception and the rest of the states include an exception only when a woman's life is in danger.[14]

- In 2003, the President signed the Partial-Birth Abortion Ban Act of 2003, which banned "partial-birth" abortions with no health exception. This legislation was upheld by the Supreme Court in the April 2007 *Gonzales v. Carhart* decision. The procedure banned by this Act is sometimes medically defined as intact dilation and extraction.[15] Following the high court ruling, state legislatures have been reviving their bans on late-term abortion procedures previously blocked by lower courts.

- Complications from abortions are rare, with less than 0.3% of abortion patients in the United States experiencing a major complication requiring hospitalization.[16] The annual risk of death associated with abortion has been approximately one death per 100,000 legal abortions.[17]

- Research has shown that both medical and surgical abortions performed in the first trimester are not significantly associated with later infertility, ectopic pregnancy, spontaneous abortion, or preterm or low-birth-weight deliveries[18,19,20] and no greater risk of breast cancer.[21,22,23]

Abortion Financing

The cost of an abortion varies depending on factors such as location, facility, timing, and type of procedure. In 2005, a nonhospital abortion at 10 weeks' gestation ranged from $90 to $1,800 (average: $430), whereas an abortion at 20 weeks' gestation ranged from $350 to $4,520 (average: $1,260).[24] Costs are higher for a medical abortion than a first-trimester surgical abortion.[25]

Medicaid

- Federal law requires that states cover abortions under Medicaid in the event of rape, incest, and life endangerment, but bans the use of federal Medicaid funds for any other abortions.

- Based on these restrictions, 32 states and DC fund abortions through Medicaid only in the cases of rape, incest, or life endangerment.[26] SD covers abortions only in the cases of life endangerment, which does not comply with federal requirements under the Hyde Amendment. IN, UT and WI have expanded coverage to women whose physical health is jeopardized, and IA, MS, UT and VA also include fetal abnormality cases.

- Seventeen states (AK, AZ, CA, CT, HI, IL, MD, MA, MN, MT, NJ, NM, NY, OR, VT, WA, WV) use their own funds to cover all or most "medically necessary" abortions sought by low-income women under Medicaid.[27]

Private Insurance

- Five states (ID, KY, MO, ND, OK) restrict insurance coverage of abortion services in private plans: OK limits coverage to life endangerment, rape, or incest circumstances; and the other four states limit coverage to cases of life endangerment.[28]

- Twelve states (CO, IL, KY, MA, MS, NE, ND, OH, PA, RI, SC, VA) restrict abortion coverage in insurance plans for public employees, with CO and KY restricting insurance coverage of abortion under any circumstances.[29]

- U.S. laws also ban federal funding of abortions for Federal employees and their dependents, Native Americans covered by the Indian Health Service, military personnel and their dependents, and women with disabilities covered by Medicare.

Availability of and Access to Abortion Services

- 1,787 facilities provided abortions in 2005 in the United States, a 2% decline from the year 2000.[30]

- 87% of U.S. counties have no abortion provider, and 35% of women of reproductive age (15–44) live in these counties.[31] Women in the Midwest and South are more likely to live in a county without a provider (50% and 47%, respectively) than women in the Northeast and West (17% and 15%, respectively).

- Over half of abortion providers (57%) performed early medical abortions in 2005, up from 33% in 2001.[32] More than half of early medical abortions were provided at abortion clinics.

- Most abortion providers performed abortions within the first eight weeks. Forty percent performed early abortion within first four weeks' gestation, whereas 8% of abortion providers performed abortions at 24 weeks.[33]

- In recent years, 28 states have adopted laws and regulations specific to abortion clinics and providers. These laws involve special requirements for abortion providers to have health facility licenses and ambulatory surgical center licenses, or requirements that abortions after a specified gestation age be performed in a hospital, or that providers have admitting privileges in local hospitals.[34] These policies can make it more difficult for providers to offer abortion services to women.

- The Federal Freedom of Access to Clinic Entrances (FACE) Act was passed in 1994 to prohibit acts of physical or psychological intimidation to persons seeking or providing reproductive health services. Fifteen states (CA, CO, KS, ME, MD, MA, MI, MN, MT, NV, NY, NC, OR, WA, WI) and DC go beyond the FACE protections and prohibit certain specified actions aimed at abortion providers, such as threatening or intimidating staff, property damage, and telephone harassment.[35]

- Twenty-four states have passed requirements for women to wait a specified time (usually 24 hours) between receiving counseling and undergoing an abortion.[36] As a result, women must make two visits to the clinic, which can be difficult for those who live far from the clinic. Eight percent of women travel more than 100 miles to access abortion services and 19% travel between 50 and 100 miles.[37]

- Thirty-five states have adopted "parental involvement" laws that require notification and/or consent of one or both parents before a minor has an abortion.[38] Most states with these laws apply them to girls under age 18, although several set the level to 16 or 17.

Endnotes

1. Ventura SJ et al. Estimated pregnancy rates by outcome for the United States, 1990–2004. *CDC National Vital Health Statistics,* 2008.

2. Owings MF & Kozak LJ. Ambulatory and inpatient procedures in the United States, 1996. *CDC National Vital Health Statistics,* 1998.

3. Jones RK et al. Abortion in the United States: Incidence and access to services, 2005. *Perspectives on Sexual and Reproductive Health,* 40(1), 2008.

4. Finer LB & Henshaw SK. Disparities in rates of unintended pregnancy in the United States, 1994 and 2001. *Perspectives on Sexual and Reproductive Health,* 38(2), 2006.

5. Jones RK et al. Abortion in the United States: Incidence and access to services, 2005. *Perspectives on Sexual and Reproductive Health,* 40(1), 2008.

6. Guttmacher Institute. Henshaw SK adjustments to Strauss LT et al. Abortion surveillance—United States, 2004. *MMWR,* 56(SS-9), 2007.

7. Jones RK et al. Patterns in the socioeconomic characteristics of women obtaining abortions in 2000–2001. *Perspectives on Sexual and Reproductive Health,* 34(5), 2002.

8. Ibid.

9. Ibid.

10. Ibid.

11. Jones RK et al. Abortion in the United States: Incidence and access to services, 2005. *Perspectives on Sexual and Reproductive Health,* 40(1), 2008.

12. Virk J, Zhang J et al. Medical abortion and the risk of subsequent adverse pregnancy outcomes. *NEJM,* 357(7), 2007.

13. Jones RK et al. Abortion in the United States: Incidence and access to services, 2005. *Perspectives on Sexual and Reproductive Health,* 40(1), 2008.

14. Guttmacher Institute. Bans on "partial-birth" abortions. *State Policies in Brief,* 2008.

15. Gostin LO. Abortion politics: Clinical freedom, trust in the Judiciary, and the autonomy of women. *JAMA,* 298(13), 2007.

16. Henshaw SK, Unintended pregnancy and abortion: a public health perspective, in: Paul M et al., eds., *A Clinician's Guide to Medical and Surgical Abortion,* 1999.

17. Strauss LT et al. Abortion surveillance—United States, 2004. *MMWR,* 56(SS-9), 2007.

18. Virk J, Zhang J et al. Medical abortion and the risk of subsequent adverse pregnancy outcomes. *NEJM,* 357(7), 2007.

19. Atrash HK, Strauss LT et al. The relation between induced abortion and ectopic pregnancy. *Obstet Gynecol,* 89(4), 1997.

20. Chen A et al. Mifepristone-induced early abortion and outcome of subsequent wanted pregnancy. *Am J Epi,* 160(2), 2004.

21. Beral V et al. Breast cancer and abortion: Collaborative reanalysis of data from 53 epidemiological studies. *Lancet,* 363(9414), 2004.

22. Michels K et al. Induced and spontaneous abortion and incidence of breast cancer among young women. *Arch Intern Med,* 167(8), 2007.

23. Melbywe M et al. Induced abortion and the risk of breast cancer. *NEJM,* 336(2), 1997.

24. Jones RK et al. Abortion in the United States: Incidence and access to services, 2005. *Perspectives on Sexual and Reproductive Health,* 40(1), 2008.

25. Boonstra H. Mifepristone in the United States: Status and future. *The Guttmacher Report on Public Policy,* 5(3), 2002.

26. Guttmacher Institute. State funding of abortion under Medicaid. *State Policies in Brief,* 2008.

27. Ibid.

28. Guttmacher Institute. Restricting insurance coverage of abortion. *State Policies in Brief,* 2008.

29. Ibid.

30. Jones RK et al. Abortion in the United States: Incidence and access to services, 2005. *Perspectives on Sexual and Reproductive Health,* 40(1), 2008.

31. Ibid.

32. Ibid.

33. Ibid.

34. Center for Reproductive Rights. *Targeted Regulation of Abortion Providers,* 2007.

35. Guttmacher Institute. Protecting access to clinics. *State Policies in Brief,* 2008.

36. Guttmacher Institute. Counseling and waiting periods for abortion. *State Policies in Brief,* 2008.

37. Jones RK et al. Abortion in the United States: Incidence and access to services, 2005. *Perspectives on Sexual and Reproductive Health,* 40(1), 2008.

38. Guttmacher Institute. Parental involvement in minors' abortions. *State Policies in Brief,* 2008.

Additional copies of this publication (#3269-02) are available on the Kaiser Family Foundation's website at www.kff.org.

Part Two

Understanding Pregnancy-Related Changes and Fetal Development

Chapter 8

Are You Pregnant?

Chapter Contents

Section 8.1

Signs of Pregnancy

From "Pregnancy," by the National Institute of Child Health
and Human Development (NICHD, www.nichd.nih.gov), part of
the National Institutes of Health, February 5, 2008.

What is pregnancy?

Pregnancy is the term used to describe when a woman has a growing fetus inside of her. In most cases, the fetus grows in the uterus.

Human pregnancy lasts about 40 weeks, or just more than 9 months, from the start of the last menstrual period to childbirth.

What are the signs of pregnancy?

The primary sign of pregnancy is missing one or more consecutive menstrual periods. However, because many women experience menstrual irregularities that may cause missed periods, women who miss a period should see their health care provider to find out whether they are pregnant or whether there is another health problem.

Others signs and symptoms of pregnancy may include:

- nausea or vomiting, morning sickness;
- sore breasts or nipples;
- fatigue;
- headaches;
- food cravings or aversions;
- mood swings; and
- frequent urination.

How do I know I'm pregnant?

A pregnancy test is the best way to determine if you are pregnant. Home pregnancy test kits are available over the counter and are considered highly accurate. A health care provider can also do a pregnancy test.

NICHD research in the 1970s found that high levels of the hormone human chorionic gonadotropin (HCG) in the urine were associated with pregnancy. This research led to the development of the home pregnancy test that is commercially available today.

If you think you may be pregnant, or have a positive home pregnancy test, see a health care provider.

What is prenatal care and why is it important?

Prenatal care is the care woman gets during a pregnancy. Getting early and regular prenatal care is important for the health of both mother and the developing baby.

In addition, health care providers are now recommending a woman see a health care provider for preconception care, before she is even trying to get pregnant.

Health care providers recommend women take the following steps to ensure the best health outcome for mother and baby:

- getting at least 400 micrograms of folic acid every day to help prevent many types of neural tube defects. Health care providers recommend taking folic acid both before and during pregnancy.

- being properly vaccinated for certain diseases (such as chickenpox and rubella) that could harm a developing fetus—it is important to have the vaccinations before becoming pregnant.

- maintaining a healthy weight and diet and getting regular physical activity before, during, and after pregnancy.

- avoiding smoking, alcohol, or drug use before, during, and after pregnancy.

What is a high-risk pregnancy?

All pregnancies involve a certain degree of risk to both mother and baby. But, factors present before pregnancy or that develop during pregnancy can place the mother and baby at higher risk for problems. Women with high-risk pregnancies may need care from specialists or a team of health care providers to help promote healthy pregnancy and birth.

Factors present before pregnancy that can increase risk may include:

- young or old maternal age;

- being overweight or underweight;

- having had problems in previous pregnancies, such as miscarriage, stillbirth, or preterm labor or birth; and

- pre-existing health conditions, such as high blood pressure, diabetes, or HIV/AIDS [human immunodeficiency virus/acquired immunodeficiency syndrome].

During pregnancy, problems may also develop even in a woman who was previously healthy. These may include (but are not limited to) gestational diabetes or preeclampsia/eclampsia.

Getting good prenatal care and seeing a health care provider regularly during pregnancy are important ways to promote a healthy pregnancy.

Section 8.2

Understanding Home Pregnancy Tests

From "Pregnancy Tests: Frequently Asked Questions," by the Office of Women's Health (www.womenshealth.gov), March 20, 2009.

How do pregnancy tests work?

All pregnancy tests work by detecting a certain hormone in the urine or blood that is only there when a woman is pregnant. This hormone is called human chorionic gonadotropin, or hCG. It is also called the pregnancy hormone.

hCG is made when a fertilized egg implants in the uterus. This usually happens about six days after the egg and sperm merge. But studies show that in up to 10 percent of women, implantation does not occur until much later, after the first day of the missed period. The amount of hCG rapidly builds up in your body with each passing day you are pregnant.

Are there different types of pregnancy tests?

Yes. There are two types of pregnancy tests. One tests the blood for the pregnancy hormone, hCG. You need to see a doctor to have a blood test. The other checks the urine for the hCG hormone. You can do a urine test at a doctor's office or at home with a home pregnancy test (HPT).

These days, many women first use an HPT to find out if they are pregnant. HPTs are inexpensive, private, and easy to use. HPTs also are highly accurate if used correctly and at the right time. HPTs will be able to tell if you're pregnant about one week after a missed period.

Doctors use two types of blood tests to check for pregnancy. Blood tests can pick up hCG earlier in a pregnancy than urine tests can. Blood tests can tell if you are pregnant about six to eight days after you ovulate (or release an egg from an ovary). A quantitative blood test (or the beta hCG test) measures the exact amount of hCG in your blood. So it can find even tiny amounts of hCG. This makes it very accurate. A qualitative hCG blood test just checks to see if the pregnancy hormone is present or not. So this test gives a yes or no answer. The qualitative hCG blood test is about as accurate as a urine test.

How do you do a home pregnancy test?

There are many different types of home pregnancy tests (HPTs). Most drugstores sell HPTs over the counter. They are inexpensive. But the cost depends on the brand and how many tests come in the box.

Most HPTs work in a similar way. Many instruct the user to hold a stick in the urine stream. Others involve collecting urine in a cup and then dipping the stick into it. At least one brand tells the woman to collect urine in a cup and then use a dropper to put a few drops of the urine into a special container. Then the woman needs to wait a few minutes. Different brands instruct the woman to wait different amounts of time. Once the time has passed, the user should inspect the result window. If a line or plus symbol appears, you are pregnant. It does not matter how faint the line is. A line, whether bold or faint, means the result is positive. New digital tests show the words "pregnant" or "not pregnant."

Most tests also have a control indicator in the result window. This line or symbol shows whether the test is working properly. If the control indicator does not appear, the test is not working properly. You should not rely on any results from an HPT that may be faulty.

Most brands tell users to repeat the test in a few days, no matter what the results. One negative result (especially soon after a missed period) does not always mean you're not pregnant. All HPTs come with written instructions. Most tests also have toll-free phone numbers to call in case of questions about use or results.

How accurate are home pregnancy tests?

Home pregnancy tests (HPTs) can be quite accurate. But the accuracy depends on the following factors:

- **How you use them:** Be sure to check the expiration date and follow the instructions. Wait ten minutes after taking the test to check the results window. Research suggests that waiting 10 minutes will give the most accurate result.

- **When you use them:** The amount of hCG or pregnancy hormone in your urine increases with time. So, the earlier after a missed period you take the test, the harder it is to spot the hCG. Many HPTs claim to be 99 percent accurate on the first day of your missed period. But research suggests that most HPTs do not always detect the low levels of hCG usually present this early in pregnancy. And when they do, the results are often very faint. Most HPTs can accurately detect pregnancy one week after a missed period. Also, testing your urine first thing in the morning may boost the accuracy.

- **Who uses them:** Each woman ovulates at a different time in her menstrual cycle. Plus, the fertilized egg can implant in a woman's uterus at different times. hCG only is produced once implantation occurs. In up to 10 percent of women, implantation does not occur until after the first day of a missed period. So, HPTs will be accurate as soon as one day after a missed period for some women but not for others.

- **The brand of test:** Some HPTs are more sensitive than others. So, some tests are better than others at spotting hCG early on.

How soon after a missed period can I take a home pregnancy test and get an accurate result?

Many home pregnancy tests (HPTs) claim to be 99 percent accurate on the first day of your missed period. But research suggests that most HPTs do not always spot pregnancy that early. And when they do, the results are often so faint they are misunderstood. If you can wait one week after your missed period, most HPTs will give you an accurate answer. Ask your doctor for a more sensitive test if you need to know earlier.

My home pregnancy test says I am pregnant. What should I do next?

If a home pregnancy test is positive and shows that you are pregnant, you should call your doctor right away. Your doctor can use a more sensitive test along with a pelvic exam to tell for sure if you're pregnant. Seeing your doctor early on in your pregnancy will help you and your baby stay healthy.

My home pregnancy test says that I am not pregnant. Might I still be pregnant?

Yes. Most home pregnancy tests (HPTs) suggest women take the test again in a few days or a week if the result is negative.

Each woman ovulates at a different time in her menstrual cycle. Plus, the fertilized egg can implant in a woman's uterus at different times. So, the accuracy of HPT results varies from woman to woman.

Other things can also affect the accuracy. Sometimes women get false negative results when they test too early in the pregnancy. This means that the test says you are not pregnant when you are. Other times, problems with the pregnancy can affect the amount of hCG in the urine.

If your HPT is negative, test yourself again in a few days or one week. If you keep getting a negative result but think you are pregnant, talk with your doctor right away.

Can anything affect home pregnancy test results?

Most medicines should not affect the results of a home pregnancy test (HPT). This includes over-the-counter and prescription medicines, including birth control pills and antibiotics. Only medicines that have the pregnancy hormone hCG in them can give a false positive test result. A false positive is when a test says you are pregnant when you're not. Sometimes medicines containing hCG are used to treat infertility (not being able to get pregnant).

Alcohol and illegal drugs do not affect HPT results. But do not use these substances if you are trying to become pregnant or are sexually active and could become pregnant.

For More Information

For more information on pregnancy tests, contact the National Women's Health Information Center (800-994-9662) or the following organizations:

American College of Obstetricians and Gynecologists
409 12th Street, SW
P.O. Box 96920
Washington, DC 20090-6920
Phone: 202-638-5577
Website: www.acog.org

American Pregnancy Association
1425 Greenway Drive
Irving, TX 75038
Phone: 972-550-0140
Fax: 972-550-0800
Website: www.americanpregnancy.org
E-mail: questions@americanpregnancy.org

Planned Parenthood Federation of America
434 West 33rd Street
New York, NY 10001
Toll-Free: 800-230-7526
Phone: 212-541-7800
Fax: 212-245-1845
Website: www.plannedparenthood.org

U.S. Food and Drug Administration
10903 New Hampshire Avenue
Silver Spring, MD 20903
Toll-Free: 888-463-6332
Website: www.fda.gov

Section 8.3

Calculating Your Dates:
Gestation, Conception, and Due Date

"Calculating Your Dates: Gestation, Conception & Due Date,"
© 2008 American Pregnancy Association (www.americanpregnancy.org).
Reprinted with permission.

Gestational age, or the age of the baby, is calculated from the first day of the mother's last menstrual period. Since the exact date of conception is almost never known, the first day of the last menstrual period is used to measure how old the baby is.

Calculating Gestational Age

Last menstrual period: If the mother has a regular period and knows the first day of her last menstrual period, gestational age can be calculated from this date. Gestational age is calculated from the first day of the mother's last menstrual period and not from the date of conception.

Ultrasound: The baby can be measured as early as five or six weeks after the mother's last menstrual period. Measuring the baby using ultrasound is most accurate in early pregnancy. It becomes less accurate later in pregnancy. The best time to estimate gestational age using ultrasound is between the 8th and 18th weeks of pregnancy. The most accurate way to determine gestational age is using the first day of the woman's last menstrual period and confirming this gestational age with the measurement from an ultrasound exam.

Calculating Conception Date

In a typical pregnancy: For a woman with a regular period, conception typically occurs about 11–21 days after the first day of the last period. Most women do not know the exact date of conception, and their conception date is merely an estimate based on the first day of their last period.

Special cases: Women who undergo special procedures such as artificial insemination or in vitro fertilization typically know the exact date of conception.

Calculating Due Date

Estimated due date: Based on the last menstrual period, the estimated due date is 40 weeks from the first day of the period. This is just an estimate since only about 5% of babies are born on their estimated due date.

Difficulties in Determining Gestational Age

Last menstrual period: For women who have irregular menstrual periods or women who cannot remember the first day of their last menstrual period, it can be difficult to determine gestational age using this method. In these cases, an ultrasound exam is often required to determine gestational age.

Baby's growth: In some cases it is difficult to determine the gestational age because the baby is unusually large or small. Also, in some cases the size of the uterus in early pregnancy or the height of the uterus in later pregnancy does not match the first day of the last menstrual period. In these cases as well, it is difficult to obtain an accurate gestational age.

Chapter 9

Physical Changes during Pregnancy

Chapter Contents

Section 9.1

Common Pregnancy Discomforts

The text in this section is from "Pregnancy Basics," by the Office of Women's Health (www.womenshealth.gov), part of the U.S. Department of Health and Human Services, March 2007. Figure 9.1 is from *The Healthy Woman: A Complete Guide for All Ages,* U.S. Department of Health and Human Services, Office on Women's Health, 2008.

Everyone expects pregnancy to bring an expanding waistline. But many women are surprised by the other body changes that pop up. Get the lowdown on stretch marks, weight gain, heartburn, and other "joys" of pregnancy. Find out what you can do to feel better.

Body Changes

Aches, Pains, and Backaches

As your uterus expands, pains in the back, abdomen, groin area, and thighs often appear. Many women also have backaches and aching near the pelvic bone due the pressure of the baby's head, increased weight, and loosening joints.

To ease some of these aches and pains try:

- lying down;
- resting; and
- applying heat.

If you are worried or the pains do not get better, call your doctor.

Breast Changes

A woman's breasts increase in size and fullness during pregnancy. As the due date approaches, hormone changes will cause your breasts to get even bigger in preparation for breastfeeding. Your breasts may feel full and heavy, and they might be tender or uncomfortable.

In the third trimester, some pregnant women begin to leak colostrum from their breasts. Colostrum is the first milk that your breasts produce for the baby. It is a thick, yellowish fluid containing antibodies that protect newborns from infection. If leaking becomes embarrassing, put nursing pads inside your bra.

Try to these tips to stay comfortable:

- Wear a soft, comfortable maternity or nursing bra with extra support.

- Wash your nipples with water instead of soap. Soap can dry and irritate nipples. If you have cracked nipples, use a heavy moisturizing cream that contains lanolin.

Dizziness

Many pregnant women complain of dizziness and lightheadedness throughout their pregnancies. Fainting is rare but does happen even in some healthy pregnant women. There are many reasons for these

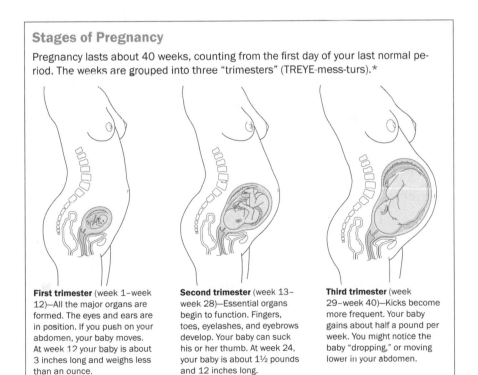

Stages of Pregnancy

Pregnancy lasts about 40 weeks, counting from the first day of your last normal period. The weeks are grouped into three "trimesters" (TREYE-mess-turs).*

First trimester (week 1–week 12)—All the major organs are formed. The eyes and ears are in position. If you push on your abdomen, your baby moves. At week 12 your baby is about 3 inches long and weighs less than an ounce.

Second trimester (week 13–week 28)—Essential organs begin to function. Fingers, toes, eyelashes, and eyebrows develop. Your baby can suck his or her thumb. At week 24, your baby is about 1½ pounds and 12 inches long.

Third trimester (week 29–week 40)—Kicks become more frequent. Your baby gains about half a pound per week. You might notice the baby "dropping," or moving lower in your abdomen.

*According to the American College of Obstetricians and Gynecologists.

***Figure 9.1.** Body changes during pregnancy.*

symptoms. The growth of more blood vessels in early pregnancy, the pressure of the expanding uterus on blood vessels, and the body's increased need for food all can make a pregnant woman feel lightheaded and dizzy.

To feel better follow these tips:

- Stand up slowly.
- When you're feeling lightheaded, lay down on your left side.
- Avoid sitting or standing in one position for a long time.
- Eat healthy snacks or small meals frequently.
- Don't get overheated.
- Call your doctor as soon as possible if you faint. Dizziness or lightheadedness can be discussed at regular prenatal visits.

Hemorrhoids

Up to 50% of pregnant women get hemorrhoids. Hemorrhoids are swollen and bulging veins in the rectum. They can cause itching, pain, and bleeding.

Hemorrhoids are more common during pregnancy for many reasons. During pregnancy there is a huge increase in the amount of blood in the body. This can cause veins to enlarge. The expanding uterus also puts pressure on the veins in the rectum. Plus, constipation can make hemorrhoids worse. Hemorrhoids usually improve after delivery.

Follow these tips to help prevent and relieve hemorrhoids:

- Drink lots of fluids.
- Eat plenty of fiber-rich foods like whole grains, raw or cooked leafy green vegetables, and fruits.
- Try not to strain for bowel movements.
- Talk with your doctor before taking any laxative.
- Talk to your doctor about using witch hazel or ice packs to soothe hemorrhoids.

Leg Cramps

At different times during your pregnancy, you might have cramps in your legs or feet. They usually happen at night. This is due to a change in the way your body processes, or metabolizes, calcium.

Try these tips to prevent and ease leg cramps:

- Eat lots of low-fat calcium-rich foods.

- Get regular mild exercise, like walking.

- Ask your doctor if you should be taking a prenatal vitamin containing calcium.

- Gently stretch the muscle to relieve leg and foot cramps. If you have a sudden leg cramp, flex your foot toward your body.

- Use heating pads or warm, moist towels to help relax the muscles and ease leg and foot cramps.

Nasal Problems

Nosebleeds and nasal stuffiness are common during pregnancy. They are caused by the increased amount of blood in your body and hormones acting on the tissues of your nose.

To ease nosebleeds blow gently when you blow your nose. Stop nosebleeds by squeezing your nose between your thumb and finger for a few minutes. If you have nosebleeds that do not stop in a few minutes or happen often, see your doctor.

Drinking extra water and using a cool mist humidifier in your bedroom may help relieve nasal stuffiness. Talk with your doctor before taking any over-the-counter or prescription medicines for colds or nasal stuffiness.

Shortness of Breath

As the baby grows, your expanding uterus will put pressure on all of your organs, including your lungs. You may notice that you are short of breath or might not be able to catch your breath.

Tips to ease breathing include:

- Take deep, long breaths.

- Maintain good posture so your lungs have room to expand.

- Use an extra pillow and try sleeping on your side to breathe easier at night.

Swelling

Most women develop mild swelling in the face, hands, or ankles at some point in their pregnancies. As the due date approaches, swelling often becomes more noticeable. If you have rapid, significant weight gain or your hands or feet suddenly get very puffy, call your doctor as soon as possible. It could be a sign of high blood pressure called pre-eclampsia or toxemia.

To keep swelling to a minimum:

- Drink 8 to 10 eight-ounce glasses of fluids (water is best) daily.
- Avoid caffeine.
- Try to avoid very salty foods.
- Rest when you can with your feet elevated.
- Ask your doctor about using support hose.

Teeth and Gum Problems

A pregnant woman's teeth and gums need special care. Pregnant women with gum disease are much more likely to have premature babies with low birthweight. This may result from the transfer of bacteria in the mother's mouth to the baby during pregnancy. The microbes can reach the baby through the placenta (a temporary organ joining the mother and fetus which supplies the fetus with blood and nutrients), through the amniotic fluid (fluid around the fetus), and through the layer of tissues in the mother's stomach.

Every expectant mother should have a complete oral exam prior to or very early in pregnancy. All needed dental work should be managed early, because having urgent treatment during pregnancy can present risks. Interventions can be started to control risks for gum inflammation and disease. This also is the best time to change habits that may affect the health of teeth and gums, and the health of the baby.

Remember to tell your dentist that you are pregnant! You can ease bleeding gums by brushing with a soft-bristled toothbrush and flossing at least twice a day. Get more details on taking care of your teeth and gums during pregnancy.

Varicose Veins

During pregnancy there is a huge increase in the amount of blood in the body. This can cause veins to enlarge. Plus, pressure on the large veins behind the uterus causes the blood to slow in its return to the heart. For these reasons, varicose veins in the legs and anus (hemorrhoids) are more common in pregnancy.

Varicose veins look like swollen veins raised above the surface of the skin. They can be twisted or bulging and are dark purple or blue in color. They are found most often on the backs of the calves or on the inside of the leg.

Try these tips to reduce the chances of varicose veins:

- Avoid tight knee-highs or garters.
- Sit with your legs and feet raised when possible.

Digestive Difficulties

Constipation

Many pregnant women complain of constipation. High levels of hormones in your pregnant body slow down digestion and relax muscles in the bowels leaving many women constipated. Plus, the pressure of the expanding uterus on the bowels boosts the chances for constipation.

Try these tips to stay more regular:

- Eat fiber-rich foods like fresh or dried fruit, raw vegetables, and whole-grain cereals and breads daily.
- Drink eight to 10 glasses of water everyday.
- Avoid caffeinated drinks (coffee, tea, colas, and some other sodas), since caffeine makes your body lose fluid needed for regular bowel movements.
- Get moving. Mild exercise like walking may also ease constipation.

Heartburn and Indigestion

Almost every pregnant woman experiences indigestion and heartburn. Hormones and the pressure of the growing uterus cause this discomfort. Pregnancy hormones slow down the muscles of the digestive tract. So food tends to move more slowly and digestion is sluggish. This causes many pregnant women to feel bloated.

Hormones also relax the valve that separates the esophagus from the stomach. This allows food and acids to come back up from the stomach to the esophagus. The food and acid causes the burning feeling of heartburn. As your baby gets bigger, the uterus pushes on the stomach making heartburn more common in later pregnancy.

Try these tips to prevent and ease indigestion and heartburn:

- Avoid greasy and fried foods.

- Eat six to eight small meals instead of three large meals.

- Don't gain more than the recommended amount of weight.

- Take small sips of milk or eat small pieces of chipped ice to soothe burning.

- Eat slowly.

- Ask your doctor if you can take an antacid medicine.

Stretch Marks and Other Skin Changes

Stretch Marks

Worried about the dreaded stretch marks of pregnancy? Just about all pregnant women are. The good news is that only about half of pregnant women get stretch marks.

Stretch marks are red, pink, or purple streaks in the skin. Most often they appear on the thighs, buttocks, abdomen, and breasts. These scars are caused by the stretching of the skin, and usually appear in the second half of pregnancy.

The color of stretch marks depends on a woman's skin color. They can be pink, reddish brown, or dark brown streaks. While creams and lotions can keep your skin well moisturized, they do not prevent stretch marks from forming. Most stretch marks fade after delivery to very light lines.

Other Skin Changes

Some women notice other skin changes during pregnancy. For many women, the nipples become darker and browner during pregnancy. Many pregnant women also develop a dark line (called the linea nigra) on the skin that runs from the belly button down to the pubic hairline.

Blotchy brown pigmentations on the forehead, nose, and cheeks are also common. These spots are called melasma or chloasma and are more common in darker-skinned women. Most of these skin changes are caused by pregnancy hormones and will fade or disappear after delivery.

Tingling and Itching

Tingling and numbness of the fingers and a feeling of swelling in the hands are common during pregnancy. These symptoms are due to swelling of tissues in the narrow passages in your wrists, and they should disappear after delivery.

About 20 percent of pregnant women feel itchy during pregnancy. Usually women feel itchy in the abdomen. But red, itchy palms and soles of the feet are also common complaints. Pregnancy hormones and stretching skin are probably to blame for most of your discomfort.

Usually the itchy feeling goes away after delivery. In the meantime, try these tips to feel better:

- Use thick moisturizing creams instead of lotions on your skin.
- Use gentle soaps.
- Avoid hot showers or baths that can dry your skin.
- Avoid itchy fabrics and clothes.
- Try not to get overheated. Heat can make the itching worse.

Rarely, itchiness can be a sign of a serious condition called cholestasis of pregnancy. If you have nausea, loss of appetite, vomiting, jaundice, or fatigue with itchiness, call your doctor. Cholestasis of pregnancy is a serious liver problem.

Sleeping Troubles

During your pregnancy, you might feel tired even after you've had a lot of sleep. Many women find they're particularly exhausted in the first trimester. Don't worry, this is normal! This is your body's way of telling you that you need more rest.

In the second trimester, tiredness is usually replaced with a feeling of well being and energy. But in the third trimester, exhaustion often sets in again. As you get larger, sleeping may become more difficult. The baby's movements, bathroom runs, and an increase in the body's metabolism might interrupt or disturb your sleep. Leg cramping can also interfere with a good night's sleep.

Try these tips to feel and sleep better:

- When you're tired, get some rest.
- Try to get about 8 hours of sleep every night, and a short nap during the day.
- If you feel stressed, try to find ways to relax.
- Sleep on your left side. This will relieve pressure on blood vessels that supply oxygen and nutrients to the fetus.

- If you have high blood pressure during pregnancy, always lay on your left side when you're lying down.
- Avoid eating large meals 3 hours before going to bed.
- Get some mild exercise like walking.
- Avoid long naps during the day.

Weight Gain

The amount of weight you need to gain during pregnancy depends upon how much you weighed before you became pregnant. According to the American College of Obstetricians and Gynecologists (ACOG) women who have a normal weight before getting pregnant should gain 25 to 35 pounds. Women who are underweight before pregnancy should gain 28 to 40 pounds. And women who are overweight should gain 15 to 25 pounds.

Research shows that women who gain more than the recommended amount during pregnancy have a higher chance of being obese 10 years later. Ask your doctor how much weight gain during pregnancy is healthy for you.

Is It Safe to Have Sex?

Unless your doctor tells you otherwise, sexual intercourse is safe throughout your pregnancy. For many women, pregnancy increases their sex drive. For others, it has the opposite effect. And almost all women need to try different positions when they start to get large bellies.

If you have problems during your pregnancy or have had miscarriages in the past your doctor may suggest you avoid sexual intercourse. Call your doctor if you have any of the following problems during or after sexual intercourse:

- pain in the vagina or abdomen;
- bleeding from the vagina; or
- leaking of fluid from the vagina.

When to Call the Doctor

When you are pregnant you should not hesitate to call your doctor or midwife if something is bothering or worrying you. Sometimes physical changes can be signs of a problem.

Call your doctor or midwife immediately if you:

- are bleeding or leaking fluid from the vagina;
- have sudden or severe swelling in the face, hands, or fingers;
- get severe or long-lasting headaches;
- have discomfort, pain, or cramping in the abdomen;
- have a fever or chills;
- are vomiting or have persistent nausea;
- feel discomfort, pain, or burning with urination;
- have problems seeing or blurred vision;
- feel dizzy;
- sense a change in your baby's movement; and
- suspect your baby is moving less than normally after 28 weeks of pregnancy (if you count less than 10 movements in 2 hours or less).

Section 9.2

Back Pain during Pregnancy

Most women have back pain at some point during pregnancy. The pain can be mild or severe, but it can usually be treated. In some cases, it can be prevented.

Why do pregnant women have back pain?

Pregnancy hormones loosen all of your joints. Your growing abdomen changes your posture. These changes can increase the normal curves that are in your back which can cause back pain. Later in pregnancy the looser joints in the pelvis move more from the growing weight of your baby and this can cause general pain in your lower back and sometimes shooting pain in your buttock or upper legs.

What makes the pain worse?

Lying on your back, sitting upright in a chair, rolling over at night, or getting out of bed or out of a chair can cause back pain to be worse.

How can I avoid and reduce back pain?

- Avoid sitting for long periods of time. Change positions and move frequently.

- Avoid bending, arching, and twisting motions; you will feel less discomfort.

- When lifting heavy things, keep your back straight and use your leg muscles instead of your back when picking things up.

- Whenever you are sitting, put your feet up on a stool or box so your hips tilt forward and the curve in your lower back flattens out.

- Many women get pain relief from using moist heat or cold packs, getting a massage, or sitting in a warm bath.

- Some women find wearing supportive, low-heeled shoes or an abdominal support binder can also help.

- Gentle exercise, along with walking 20 minutes most days, can relieve or lessen back pain. Exercise helps strengthen the back muscles, decrease muscle tightness and spasm, and keep the joints in good position.

- Sleeping on your side with a body pillow in your arms and between your knees may help as well.

What strengthening exercises are helpful?

The following text has exercises that will strengthen the back muscles. The exercises can be held for 3–5 seconds and repeated 10–30 times. Be sure not to hold your breath when you are doing them.

What stretches are recommended?

Stretching the back and hamstring muscles after a warm shower or short walk can help reduce back pain. Hold each stretch for 20 seconds, and repeat 2–3 times. See the following text for directions.

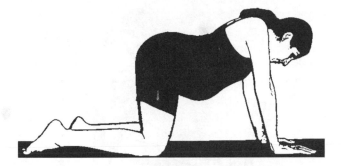

Figure 9.2. Pelvic tilt start position: Note arch in lower back. Kneel on your hands and knees; you'll notice an arch in your lower back. Tilt your pelvis backwards, so you flatten your back, keeping your buttocks relaxed.

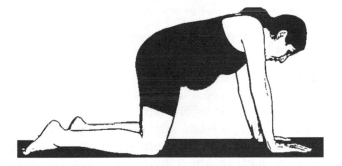

Figure 9.3. Pelvic tilt end position: Note absence of arch in lower back.

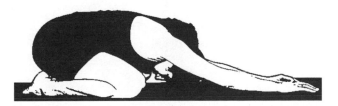

Figure 9.4. Back stretch: Kneel on your hands and knees, with your legs spread apart, and a small pillow under your belly. Sit back and reach your arms forward to feel a stretch along your spine.

91

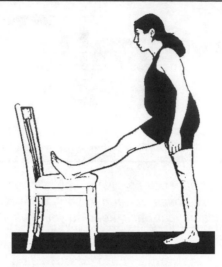

Figure 9.5. Hamstring stretch: Face a chair and place one foot on it. Keep your back straight as you gently lean forward to stretch the back of the thigh.

What is sciatica?

The sciatic nerve is a large nerve that runs down the back across the buttocks and down the back of your legs. Sciatica is pain in the sciatic nerve which is caused by pressure on the nerve. The symptoms of sciatica that are different from normal back pain in pregnancy are: pain down the buttock and back of your leg past your knee, tingling, numbness, or if you have trouble moving your leg. The treatment for sciatica is the same as the treatment for back pain but your health care provider may also suggest bedrest and physical therapy. Sciatic pain usually goes away in 1 to 2 weeks.

Chapter 10

Pregnancy, Pelvic Floor Disorders, and Bladder Control

Chapter Contents

Section 10.1

Pregnancy Increases Risk of Pelvic Floor Problems

From "Pelvic Floor Disorders," by the National Institute of Child Health and Human Development (NICHD, www.nichd.nih.gov), part of the National Institutes of Health, January 10, 2007.

What are pelvic floor disorders?

The term "pelvic floor" refers to the group of muscles that form a sling or hammock across the opening of a woman's pelvis. These muscles, together with their surrounding tissues, keep all of the pelvic organs in place so that the organs can function correctly.

A pelvic floor disorder occurs when the pelvic muscles and connective tissue in the pelvis weaken or are injured.

An estimated one-third of all U.S. women are affected by one type of pelvic floor disorder in her lifetime. Disorders may result from pelvic surgery, radiation treatments, and, in some cases, pregnancy or vaginal delivery of a child.

What are the most common pelvic floor disorders?

There are a variety of problems related to the pelvic floor. The most common include the following:

- **Pelvic organ prolapse:** A "prolapse" occurs when the pelvic muscles and tissue become weak and can no longer hold the organs in place correctly. In uterine prolapse, the uterus can press down on the vagina, causing it to invert, or even to come out through the vaginal opening. In vaginal prolapse, the top of the vagina loses support and can drop through the vaginal opening. Some symptoms of pelvic organ prolapse may include:

  - a feeling of heaviness or fullness or as if something falling out of the vagina;

  - some women also feel a pulling or aching or a "bulge" in the lower abdomen or pelvis; and

94

- prolapse may also cause a kinking in the urethra, making it harder for a woman to empty her bladder completely, or causing frequent urinary tract infections.

- **Urinary incontinence:** This can occur when the bladder drops down into the vagina. Because the bladder is not in its proper place, a key symptom of urinary incontinence is urine leaking without a woman's control. Other symptoms might include urgency to urinate, frequent urination, and painful urination.

- **Anal incontinence:** This can occur when the rectum bulges into or out of the vagina, making it difficult to control the bowels. It can also occur when there is damage to the anal sphincter, the ring of muscles that keep the anus closed.

What are the treatments for pelvic floor disorders?

Many women don't need treatment for their pelvic floor disorder. In other cases, treatment for symptoms includes changes in diet, weight control, and other lifestyle changes. Treatment may also include surgery, medication, and use of a device placed in the vagina called a pessary that helps support the pelvic organs.

Exercises for the pelvic floor muscles (known as Kegel exercises) can often help strengthen the muscles around the openings of the urethra, vagina, and rectum. Treatments for incontinence can also include medication and bladder or bowel control training.

Section 10.2

Pregnancy and Bladder Control

From "Pregnancy, Childbirth, and Bladder Control," by the National Institute of Diabetes and Digestive and Kidney Diseases (NIDDK, www.niddk.nih.gov), part of the National Institutes of Health, May 2002. Reviewed by David A. Cooke, MD, FACP, March 31, 2009.

Do pregnancy and childbirth affect bladder control?

Yes. But don't panic. If you lose bladder control after childbirth, the problem often goes away by itself. Your muscles may just need time to recover.

When do you need medical help?

If you still have a problem after six weeks, talk to your doctor. Without treatment, lost bladder control can become a long-term problem. Accidental leaking can also signal that something else is wrong in your body.

Bladder control problems do not always show up right after childbirth. Some women do not begin to have problems until later, often in their 40s.

You and your health care team must first find out why you have lost bladder control. Then you can discuss treatment.

After treatment, most women regain or improve their bladder control. Regaining control helps you enjoy a healthier and happier life.

Can you prevent bladder problems?

Yes. Women who exercise certain pelvic muscles have fewer bladder problems later on. These muscles are called pelvic floor muscles. If you plan to have a baby, talk to your doctor. Ask if you should do pelvic floor exercises. Exercises after childbirth also help prevent bladder problems in middle age.

Ask your health care team how to do pelvic exercises.

How does bladder control work?

Your bladder is a muscle shaped like a balloon. While the bladder stores urine, the bladder muscle relaxes. When you go to the bathroom, the bladder muscle tightens to squeeze urine out of the bladder.

More muscles help with bladder control. Two sphincter muscles surround the tube that carries urine from your bladder down to an opening in front of the vagina. The tube is called the urethra. Urine leaves your body through this tube. The sphincters keep the urethra closed by squeezing like rubber bands.

Pelvic floor muscles under the bladder also help keep the urethra closed.

When the bladder is full, nerves in your bladder signal the brain. That's when you get the urge to go to the bathroom. Once you reach the toilet, your brain sends a message down to the sphincter and pelvic floor muscles. The brain tells them to relax. The brain signal also tells the bladder muscles to tighten up. That squeezes urine out of the bladder.

Strong sphincter (bladder control) muscles prevent urine leakage in pregnancy and after childbirth. You can exercise these muscles to make them strong. Talk to your doctor about learning how to do pelvic floor exercises.

What do pregnancy and childbirth have to do with bladder control?

The added weight and pressure of pregnancy can weaken pelvic floor muscles. Other aspects of pregnancy and childbirth can also cause problems, such as:

- changed position of bladder and urethra;

- vaginal delivery;

- episiotomy (the cut in the muscle that makes it easier for the baby to come out); and

- damage to bladder control nerves.

Which professionals can help you with bladder control?

Professionals who can help you with bladder control include:

- your primary care doctor;

97

- a gynecologist: a women's doctor;
- a urogynecologist: an expert in women's bladder problems;
- a urologist: an expert in bladder problems;
- a specialist in female urology;
- a nurse or nurse practitioner; and
- a physical therapist.

Chapter 11

Pregnancy and Bone Health

Both pregnancy and breastfeeding cause changes and place extra demands on a woman's body. Some of these may have an effect on her bones. The good news is that most women do not experience bone problems during pregnancy and breastfeeding. And if their bones are affected during these times, the problem is often easily corrected. Nevertheless, taking care of one's bone health is especially important during pregnancy and when breastfeeding—for the good health of both the mother and her baby.

Pregnancy and Bone Health

During pregnancy, the baby growing in its mother's womb needs plenty of calcium to develop its skeleton. This need is especially great during the last three months of the pregnancy. If the mother does not get enough calcium, her baby will draw what it needs from its mother's bones. So, it is disconcerting to realize that most women of child-bearing years are not in the habit of getting enough calcium. Fortunately (unless a mother is still a teenager), pregnancy appears to help protect a woman's calcium reserves in several ways:

- Pregnant women absorb calcium better from food and supplements than women who are not pregnant. This is especially true

From "Pregnancy, Breastfeeding, and Bone Health," by the National Institute of Arthritis and Musculoskeletal and Skin Diseases (NIAMS, www.niams .nih.gov), part of the National Institutes of Health, June 2005.

during the last half of pregnancy, when the baby is growing quickly and has the greatest need for calcium.

• During pregnancy, women produce more estrogen, a hormone that protects bones.

• Any bone mass lost during pregnancy is typically restored within several months after the baby's delivery (or several months after breastfeeding is stopped).

Some studies suggest that pregnancy may be good for bone health overall. There is some evidence that the more times a woman has been pregnant (for at least 28 weeks), the greater her bone density and the lower her risk of fracture.

In some cases, women develop osteoporosis during pregnancy and/ or breastfeeding, although this is rare. Osteoporosis is bone loss that is serious enough to result in fragile bones and increased risk of fracture.

In many cases, women who develop osteoporosis during pregnancy and breastfeeding will recover lost bone after their pregnancy ends or they stop breastfeeding. It is less clear whether teenage mothers recover lost bone and are able to go on to optimize their bone mass.

Teenage mothers may be at especially high risk for bone loss during pregnancy and for osteoporosis later in life. Unlike older women, these mothers are still building much of their total bone mass during their teenage years. The unborn baby's need to develop its skeleton may compete with the teenage mother's need for calcium to build her own bones, compromising her ability to achieve optimal bone mass that will help protect her from osteoporosis later in life. Pregnant teens should be especially careful to get enough calcium during and after their babies are born to minimize any bone loss.

Breastfeeding and Bone Health

Breastfeeding also has an effect on a mother's bones. Studies have shown that women often lose three to five percent of their bone mass during breastfeeding, although it is rapidly recovered after weaning. This bone loss may be caused by the growing baby's increased need for calcium, which is drawn from the mother's bones. The amount of calcium the mother needs depends on the amount of breast milk produced and how long breastfeeding continues. Bone loss may also occur during breastfeeding because the mother produces less estrogen—the hormone that protects bones. The good news is that like the bone lost during pregnancy, bone lost during breastfeeding is usually recovered within six months after breastfeeding ends.

Tips to Keep Bones Healthy during Pregnancy, Breastfeeding, and Beyond

Taking care of your bones is important throughout life, including before, during, and after pregnancy and breastfeeding. A balanced diet with adequate calcium, regular exercise, and a healthy lifestyle are good for mothers and their babies.

Calcium: Although this important mineral is important throughout your lifetime, your body's demand for it is greater during pregnancy and breastfeeding, because both you and your baby need it. The National Academy of Sciences recommends that women who are pregnant or breastfeeding consume 1,000 mg (milligrams) of calcium each day. For pregnant teens, the recommended intake is even higher: 1,300 mg a day.

Good sources of calcium include:

- low-fat dairy products, such as milk, yogurt, cheese, and ice cream;
- dark green, leafy vegetables, such as broccoli, collard greens, and bok choy;
- canned sardines and salmon with bones;
- tofu, almonds, corn tortillas; and
- foods fortified with calcium, such as orange juice, cereals, and breads.

In addition, your doctor will probably prescribe a vitamin and mineral supplement to take during your pregnancy and while breastfeeding to ensure that you get enough of this important mineral.

Exercise: Like muscles, bones respond to exercise by becoming stronger. Regular exercise, especially weight-bearing exercise that forces you to work against gravity, helps build and maintain strong bones. Examples of weight-bearing exercise include walking, climbing stairs, dancing, and lifting weights. Being active and exercising during pregnancy can benefit your health in other ways, too. According to the American College of Obstetricians and Gynecologists, it can:

- help reduce backaches, constipation, bloating, and swelling;

- help prevent or treat gestational diabetes;
- increase energy;
- improve mood;
- improve posture;
- promote muscle tone, strength, and endurance;
- help you sleep better; and
- help you get back in shape after your baby is born.

It is important to talk to your doctor about your plans before you begin or resume an exercise program.

Healthy lifestyle: Smoking is bad for your baby, bad for your bones, and bad for your heart and lungs. Talk to your doctor about quitting. He or she can suggest resources to help you. Alcohol also is bad for pregnant and breastfeeding women and their babies, and excess alcohol is bad for bones. So, be sure to follow your doctor's orders to avoid alcohol during this important time.

Chapter 12

Carpal Tunnel Syndrome More Common during Pregnancy

What is carpal tunnel syndrome (CTS)?

Carpal tunnel syndrome (CTS) is the name for a group of problems that includes swelling, pain, tingling, and loss of strength in your wrist and hand. Your wrist is made of small bones that form a narrow groove or carpal tunnel. Tendons and a nerve called the median nerve must pass through this tunnel from your forearm into your hand. The median nerve controls the feelings and sensations in the palm side of your thumb and fingers. Sometimes swelling and irritation of the tendons can put pressure on the wrist nerve causing the symptoms of CTS. A person's dominant hand is the one that is usually affected. However, nearly half of CTS sufferers have symptoms in both hands.

CTS has become more common in the United States and is quite costly in terms of time lost from work and expensive medical treatment. The U.S. Department of Labor reported that in 2003 the average number of missed days of work due to CTS was 23 days, costing over $2 billion a year. It is thought that about 3.7 percent of the general public in this country suffer from CTS.

What are the symptoms of CTS?

Typically, CTS begins slowly with feelings of burning, tingling, and numbness in the wrist and hand. The areas most affected are the

"Frequently Asked Questions about Carpal Tunnel Syndrome," by the Office of Women's Health (www.womenshealth.gov), part of the U.S. Department of Health and Human Services, June 1, 2005.

thumb, index, and middle fingers. At first, symptoms may happen more often at night. Many CTS sufferers do not make the connection between a daytime activity that might be causing the CTS and the delayed symptoms. Also, many people sleep with their wrist bent, which may cause more pain and symptoms at night. As CTS gets worse, the tingling may be felt during the daytime too, along with pain moving from the wrist to your arm or down to your fingers. Pain is usually felt more on the palm side of the hand.

Another symptom of CTS is weakness of the hands that gets worse over time. Some people with CTS find it difficult to grasp an object, make a fist, or hold onto something small. The fingers may even feel like they are swollen even though they are not. Over time, this feeling will usually happen more often.

If left untreated, those with CTS can have a loss of feeling in some fingers and permanent weakness of the thumb. Thumb muscles can actually waste away over time. Eventually, CTS sufferers may have trouble telling the difference between hot and cold temperatures by touch.

What causes CTS and who is more likely to develop it?

Women are three times more likely to have CTS than men. Although there is limited research on why this is the case, scientists have several ideas. It may be that the wrist bones are naturally smaller in most women, creating a tighter space through which the nerves and tendons must pass. Other researchers are looking at genetic links that make it more likely for women to have musculoskeletal injuries such as CTS. Women also deal with strong hormonal changes during pregnancy and menopause that make them more likely to suffer from CTS. Generally, women are at higher risk of CTS between the ages of 45 and 54. Then, the risk increases for both men and women as they age.

There are other factors that can cause CTS, including certain health problems and, in some cases, the cause is unknown.

These are some of the things that might raise your chances of developing CTS:

- **Genetic predisposition:** The carpal tunnel is smaller in some people than others.

- **Repetitive movements:** People who do the same movements with their wrists and hands over and over may be more likely to develop CTS. People with certain types of jobs are more likely to have CTS, including manufacturing and assembly line workers, grocery store checkers, violinists, and carpenters. Some hobbies and sports that use repetitive hand movements can also cause CTS, such as golfing, knitting, and gardening. Whether or not long-term typing or computer use causes CTS is still being debated. Limited research points to a weak link, but more research is needed.

- **Injury or trauma:** A sprain or a fracture of the wrist can cause swelling and pressure on the nerve, increasing the risk of CTS. Forceful and stressful movements of the hand and wrist can also cause trauma, such as strong vibrations caused by heavy machinery or power tools.

- **Pregnancy:** Hormonal changes during pregnancy and build-up of fluid can put pregnant women at greater risk of getting CTS, especially during the last few months. Most doctors treat CTS in pregnant women with wrist splits or rest, rather than surgery, as CTS almost always goes away following childbirth.

Chapter 13

Vision and Oral Changes

Chapter Contents

Section 13.1

Pregnancy and Your Vision

Pregnancy brings an increase in hormones that may cause changes in vision. In most cases, these are temporary eye conditions that will return to normal after delivery. It's important for expectant mothers to be aware of vision changes during pregnancy and know what symptoms indicate a serious problem.

Refractive Changes

During pregnancy, changes in hormone levels can alter the strength you need in your eyeglasses or contact lenses. Though this is usually nothing to worry about, it's a good idea to discuss any vision changes with an eye doctor who can help you decide whether or not to change your prescription. The doctor may simply tell you to wait a few weeks after delivery before making a change in your prescription.

Dry Eyes

Some women experience dry eyes during pregnancy. This is usually temporary and goes away after delivery. The good news is that lubricating or rewetting eye drops are perfectly safe to use while you are pregnant or nursing. They can lessen the discomfort of dry eyes. It's also good to know that contact lenses, contact lens solutions, and enzymatic cleaners are safe to use while you are pregnant. To reduce the irritation caused by a combination of dry eyes and contact lenses, try cleaning your contact lenses with an enzymatic cleaner more often. If dry, irritated eyes make wearing contacts too uncomfortable, don't worry. Your eyes will return to normal within a few weeks after delivery.

Puffy Eyelids

Puffiness around the eyes is another common side effect of certain hormonal changes women may have while pregnant. Puffy eyelids may interfere with side vision. As a rule of thumb, don't skimp on your water intake and stick to a moderate diet, low in sodium and caffeine. These healthy habits can help limit water retention and boost your overall comfort.

Migraine Headaches

Migraine headaches linked to hormonal changes are very common among pregnant women. In some cases, painful migraine headaches make eyes feel more sensitive to light. If you are pregnant and suffering from migraines, be sure to talk to your doctor before taking any prescription or non-prescription migraine headache medications.

Prenatal care helps keep both you and your unborn child healthy. Be sure to tell your doctor if you are having any problems. Keep your eye doctor up-to-date about your overall health. Tell him or her about any pre-existing conditions, and about any prescription and non-prescription medications you are taking.

Diabetes

Women who are diabetic before their pregnancy and those who develop gestational diabetes need to watch their vision closely. Blurred vision in such cases may indicate elevated blood sugar levels.

High Blood Pressure

In some cases, a woman may have blurry vision or spots in front of her eyes while pregnant. These symptoms can be caused by an increase in blood pressure during pregnancy. At excessive levels, high blood pressure can even cause retinal detachment.

Glaucoma

Women being treated for glaucoma should tell their eye doctor right away if they are pregnant or intend to become pregnant. While many glaucoma medications are safe to take during pregnancy, certain glaucoma medications such as carbonic anhydrase inhibitors can be harmful to the developing baby.

Just because you are expecting a baby doesn't mean you have to put off your regular eye exam! You can have your eyes safely dilated while you are pregnant. If you suffer from any pre-existing eye conditions, like glaucoma, high blood pressure, or diabetes, it's very important to tell your eye doctor that you are pregnant. Your eye doctor may watch closely for changes in your vision during this exciting time in your life.

Section 13.2

Pregnancy and Oral Health

"How Does Pregnancy Affect My Oral Health?" reprinted with permission from *General Dentistry,* March 2007. © Academy of General Dentistry. All rights reserved. On the Web at www.agd.org. License # AGD-5542-MES.

It's a myth that calcium is lost from a mother's teeth and "one tooth is lost with every pregnancy." But you may experience some changes in your oral health during pregnancy. The primary changes are due to a surge in hormones—particularly an increase in estrogen and progesterone—can exaggerate the way gum tissues react to plaque.

How does a build-up of plaque affect me?

If the plaque isn't removed, it can cause gingivitis—red, swollen, tender gums that are more likely to bleed. So-called "pregnancy gingivitis" affects most pregnant women to some degree, and generally begins to surface as early as the second month. If you already have gingivitis, the condition is likely to worsen during pregnancy. If untreated, gingivitis can lead to periodontitis, a more serious form of gum disease.

Pregnant women are also at risk for developing pregnancy tumors, inflammatory, non-cancerous growths that develop when swollen gums become irritated. Normally, the tumors are left alone and will usually shrink on their own after the baby's birth. But if a tumor is uncomfortable and interferes with chewing, brushing or other oral hygiene procedures, the dentist may decide to remove it.

How can I prevent these problems?

You can prevent gingivitis by keeping your teeth clean, especially near the gumline. You should brush with fluoride toothpaste at least twice a day and after each meal when possible. You should also floss thoroughly each day. If brushing causes morning sickness, rinse your mouth with water or with antiplaque and fluoride mouthwashes. Good nutrition—particularly plenty of vitamin C and B_{12}—help keep the oral cavity healthy and strong. More frequent cleanings from the dentist will help control plaque and prevent gingivitis. Controlling plaque also will reduce gum irritation and decrease the likelihood of pregnancy tumors.

Could gingivitis affect my baby's health?

Research suggests a link between preterm, low birthweight babies and gingivitis. Excessive bacteria can enter the bloodstream through your gums. If this happens, the bacteria can travel to the uterus, triggering the production of chemicals called prostaglandins, which are suspected to induce premature labor.

When should I see my dentist?

If you're planning to become pregnant or suspect you're pregnant, you should see a dentist right away. Otherwise, you should schedule a checkup in your first trimester for a cleaning. Your dentist will assess your oral condition and map out a dental plan for the rest of your pregnancy. A visit to the dentist also is recommended in the second trimester for a cleaning, to monitor changes and to gauge the effectiveness of your oral hygiene. Depending on the patient, another appointment may be scheduled early in the third trimester, but these appointments should be kept as brief as possible.

Are there any dental procedures I should avoid?

Non-emergency procedures generally can be performed throughout pregnancy, but the best time for any dental treatment is the fourth through sixth month. Women with dental emergencies that create severe pain can be treated during any trimester, but your obstetrician should be consulted during emergencies that require anesthesia or when medication is being prescribed. Only X-rays that are needed for emergencies should be taken during pregnancy. Lastly, elective procedures that can be postponed should be delayed until after the baby's birth.

Chapter 14

Emotional Concerns and Pregnancy

Chapter Contents

Section 14.1

Depression and Pregnancy

From "Pregnant and Depressed?" by the Office of Women's Health (www.womenshealth.gov), part of the U.S. Department of Health and Human Services, March 2007.

Hormones, body changes, and new emotions make you vulnerable to emotional ups and downs during and after pregnancy. Learn to spot the signs of depression so you can take care of you and your baby.

What is depression?

Depression can be described as feeling sad, blue, unhappy, miserable, or down in the dumps. Most of us feel this way at one time or another for short periods. But true clinical depression is a mood disorder in which feelings of sadness, loss, anger, or frustration interfere with everyday life for an extended time.

Depression can be mild, moderate, or severe. The degree of depression, which your doctor can determine, influences how you are treated.

How common is depression during and after pregnancy?

Depression that occurs during pregnancy or within a year after delivery is called perinatal depression. The exact number of women with depression during this time is unknown. But researchers believe that depression is one of the most common complications during and after pregnancy. Often, the depression is not recognized or treated, because some normal pregnancy changes cause similar symptoms and are happening at the same time. Tiredness, problems sleeping, stronger emotional reactions, and changes in body weight may occur during pregnancy and after pregnancy. But these symptoms may also be signs of depression.

What causes depression?

There may be a number of reasons why a woman gets depressed. Hormone changes or a stressful life event, such as a death in the family, can cause chemical changes in the brain that lead to depression. Depression is also an illness that runs in some families. Other times, it's not clear what causes depression.

During pregnancy: During pregnancy, these factors may increase a woman's chance of depression:

- history of depression or substance abuse;
- family history of mental illness;
- little support from family and friends;
- anxiety about the fetus;
- problems with previous pregnancy or birth;
- marital or financial problems; and
- young age (of mother).

After pregnancy: Depression after pregnancy is called postpartum depression or peripartum depression. After pregnancy, hormonal changes in a woman's body may trigger symptoms of depression. During pregnancy, the amount of two female hormones, estrogen and progesterone, in a woman's body increases greatly. In the first 24 hours after childbirth, the amount of these hormones rapidly drops back down to their normal non-pregnant levels. Researchers think the fast change in hormone levels may lead to depression, just as smaller changes in hormones can affect a woman's moods before she gets her menstrual period.

Occasionally, levels of thyroid hormones may also drop after giving birth. The thyroid is a small gland in the neck that helps to regulate your metabolism (how your body uses and stores energy from food). Low thyroid levels can cause symptoms of depression including depressed mood, decreased interest in things, irritability, fatigue, difficulty concentrating, sleep problems, and weight gain. A simple blood test can tell if this condition is causing a woman's depression. If so, thyroid medicine can be prescribed by a doctor.

Other factors that may contribute to postpartum depression include:

- feeling tired after delivery, broken sleep patterns, and not enough rest often keeps a new mother from regaining her full strength for weeks;
- feeling overwhelmed with a new, or another, baby to take care of and doubting your ability to be a good mother;

115

- feeling stress from changes in work and home routines. Sometimes, women think they have to be "super mom" or perfect, which is not realistic and can add stress;

- having feelings of loss—loss of identity of who you are, or were, before having the baby, loss of control, loss of your pre-pregnancy figure, and feeling less attractive; and

- having less free time and less control over time. Having to stay home indoors for longer periods of time and having less time to spend with your partner and loved ones.

What are warning signs of depression?

Any of these symptoms during and after pregnancy that last longer than 2 weeks are signs of depression:

- feeling restless or irritable;

- feeling sad, hopeless, and overwhelmed;

- crying a lot;

- having no energy or motivation;

- eating too little or too much;

- sleeping too little or too much;

- trouble focusing, remembering, or making decisions;

- feeling worthless and guilty;

- loss of interest or pleasure in activities;

- withdrawal from friends and family; and

- having headaches, chest pains, heart palpitations (the heart beating fast and feeling like it is skipping beats), or hyperventilation (fast and shallow breathing).

After pregnancy, signs of depression may also include being afraid of hurting the baby or oneself and not having any interest in the baby.

What's the difference between "baby blues," postpartum depression, and postpartum psychosis?

The baby blues can happen in the days right after childbirth and normally go away within a few days to a week. A new mother can have sudden mood swings, sadness, crying spells, loss of appetite, sleeping problems, and feel irritable, restless, anxious, and lonely. Symptoms are not severe and treatment isn't needed. But there are things you can do to feel better. Nap when the baby does. Ask for help from your spouse, family members, and friends. Join a support group of new moms or talk with other moms.

Postpartum depression can happen anytime within the first year after childbirth. A woman may have a number of symptoms such as sadness, lack of energy, trouble concentrating, anxiety, and feelings of guilt and worthlessness. The difference between postpartum depression and the baby blues is that postpartum depression often affects a woman's well-being and keeps her from functioning well for a longer period of time. Postpartum depression needs to be treated by a doctor. Counseling, support groups, and medicines are things that can help.

Postpartum psychosis is rare. It occurs in 1 or 2 out of every 1,000 births and usually begins in the first 6 weeks postpartum. Women who have bipolar disorder or another psychiatric problem called schizo-affective disorder have a higher risk for developing postpartum psychosis. Symptoms may include delusions, hallucinations, sleep disturbances, and obsessive thoughts about the baby. A woman may have rapid mood swings, from depression to irritability to euphoria.

What should I do if I show signs of depression during or after pregnancy?

Some women don't tell anyone about their symptoms because they feel embarrassed, ashamed, or guilty about feeling depressed when they are supposed to be happy. They worry that they will be viewed as unfit parents. Perinatal depression can happen to any woman. It does not mean you are a bad or "not together" mom. You and your baby don't have to suffer. There is help.

There are different types of individual and group talk therapies that can help a woman with perinatal depression feel better and do better as a mom and as a person. Limited research suggests that many women with perinatal depression improve when treated with antidepressant medicine. Your doctor can help you learn more about these options and decide which approach is best for you and your baby. The next section contains more detailed information about available treatments.

Speak to your doctor or midwife if you are having symptoms of depression while you are pregnant or after you deliver your baby. Your doctor or midwife can give you a questionnaire to test for depression and can also refer you to a mental health professional who specializes in treating depression.

Here are some other helpful tips:

- Try to get as much rest as you can. Try to nap when the baby naps.

- Stop putting pressure on yourself to do everything. Do as much as you can and leave the rest!

- Ask for help with household chores and nighttime feedings. Ask your husband or partner to bring the baby to you so you can breastfeed. If you can, have a friend, family member, or professional support person help you in the home for part of the day.

- Talk to your husband, partner, family, and friends about how you are feeling.

- Do not spend a lot of time alone. Get dressed and leave the house.

- Run an errand or take a short walk.

- Spend time alone with your husband or partner.

- Talk with other mothers, so you can learn from their experiences.

- Join a support group for women with depression. Call a local hotline or look in your telephone book for information and services.

- Don't make any major life changes during pregnancy. Major changes can cause unneeded stress. Sometimes big changes cannot be avoided. When that happens, try to arrange support and help in your new situation ahead of time.

How is depression treated?

There are two common types of treatment for depression.

- **Talk therapy:** This involves talking to a therapist, psychologist, or social worker to learn to change how depression makes you think, feel, and act.

- **Medicine:** Your doctor can give you an antidepressant medicine to help you. These medicines can help relieve the symptoms of depression.

Women who are pregnant or breastfeeding should talk with their doctors about the advantages and risks of taking antidepressant medicines. Some women are concerned that taking these medicines may harm the baby. A mother's depression can affect her baby's development, so getting treatment is important for both mother and baby. The risks of taking medicine have to be weighed against the risks of depression. It is a decision that women need to discuss carefully with their doctors. Women who decide to take antidepressant medicines should talk to their doctors about which antidepressant medicines are safer to take while pregnant or breastfeeding.

Can untreated depression harm my baby?

Depression not only hurts the mother, but also affects her family. Some researchers have found that depression during pregnancy can raise the risk of delivering an underweight baby or a premature infant. Some women with depression have difficulty caring for themselves during pregnancy. They may have trouble eating and won't gain enough weight during the pregnancy; have trouble sleeping; may miss prenatal visits; may not follow medical instructions; have a poor diet; or may use harmful substances, like tobacco, alcohol, or illegal drugs.

Postpartum depression can affect a mother's ability to parent. She may lack energy, have trouble concentrating, be irritable, and not be able to meet her child's needs for love and affection. As a result, she may feel guilty and lose confidence in herself as a mother, which can worsen the depression. Researchers believe that postpartum depression can affect the infant by causing delays in language development, problems with emotional bonding to others, behavioral problems, lower activity levels, sleep problems, and distress. It helps if the father or another caregiver can assist in meeting the needs of the baby and other children in the family while mom is depressed.

All children deserve the chance to have a healthy mom. All moms deserve the chance to enjoy their life and their children. Don't suffer alone. If you are experiencing symptoms of depression during pregnancy or after having a baby, please tell a loved one and call you doctor or midwife right away.

Section 14.2

Stopping Antidepressant Use May Pose Risks to Pregnant Women

From "Stopping Antidepressant Use While Pregnant May Pose Risks,"
by the National Institute of Mental Health (NIMH, www.nimh.nih.gov),
part of the National Institutes of Health, February 1, 2006.

Pregnant women who discontinue antidepressant medications may significantly increase their risk of relapse during pregnancy, a new study funded by the National Institute of Health's National Institute of Mental Health found.

Women in the study who stopped taking antidepressants while pregnant were five times more likely than those who continued use of these medications to experience episodes of depression during pregnancy, reported Lee Cohen, MD, of Massachusetts General Hospital and colleagues in the February 1 [2006] issue of the *Journal of the American Medical Association*.

Depression is a disabling disorder that has been estimated to affect approximately 10 percent of pregnant women in the United States. Recently there has been concern about the use of antidepressants during pregnancy; however what has not been addressed is the risk of depression recurrence should someone discontinue antidepressant use. This study sheds light on the risk of relapse associated with discontinuing antidepressant therapy during pregnancy.

In the study, Cohen and colleagues enrolled pregnant women already taking antidepressants and then noted how many of the women decided to stop taking their medications. They then assessed the risk of relapse for the women who stopped versus maintained antidepressant therapy.

Contrary to the belief that hormonal changes shield pregnant women from depression, this study demonstrates that pregnancy itself is not protective. Among the pregnant women who stopped taking antidepressants, 68 percent relapsed during pregnancy compared to 26 percent who relapsed despite continuing their antidepressants. Among the women who discontinued use and relapsed, 50 percent experienced a relapse during the first trimester, and 90 percent did so by the end of the second trimester.

This study demonstrates the importance of weighing the risks not only of antidepressant use, but also the risk of relapse should antidepressants be discontinued. It highlights the importance of women discussing with their physicians their own individual risks verses benefits of continuing antidepressant use during pregnancy.

Section 14.3

Abuse during Pregnancy Affects One in Five Pregnant Women

"Abuse During Pregnancy," © 2008 University of Pittsburgh Medical Center (www.upmc.com). Reprinted with permission.

Abuse during pregnancy is more common than most people think. About one in five women may suffer abuse when they are pregnant. Abuse can start during pregnancy or get worse.

What Is Abuse?

Abuse includes physical hurting, like slapping, hitting, kicking, and punching. But it also can include verbal hurting, like being called names and being accused of doing things you have not done. Abuse can also include being forced to have sex against your wishes or being made to do things sexually you do not want to do.

Abuse can include threats and control. The abuser may try to make you behave in a certain way and may say something bad will happen to you if you don't. The abuser may try to keep you from seeing your family and friends. He or she may make you explain in detail what you do each day, where you go, and whom you see and talk to.

Women who are abused during pregnancy often feel confused and embarrassed. They ask themselves, "How can this be happening to me?" There is nothing to be embarrassed about. The abuser is to blame. Abuse is never your fault.

What Sparks Abuse during Pregnancy?

Adjusting and adapting to a pregnancy and a new baby can be very stressful for both partners. Some reasons why abuse happens during pregnancy may include the following:

- Your partner is angry because the pregnancy was unplanned.
- Your partner feels anxious and angry because the baby you are having has come too soon after the last baby.
- Your partner feels jealous of the baby.

Remember: There is no excuse for abuse!

Results of Abuse

Abuse affects your mind and body. Here are some of the effects it can have:

- You may have anemia (too few red blood cells), because you are not eating right or getting enough vitamins and iron.
- You may have bleeding during the first and second trimesters.
- You may not gain enough weight during the pregnancy.
- You may have more infections.
- Your baby may be too small at birth or may be born too early.
- Your baby may have problems after birth.
- You may feel depressed (sad and blue).
- You may feel anxious, upset, lonely, and worthless.
- You may not like yourself.
- You may be at risk for unhealthy behaviors, such as smoking or abusing drugs and alcohol during the pregnancy.
- You may not receive important regular prenatal care.

Are You Being Abused?

Many women don't want to accept the reality that they are being abused. Many just don't realize that their partner's actions are abusive. Here's how to know if you're being abused:

Does your partner:

- physically hurt you by hitting, slapping, grabbing, or kicking you?
- threaten you or talk about killing himself, you, and/or your children?
- seem depressed and hopeless about feeling better?
- keep weapons (guns, knives) in the house?
- keep track of all your time, where you go, and your relationships with others?
- tell you that there will be no future if you leave?
- use alcohol and/or drugs?
- threaten to hurt your pets or destroy your belongings?
- seem to be more violent as time goes on?

If you answered "yes" to three or more of these questions, you are probably being abused. You may be at high risk for being hurt or even killed by your partner.

Planning for Your Safety

Consider obtaining a Protection From Abuse (PFA) order. The PFA is a legal document granted by the court that prohibits your abuser from any form of contact with you.

Here are ways to plan for your safety so you can act quickly if you need to get away:

- Think of a safe place you and your children can go. Talk to someone you trust about your plans.
- Practice how to get out of your home safely through doors, windows, stairwells, elevators, and fire escapes.
- Remove all weapons from the home, if you can do this safely.
- Learn the phone numbers for the local police and women's shelter.
- Keep an extra set of car keys or money for a bus or cab in a safe place. Make sure you can get to them quickly.
- If you are planning to leave permanently, it will help if you have money, keys, extra clothing, and important papers ready to take with you.

At the time of a violent argument:

- Avoid a room with only one exit.

- If you are in danger, scream so that your neighbors can hear you.

- If you must leave the children in the home, call police immediately after you get to a place that is safe.

- If you have left after a violent argument, check yourself and your children for injuries, and go to the nearest hospital for care.

Effects on Children

Children who grow up in the midst of violence and abuse often are deeply affected by what they witness. Protect your children, and protect yourself. Keep in mind that a partner who abuses women during pregnancy is more likely to hurt children. Seek help for your children and yourself if you are being abused.

How to Get Help

Contact your local women's shelter, or talk to your doctor, nurse, midwife, or social worker about what is happening to you. These staff members know about abuse and are trained to help you in this situation. All information you give is confidential.

For confidential help and information, call toll-free 800-799-SAFE (7233). If you are hearing impaired, call (TDD) 800-787-3224.

Chapter 15

The Three Trimesters of Pregnancy: You and Your Baby

Pregnancy lasts about 40 weeks, counting from the first day of your last normal period. The weeks are grouped into three trimesters.

First Trimester (Week 1–Week 12)

During the first trimester your body undergoes many changes. Hormonal changes affect almost every organ system in your body. These changes can trigger symptoms even in the very first weeks of pregnancy. Your period stopping is a clear sign that you are pregnant. Other changes may include:

- extreme tiredness;
- tender, swollen breasts (your nipples might also stick out);
- upset stomach with or without throwing up (morning sickness);
- cravings or distaste for certain foods;
- mood swings;
- constipation (trouble having bowel movements);
- need to pass urine more often;
- headache;

Excerpted from "Stages of Pregnancy," by the Office of Women's Health (www.womenshealth.gov), part of the U.S. Department of Health and Human Services, March 2009.

- heartburn;
- weight gain or loss.

As your body changes, you might need to make changes to your daily routine, such as going to bed earlier or eating frequent, small meals. Fortunately, most of these discomforts will go away as your pregnancy progresses. And some women might not feel any discomfort at all. If you have been pregnant before, you might feel differently this time around. Just as each woman is different, so is each pregnancy.

Second Trimester (Week 13–Week 28)

Most women find the second trimester of pregnancy easier than the first. But it is just as important to stay informed about your pregnancy during these months.

You might notice that symptoms like nausea and fatigue are going away. But other new, more noticeable changes to your body are now happening. Your abdomen will expand as the baby continues to grow. And before this trimester is over, you will feel your baby beginning to move!

As your body changes to make room for your growing baby, you may have:

- body aches, such as back, abdomen, groin, or thigh pain;
- stretch marks on your abdomen, breasts, thighs, or buttocks;
- darkening of the skin around your nipples;
- a line on the skin running from belly button to pubic hairline;
- patches of darker skin, usually over the cheeks, forehead, nose, or upper lip (patches often match on both sides of the face; this is sometimes called the mask of pregnancy);
- numb or tingling hands, called carpal tunnel syndrome;
- itching on the abdomen, palms, and soles of the feet (Call your doctor if you have nausea, loss of appetite, vomiting, jaundice or fatigue combined with itching. These can be signs of a serious liver problem);
- swelling of the ankles, fingers, and face. (If you notice any sudden or extreme swelling or if you gain a lot of weight really quickly, call your doctor right away. This could be a sign of preeclampsia.)

Third Trimester (Week 29–Week 40)

You're in the home stretch! Some of the same discomforts you had in your second trimester will continue. Plus, many women find breathing difficult and notice they have to go to the bathroom even more often. This is because the baby is getting bigger and it is putting more pressure on your organs. Don't worry; your baby is fine and these problems will lessen once you give birth.

Some new body changes you might notice in the third trimester include:

- shortness of breath;
- heartburn;
- swelling of the ankles, fingers, and face (If you notice any sudden or extreme swelling or if you gain a lot of weight really quickly, call your doctor right away. This could be a sign of preeclampsia);
- hemorrhoids;
- tender breasts, which may leak a watery pre-milk called colostrum;
- your belly button may stick out;
- trouble sleeping;
- the baby "dropping," or moving lower in your abdomen;
- contractions, which can be a sign of real or false labor.

As you near your due date, your cervix becomes thinner and softer (called effacing). This is a normal, natural process that helps the birth canal (vagina) to open during the birthing process. Your doctor will check your progress with a vaginal exam as you near your due date. Get excited—the final countdown has begun!

Your Developing Baby

First Trimester (Week 1–Week 12)

At 4 Weeks

- Your baby's brain and spinal cord have begun to form.
- The heart begins to form.

- Arm and leg buds appear.
- Your baby is now an embryo and 1/25 of an inch long.

At 8 Weeks

- All major organs and external body structures have begun to form.
- Your baby's heart beats with a regular rhythm.
- The arms and legs grow longer, and fingers and toes have begun to form.
- The sex organs begin to form.
- The eyes have moved forward on the face and eyelids have formed.
- The umbilical cord is clearly visible.
- At the end of 8 weeks, your baby is a fetus and looks more like a human. Your baby is nearly 1 inch long and weighs less than 1/8 of an ounce.

At 12 Weeks

- The nerves and muscles begin to work together. Your baby can make a fist.
- The external sex organs show if your baby is a boy or girl.
- A woman who has an ultrasound in the second trimester or later might be able to find out the baby's sex.
- Eyelids close to protect the developing eyes. They will not open again until the 28th week.
- Head growth has slowed, and your baby is much longer. Now, at about 3 inches long, your baby weighs almost an ounce.

Second Trimester (Week 13–Week 28)

At 16 Weeks

- Muscle tissue and bone continue to form, creating a more complete skeleton.
- Skin begins to form. You can nearly see through it.
- Meconium develops in your baby's intestinal tract. This will be your baby's first bowel movement.

128

- Your baby makes sucking motions with the mouth (sucking reflex).
- Your baby reaches a length of about 4 to 5 inches and weighs almost 3 ounces.

At 20 Weeks

- Your baby is more active. You might feel slight fluttering.
- Your baby is covered by fine, downy hair called lanugo and a waxy coating called vernix. This protects the forming skin underneath.
- Eyebrows, eyelashes, fingernails, and toenails have formed.
- Your baby can even scratch itself.
- Your baby can hear and swallow.
- Now halfway through your pregnancy, your baby is about 6 inches long and weighs about 9 ounces.

At 24 Weeks

- Bone marrow begins to make blood cells.
- Taste buds form on your baby's tongue.
- Footprints and fingerprints have formed.
- Real hair begins to grow on your baby's head.
- The lungs are formed, but do not work.
- The hand and startle reflex develop.
- Your baby sleeps and wakes regularly.
- If your baby is a boy, his testicles begin to move from the abdomen into the scrotum. If your baby is a girl, her uterus and ovaries are in place, and a lifetime supply of eggs have formed in the ovaries.
- Your baby stores fat and has gained quite a bit of weight. Now at about 12 inches long, your baby weighs about 1 1/2 pounds.

Third Trimester (Week 29–Week 40)

At 32 Weeks

- Your baby's bones are fully formed, but still soft.

- Your baby's kicks and jabs are forceful.
- The eyes can open and close and sense changes in light.
- Lungs are not fully formed, but practice "breathing" movements occur.
- Your baby's body begins to store vital minerals, such as iron and calcium.
- Lanugo begins to fall off.
- Your baby is gaining weight quickly, about 1/2 pound a week.
- Now, your baby is about 15 to 17 inches long and weighs about 4 to 4 1/2 pounds.

At 36 Weeks

- The protective waxy coating called vernix gets thicker.
- Body fat increases. Your baby is getting bigger and bigger and has less space to move around. Movements are less forceful, but you will feel stretches and wiggles.
- Your baby is about 16 to 19 inches long and weighs about 6 to 6 1/2 pounds.

Weeks 37–40

- By the end of 37 weeks, your baby is considered full term.
- Your baby's organs are ready to function on their own.
- As you near your due date, your baby may turn into a head-down position for birth. Most babies "present" head down.
- At birth, your baby may weigh somewhere between 6 pounds, 2 ounces and 9 pounds, 2 ounces and be 19 to 21 inches long.
- Most full-term babies fall within these ranges. But healthy babies come in many different sizes.

Part Three

Staying Healthy during Pregnancy

Chapter 16

Choosing a Pregnancy
Health Care Provider

Chapter Contents

Section 16.1

How to Choose an Obstetrician/Gynecologist

Excerpted from "Choosing a Prenatal Care Provider," by the Office of Women's Health (www.womenshealth.gov), part of the U.S. Department of Health and Human Services, March 2009.

Medical checkups and screening tests help keep you and your baby healthy during pregnancy. This is called prenatal care. It also involves education and counseling about how to handle different aspects of your pregnancy. During your visits, your doctor may discuss many issues, such as healthy eating and physical activity, screening tests you might need, and what to expect during labor and delivery.

Choosing a Prenatal Care Provider

You will see your prenatal care provider many times before you have your baby. So you want to be sure that the person you choose has a good reputation, and listens to and respects you. You also will want to find out if the doctor or midwife can deliver your baby in the place you want to give birth, such as a specific hospital or birthing center.

Health care providers that care for women during pregnancy include:

- **Obstetricians (OB)** are medical doctors who specialize in the care of pregnant women and in delivering babies. OBs also have special training in surgery so they are also able to do a cesarean delivery. Women who have health problems or are at risk for pregnancy complications should see an obstetrician. Women with the highest risk pregnancies might need special care from a maternal-fetal medicine specialist.

- **Family practice doctors** are medical doctors who provide care for the whole family through all stages of life. This includes care during pregnancy and delivery and following birth. Most family practice doctors cannot perform cesarean deliveries.

- **A certified nurse-midwife (CNM) and certified professional midwife (CPM)** are trained to provide pregnancy and postpartum care. Midwives can be a good option for healthy women at low risk for problems during pregnancy, labor, or delivery. A CNM is educated in both nursing and midwifery. Most CNMs practice in hospitals and birth centers. A CPM is required to have experience delivering babies in home settings because most CPMs practice in homes and birthing centers. All midwives should have a backup plan with an obstetrician in case of a problem or emergency.

Ask your primary care doctor, friends, and family members for provider recommendations. When making your choice, think about:

- reputation;
- personality and bedside manner;
- the provider's gender and age;
- office location and hours;
- whether you always will be seen by the same provider during office checkups and delivery;
- who covers for the provider when she or he is not available;
- where you want to deliver; and
- how the provider handles phone consultations and after-hour calls.

Section 16.2

What Is a Midwife?

"What Is a Midwife?" *Journal of Midwifery and Women's Health,*
September/October 2006. © 2006 American College of Nurse-Midwives
(www.midwife.org). Reprinted with permission.

Certified nurse-midwives (CNMs) are licensed health care providers educated in nursing and midwifery. Certified midwives (CMs) are licensed health care providers educated in midwifery. CNMs and CMs have graduated from college; they have passed a national examination; and they have a license to practice midwifery from the state they live in. Most of the midwives in the United States are CNMs or CMs.

What do midwives do?

CNMs/CMs help over 300,000 women give birth each year in the United States. Most of these births are in hospitals. CNMs/CMs also care for women who decide to have their baby in freestanding birth centers and/or at home. CNMs/CMs provide health care to women all through life, including: prenatal care, birth, care after birth, care for the new baby, annual exams, birth control planning, menopause, and health counseling.

Why would I choose a midwife for care during my pregnancy?

CNMs/CMs believe you need time and special attention so you can be healthy and able to take care of your baby. Midwives specialize in providing support, regular health care, and in helping you get any additional care needed. Midwives are experts in knowing the difference between normal changes that occur during pregnancy and symptoms that require extra attention.

What if I have a high-risk pregnancy or complication during labor?

Your CNM/CM will prescribe medicine and order treatment for any common illness that you might get during pregnancy. Midwives work with doctors who specialize in illness during pregnancy. If you have a medical problem during pregnancy or complication during labor, your midwife will work with a doctor to make sure you get the best and safest care for you and your baby. Your midwife will also work with other health care providers: nurses, social workers, nutritionists, doulas, childbirth educators, physical therapists, and other specialists to help you get the care you need.

What if I want pain medicine during labor?

If you think you want pain medicine during labor, your midwife will give you information about the medicines available so you can decide what is right for you. Midwife means "with woman." If you decide you want pain medicine during labor, your midwife can prescribe it for you.

Should I see a midwife if I am not pregnant?

Many women go to their CNM or CM for annual check ups, family planning, and to get care for common infections that happen to women. For example, your midwife can answer questions about all the methods of birth control, help you decide what is best and safest for you, and prescribe it for you.

Questions to Ask When Choosing a Health Care Provider during Pregnancy

Questions to ask any health care provider:

- Do you practice alone or with others? Do they share your beliefs and manner of practice?
- Who attends births for you when you are away? How can I reach you?
- What kind of childbirth preparation do you recommend?
- Do you provide labor support and stay with women throughout labor?
- How do you feel about doulas or family and friends being with me during labor?
- Do you allow moving around and eating or drinking during labor?
- Can I hold my baby right after birth, breastfeed, and not be separated?

- When do you recommend IVs [intravenous], fetal heart rate monitoring, Pitocin, or episiotomy?

- Do you care for women who want a vaginal birth after a previous Cesarean (C) section?

- How much do you charge? Is your care paid for by my insurance?

Questions to ask providers in free-standing birth centers:

- What are your requirements for birth in this center?

- How often do women in your birth center go to a hospital during labor?

- When do you advise women to go into the hospital?

- What are your arrangements if I have a problem that requires being in a hospital?

Questions to ask providers who attend homebirths:

- How do you handle problems during labor? When would we go to the hospital?

- What drugs and equipment do you use in the home?

- Do you have a formal agreement with an obstetrician/gynecologist to provide care if problems occur?

- Which hospital will I be transported to if a problem occurs during labor?

- Would you stay with me if we transfer?

- Are you trained in newborn resuscitation?

- How many times do you visit after my baby is born?

For More Information

- www.MyMidwife.org—A website with information on midwifery, maternity, women's health, and family-centered care. There is a "find a midwife" link, where you can search for a midwife by location.

- www.ChildbirthConnection.org—A not-for-profit organization that has worked to improve maternity care for mothers, babies, and families since 1918. They promote safe, effective, and satis-fying evidence-based maternity care.

- www.ourbodiesourselves.org—Our Bodies Ourselves (OBOS), also known as the Boston Women's Health Book Collective (BWHBC), is a nonprofit, public interest women's health educa-tion, advocacy, and consulting organization.

- www.jmwh.org—A link to other, free Share With Women col-umns.

Chapter 17

Prenatal Medical Tests and Care during Pregnancy

Every parent-to-be hopes for a healthy baby, but it can be hard not to worry: What if the baby has a serious or untreatable health problem? What would I do? Is there anything I can do to prevent problems?

Concerns like these are completely natural. Fortunately, though, a wide array of tests for pregnant women can help to reassure them and keep them informed throughout their pregnancies.

Prenatal tests can help identify health problems that could endanger both you and your unborn child, some of which are treatable. However, these tests do have limitations. As an expectant parent, it's important to educate yourself about them and to think about what you would do if a health problem is detected in either you or your baby.

Why Are Prenatal Tests Performed?

Prenatal tests can identify several different things:

- treatable health problems in the mother that can affect the baby's health;

- characteristics of the baby, including size, sex, age, and placement in the uterus;

"Prenatal Tests," July 2008, reprinted with permission from www.kidshealth .org. Copyright © 2008 The Nemours Foundation. This information was provided by KidsHealth, one of the largest resources online for medically reviewed health information written for parents, kids, and teens. For more articles like this one, visit www.KidsHealth.org, or www.TeensHealth.org.

- the chance that a baby has certain congenital, genetic, or chromosomal problems;

- certain types of fetal abnormalities, including some heart problems.

The last two items on this list may seem the same, but there's a key difference. Some prenatal tests are screening tests and only reveal the possibility of a problem. Other prenatal tests are diagnostic, which means they can determine—with a fair degree of certainty—whether a fetus has a specific problem. In the interest of making the more specific determination, the screening test may be followed by a diagnostic test.

Prenatal testing is further complicated by the fact that more abnormalities can be diagnosed in a fetus than can be treated or cured.

What Do Prenatal Tests Find?

Among other things, routine prenatal tests can determine key things about the mother's health, including:

- her blood type;

- whether she has gestational diabetes;

- her immunity to certain diseases;

- whether she has a sexually transmitted disease (STD) or cervical cancer.

All of these conditions can affect the health of the fetus.

Prenatal tests also can determine things about the fetus' health, including whether it's one of the 2% to 3% of babies in the United States that the American College of Obstetricians and Gynecologists (ACOG) says have major congenital birth defects.

Tests for Disorders

Categories of defects which can be picked up by prenatal tests include the following disorders:

Dominant Gene Disorders

In dominant gene disorders when one parent is affected, there's a 50–50 chance a child will inherit the gene from the affected parent and have the disorder.

Dominant gene disorders include:

- Achondroplasia, a rare abnormality of the skeleton that causes a form of dwarfism, can be inherited from a parent who has it, but most cases occur without a family history.

- Huntington disease, a disease of the nervous system that causes a combination of mental deterioration and a movement disorder.

Recessive Gene Disorders

Because there are so many genes in each cell, everyone carries some abnormal genes, but most people don't have a defect because the normal gene overrules the abnormal recessive one. But if a fetus has a pair of abnormal recessive genes (one from each parent), the child will have the disorder. It can be more likely for this to happen in children born to certain ethnic groups.

Recessive gene disorders include:

- cystic fibrosis, most common among people of northern European descent; this disease is life threatening and causes severe lung damage and nutritional deficiencies.

- sickle cell disease, most common among people of African descent, is a disease in which red blood cells form a "sickle" shape (rather than the typical donut shape) that can get caught in blood vessels and damage organs and tissues.

- Tay-Sachs disease, most common among people of eastern European (Ashkenazi) Jewish descent, can cause mental retardation, blindness, seizures, and death.

- beta-thalassemia, most common among people of Mediterranean descent; this disorder can cause anemia.

X-Linked Disorders

These disorders are determined by genes on the X chromosome. The X and Y chromosomes are the chromosomes that determine sex. These disorders are much more common in boys because the pair of sex chromosomes in males contains only one X chromosome (the other is a Y chromosome). If the disease gene is present on the one X chromosome, the X-linked disease shows up because there's no other paired gene to "overrule" the disease gene. One such X-linked disorder is hemophilia, which prevents the blood from clotting properly.

Chromosomal Disorders

Chromosomal disorders occur when there is an abnormality in the number or structure of chromosomes, which contain the genetic material. Some chromosomal disorders are inherited but most are caused by a random error in the genetics of the egg or sperm. The chance of a child having these disorders increases with the age of the mother. For example, according to ACOG, 1 in 1,667 live babies born to 20-year-olds have Down syndrome, which causes mental retardation and physical defects. That number changes to 1 in 378 for 35-year-olds and 1 in 106 for 40-year-olds.

Multifactorial Disorders

This final category includes disorders that are caused by a mix of genetic and environmental factors. Their frequency varies from location to location, and some can be detected during pregnancy.

Multifactorial disorders include neural tube defects, which occur when the tube enclosing the spinal cord doesn't form properly. Neural tube defects, which often can be prevented by taking folic acid (which is in prenatal vitamins) around the time of conception and during pregnancy, include:

- spina bifida. Also called "open spine," this defect happens when the lower part of the neural tube doesn't close during embryo development. The spinal cord and nerves may be covered only by skin, or may be open to the environment, leaving them unprotected.

- anencephaly. This defect occurs when the brain and head don't develop properly, and parts of the brain are completely absent or malformed.

Other multifactorial disorders include:

- congenital heart defects;
- obesity;
- diabetes;
- cancer.

Who Has Prenatal Tests?

Certain prenatal tests are considered routine—that is, almost all pregnant women receiving prenatal care get them. Other nonroutine tests are recommended only for certain women, especially those with high-risk pregnancies. These may include women who:

- are age 35 or older;
- are adolescents;
- have had a premature baby;
- have had a baby with a birth defect—especially heart or genetic problems;
- are carrying more than one baby;
- have high blood pressure, diabetes, lupus, heart disease, kidney problems, cancer, a sexually transmitted disease, asthma, or a seizure disorder;
- have an ethnic background in which genetic disorders are common (or a partner who does);
- have a family history of mental retardation (or a partner who does).

Although your health care provider (which may be your OB-GYN, family doctor, or a certified nurse-midwife) may recommend these tests, it's ultimately up to you to decide whether to have them.

Also, if you or your partner have a family history of genetic problems, you may want to consult with a genetic counselor to help you look at the history of problems in your family, and to determine the risk to your children.

To decide which tests are right for you, it's important to carefully discuss with your health care provider:

- what these tests are supposed to measure;
- how reliable they are;
- the potential risks;
- your options and plans if the results indicate a disorder or defect.

Prenatal Tests during the First Visit

During your first visit to your health care provider for prenatal care, you can expect to have a full physical, which may include a pelvic and rectal examination, and you'll undergo certain tests regardless of your age or genetic background.

You may have a urine test to check for protein, sugar, or signs of infection.

Blood tests check for:

• your blood type and Rh factor. If your blood is Rh negative and your partner's is Rh positive, you may develop antibodies that prove dangerous to your fetus. This can be prevented through a course of injections given to you;

• anemia (a low red blood cell count);

• hepatitis B, syphilis, and HIV [human immunodeficiency virus];

• immunity to German measles (rubella) and chickenpox (varicella);

• cystic fibrosis. Health care providers now routinely offer this screening even when there's no family history of the disorder.

Cervical tests (also called Pap smears) check for:

• STDs such as chlamydia and gonorrhea;

• changes that could lead to cervical cancer.

To do a Pap smear, your health care provider uses what looks like a very long mascara wand or cotton swab to gently scrape the inside of your cervix (the opening to the uterus that's located at the very top of the vagina). This may be a little uncomfortable, but it is over quickly.

Prenatal Tests Performed throughout or Later in Pregnancy

After the initial visit, your health care provider will order other tests based on, among other things, your personal medical history and risk factors, as well as the current recommendations. These tests may include:

• urine tests for sugar, protein, and signs of infection. The sugar in urine may indicate gestational diabetes—diabetes that occurs during pregnancy; the protein can indicate preeclampsia—a condition that develops in late pregnancy and is characterized by a rise in blood pressure, with fluid retention and protein in the urine.

• group B streptococcus (GBS) infection. GBS bacteria are found naturally in the vaginas of many women but can cause serious infections in newborns. This test involves swabbing the vagina and rectum, usually between the 35th and 37th weeks of pregnancy. If the test comes back positive, it is important to go to the hospital as soon as your labor begins so that intravenous antibiotics can be started in order to reduce the chance of the baby being infected.

- sickle cell trait tests for women of African or Mediterranean descent, who are at higher risk for having sickle cell anemia—a chronic blood disease—or carrying the trait, which can be passed on to their children.

Other Tests

Here are some other tests that might be performed during pregnancy.

Ultrasound

Why Is This Test Performed?

In this test, sound waves are bounced off the baby's bones and tissues to construct an image showing the baby's shape and position in the uterus. Ultrasounds were once used only in high-risk pregnancies but have become so common that they're often part of routine prenatal care.

Also called a sonogram, sonograph, echogram, or ultrasonogram, an ultrasound is used:

- to determine whether the fetus is growing at a normal rate;
- to verify the expected date of delivery;
- to record fetal heartbeat or breathing movements;
- to see whether there might be more than one fetus;
- to identify a variety of abnormalities that might affect the remainder of the pregnancy or delivery;
- to make sure the amount of amniotic fluid in the uterus is adequate;
- to indicate the position of the placenta in late pregnancy (which may be blocking the baby's way out of the uterus);
- to detect pregnancies outside the uterus;
- as a guide during other tests such as amniocentesis.

Ultrasounds also are used to detect:

- structural defects such as spina bifida and anencephaly;
- congenital heart defects;
- gastrointestinal and kidney malformations;
- cleft lip or palate.

Should I Have This Test?

Most women have at least one ultrasound. The test is considered to be safe. Some women will have multiple ultrasounds during the pregnancy, others do not have any. Ask your health care provider if he or she thinks you will have ultrasounds during your pregnancy.

When Should I Have This Test?

An ultrasound is usually performed at 18 to 20 weeks to look at your baby's anatomy. If you want to know your baby's gender, you may be able to find out during this time—that is, if the genitals are in a visible position.

Ultrasounds also can be done sooner or later and sometimes more than once, depending on the health care provider and the pregnancy. For example, some providers will order an ultrasound to date the pregnancy, usually during the first 3 months. And others may want to order one during late pregnancy to make sure the baby's turned the right way before delivery.

Women with high-risk pregnancies may need to have multiple ultrasounds using more sophisticated equipment. Results can be confirmed when needed using special three-dimensional (3-D) equipment that allows the technician to get a more detailed look at the baby.

How Is This Test Performed?

Women need to have a full bladder for a transabdominal ultrasound (an ultrasound of the belly) to be performed in the early months—you may be asked to drink a lot of water and not urinate. You'll lie on an examining table and your abdomen will be coated with a special ultrasound gel. A technician will pass a wand-like instrument called a transducer back and forth over your abdomen. You may feel some pressure as the technician presses on the bladder. High-frequency sound waves "echo" off your body (and the fetus) and create a picture of the fetus inside on a computer screen. You may want to ask to have the picture interpreted for you, even in late pregnancy—it often doesn't look like a baby to the untrained eye.

Sometimes, if the technician isn't able to see a good enough image from the ultrasound, he or she will determine that a transvaginal ultrasound is necessary. This is especially common in early pregnancy. For this procedure, your bladder should be empty. Instead of a transducer being moved over your abdomen, a slender probe called an endovaginal transducer is placed inside your vagina. This technique often provides improved images of the uterus and ovaries.

Some health care providers may have the equipment and trained personnel necessary to provide in-office ultrasounds, whereas others may have you go to a local hospital or radiology center. Depending on where you have the ultrasound done, you may be able to get a printed picture (or multiple pictures) of your baby and/or a disc of images you can view on your computer and even send to friends and family.

When Are the Results Available?

Although the technician can see the images immediately, a full evaluation by a physician may take up to 1 week.

Depending on where you have the ultrasound done, the technician may be able to tell you that day whether everything looks OK. However, most radiology centers or health care providers prefer that technicians not comment until a specialist has taken a look—even when everything is OK.

Glucose Screening

Why Is This Test Performed?

Glucose screening checks for gestational diabetes, a short-term form of diabetes that develops in some women during pregnancy. Gestational diabetes is increasing in frequency in the United States, and may occur in 3 to 8% of pregnancies. Gestational diabetes can cause health problems for the baby, especially if it is not diagnoses or treated.

Should I Have This Test?

Most women have this test in order to diagnose and treat gestational diabetes, reducing the risk to the baby.

When Should I Have This Test?

Screening for gestational diabetes usually takes place at 24 to 28 weeks. Testing may be done earlier for women who are at higher risk of having gestational diabetes, such as those who:

- have previously had a baby that weighs more than 9 pounds (4.1 kilograms);
- have a family history of diabetes;
- are obese;
- are older than age 25;
- have sugar in the urine on routine testing;
- have high blood pressure;
- have polycystic ovary syndrome.

How Is the Test Performed?

This test involves drinking a sugary liquid and then having your blood drawn after an hour. If the sugar level in the blood is high, you'll have a glucose-tolerance test, which means you'll drink a glucose solution on an empty stomach and have your blood drawn once every hour for 3 hours.

When Are the Results Available?

The results are usually available within 1 to 2 days. Ask if your health care provider will call you with the results if they are normal or only if the reading is high and you need to come in for another test.

Chorionic Villus Sampling (CVS)

Why Is This Test Performed?

Chorionic villi are tiny finger-like units that make up the placenta (a disk-like structure that sticks to the inner lining of the uterus and provides nutrients from the mother to the fetus through the umbilical cord). They have the same chromosomes and genetic makeup as the fetus.

This alternative to an amniocentesis removes some of the chorionic villi and tests them for chromosomal abnormalities, such as Down syndrome. Its advantage over an amniocentesis is that it can be performed earlier, allowing more time for expectant parents to receive counseling and make decisions. The risks of CVS are higher than with amniocentesis so the risks and benefits of the test must be weighed.

Should I Have This Test?

Your health care provider may recommend this test if you:

- are older than age 35;
- have a family history of genetic disorders (or a partner who does);
- have a previous child with a genetic disorder or had a previous pregnancy with a chromosomal abnormality;
- have had an earlier screening test that indicates that there may be a concern.

Possible risks of this test include:

- approximately 1% risk of miscarriage (the risk is higher with the transcervical method than with the transabdominal method);
- infection;
- spotting or bleeding (this is more common with the transcervical method—see below);
- birth defects when the test is done too early in pregnancy.

When Should I Have This Test?

At 10 to 12 weeks.

How Is This Test Performed?

This test is done in one of two ways:

- transcervical. Using ultrasound as a guide, a thin tube is passed from the vagina into the cervix. Gentle suction removes a sample of tissue from the chorionic villi. Some women experience cramping with the removal.
- transabdominal. A needle is inserted through the abdominal wall with ultrasound guidance, and a sample of the chorionic villi is removed. Cramping may be felt with this approach as well.

After the sample is taken, the doctor may check the fetus' heart rate. You should rest for several hours afterward.

When Are the Results Available?

Usually 1 to 2 weeks depending on what the test is being used to look for.

151

Maternal Blood Screening/Triple Screen/Quadruple Screen

Why Is This Test Performed?

Doctors use this to test to screen for Down syndrome and neural tube defects. Alpha-fetoprotein (AFP) is a protein produced by the fetus, and it appears in varying amounts in the mother's blood and the amniotic fluid at different times during pregnancy. A certain level in the mother's blood is considered normal, but higher or lower levels may indicate a problem.

This test also looks at the levels of two pregnancy hormones—estriol and human chorionic gonadotropin (HCG)—which is why it's sometimes called a "triple screen" or "triple marker." The test is called a "quadruple screen" ("quad screen") or "quadruple marker" ("quad marker") when the level of an additional substance—inhibin-A—is also measured. The greater number of markers increases the accuracy of the screening and better identifies the possibility of a problem.

This test, which also is called a multiple-marker screening or maternal serum screening, calculates a woman's individual risk based on the levels of the three (or more) substances plus:

- her age;
- her weight;
- her race;
- whether she has diabetes requiring insulin treatment;
- whether she is carrying one fetus or multiple ones.

Sometimes this test is done along with an ultrasound and blood work during the first trimester, which makes it even more accurate than the second trimester blood work alone.

It's important to note, though, that each of these screening tests determine risk only—they don't diagnose a condition.

Should I Have This Test?

All women are offered some form of this test. Some practitioners include more parts of it than others. Remember that this is a screening, not a definitive test—it indicates whether a woman is likely to be carrying an affected fetus. It's also not foolproof—Down syndrome, another chromosomal abnormality, or a neural tube defect may go undetected, and some women with abnormal levels have been found to be carrying a healthy baby. Further testing is recommended to confirm a positive result.

When Should I Have This Test?

The blood tests are typically done between 15 and 20 weeks. When first trimester screening is added, the initial tests are done at about 11 to 13 weeks.

How Is the Test Performed?

Blood is drawn from the mother. When first trimester screening is added, an ultrasound is included.

When Are the Results Available?

Usually within a week, although it may take up 2 weeks.

Amniocentesis

Why Is This Test Performed?

This test is most often used to detect:

- Down syndrome and other chromosome abnormalities;
- structural defects such as spina bifida and anencephaly;
- inherited metabolic disorders.

Late in the pregnancy, this test can reveal if a baby's lungs are strong enough to allow the baby to breathe normally after birth. This can help the health care provider make decisions about inducing labor or trying to prevent labor, depending on the situation. For instance, if a mother's water breaks early, the health care provider may want to try to hold off on delivering the baby as long as possible to allow for the baby's lungs to mature.

Other common birth defects, such as heart disorders and cleft lip and palate, can't be determined using this test.

Should I Have This Test?

Your health care provider may recommend this test if you:

- are older than age 35;
- have a family history of genetic disorders (or a partner who does);

- have a previous child with a birth defect, or had a previous pregnancy with a chromosomal abnormality or neural tube defect;

- had an abnormal screening test.

This test can be very accurate—close to 100%—but only certain disorders can be detected. The rate of miscarriage with this procedure is between 1 in 300 and 1 in 500. It also carries a low risk of uterine infection, which can also cause miscarriage, leakage of amniotic fluid, and injury to the fetus.

When Should I Have This Test?

Amniocentesis is usually performed between 15 and 20 weeks.

How Is the Test Performed?

While watching with an ultrasound, the doctor inserts a needle through the abdominal wall into the uterus to remove some (about 1 ounce) of the amniotic fluid. Some women report that they experience cramping when the needle enters the uterus or pressure while the doctor retrieves the sample.

The doctor may check the fetus' heartbeat after the procedure to make sure it's normal. Most doctors recommend rest for several hours afterward.

The cells in the withdrawn fluid are grown in a special culture and then analyzed (the specific tests conducted on the fluid depend on personal and family medical history).

When Are the Results Available?

Timing varies; depending on what is being tested for, the results are usually available within 1 to 2 weeks. Tests of lung maturity are often available within a few hours.

Nonstress Test

Why Is This Test Performed?

A nonstress test (NST) can determine if the baby is responding normally to a stimulus. Used mostly in high-risk pregnancies or when a health care provider is uncertain of fetal movement, an NST can be performed at any point in the pregnancy after the 26th to 28th week when fetal heart rate can appropriately respond by accelerating and decelerating.

This test may also be done if you've gone beyond your due date. The NST can help a doctor make sure that the baby is receiving enough oxygen and is responding to stimulation. However, an unresponsive baby isn't necessarily in danger, though further testing might be needed.

Sometimes, a biophysical profile is done, which is when an NST and ultrasound are performed, looking at the breathing, movement, amount of amniotic fluid, and tone of the fetus, in addition to the heart rate response.

Should I Have This Test?

Your health care provider may recommend this if you have a high-risk pregnancy, if there are concerns during your pregnancy, or if you have a low-risk pregnancy but are past your due date.

When Should I Have This Test?

An NST may be recommended any time after 26 to 28 weeks, depending on why it is needed.

How Is the Test Performed?

The health care provider will measure the response of the fetus' heart rate to each movement the fetus makes as reported by the mother or observed by the doctor on an ultrasound screen. If the fetus doesn't move during the test, he or she may be asleep and the health care provider may use a buzzer to wake the baby. You also may be asked to drink or eat to try to stimulate the baby more.

When Are the Results Available?

Immediately.

Contraction Stress Test

Why Is This Test Performed?

This test stimulates the uterus with Pitocin, a synthetic form of oxytocin (a hormone secreted during childbirth), to determine the effect of contractions on fetal heart rate. It may be recommended when a nonstress test or biophysical profile indicates a problem and can determine whether the baby's heart rate remains stable during contractions.

Should I Have This Test?

This test may be ordered if the nonstress test or biophysical profile indicates a problem. However, it can induce labor.

When Should I Have This Test?

Your doctor may schedule it if he or she is concerned about how the baby will respond to contractions or feels that it is the appropriate test to determine the fetal heart rate response to a stimulus.

How Is the Test Performed?

Mild contractions are brought on either by injections of Pitocin or by squeezing the mother's nipples (which causes oxytocin to be secreted). The fetus' heart rate is then monitored.

When Are the Results Available?

Immediately.

Percutaneous Umbilical Blood Sampling (PUBS)

Why Is This Test Performed?

This test obtains fetal blood by guiding a needle into the umbilical cord. It's primarily used in addition to an ultrasound and amniocentesis if your health care provider needs to quickly check your baby's chromosomes for defects or disorders or is concerned that your baby may have another problem, such as a low platelet count or a thyroid condition.

The advantage to this test is its speed. There are situations (such as when a fetus shows signs of distress) in which it's helpful to know whether the fetus has a fatal chromosomal defect. If the fetus is suspected to be anemic or to have a platelet disorder, this test is the only way to confirm this because it provides a blood sample rather than amniotic fluid. It also allows transfusion of blood or needed fluids into the baby while the needle is in place.

Should I Have This Test?

This test may be used:

• after an abnormality has been noted on an ultrasound;

- when results from other tests, such as amniocentesis, aren't conclusive;

- if the fetus may have Rh disease;

- if you've been exposed to an infectious disease that could potentially affect fetal development.

Risks are associated with this procedure, such as miscarriage or infection, so the risks and benefits should be discussed with your health care provider.

When Should I Have This Test?

After 18 weeks.

How Is the Test Performed?

A fine needle is passed through your abdomen and uterus into the umbilical cord and blood is withdrawn for testing.

When Are the Results Available?

Usually within 3 days.

Talking to Your Health Care Provider

Some prenatal tests can be stressful, and because many aren't definitive, even a negative result may not completely relieve any anxiety you might be experiencing. Because many women who have abnormal tests end up having healthy babies and because some of the problems that are detected can't be treated, some women decide not to have some of the tests.

One important thing to consider is what you'll do in the event that a birth defect or chromosomal abnormality is discovered. Your health care provider or a genetic counselor can help you establish priorities, give you the facts, and discuss your options.

It's also important to remember that tests are offered to women—they are not mandatory. You should feel free to ask your health care provider why he or she is ordering a certain test, what the risks and benefits are, and, most important, what the results will—and won't—tell you.

If you think that your health care provider isn't answering your questions adequately, you should say so. Things you might want to ask include:

- How accurate is this test?
- What are you looking to get from these test results?/What do you hope to learn?
- How long before I get the results?
- Is the procedure painful?
- Is the procedure dangerous to me or the fetus?
- Do the potential benefits outweigh the risks?
- What could happen if I don't undergo this test?
- How much will the test cost?
- Will the test be covered by insurance?
- What do I need to do to prepare?

You also can ask your health care provider for literature about each type of test.

Preventing Birth Defects

The best thing that mothers-to-be can do to avoid birth defects and problems with the pregnancy is to take care of their bodies by:

- not smoking (and avoiding secondhand smoke);
- avoiding alcohol and other drugs;
- checking with the doctor about the safety of prescription and over-the-counter medications;
- avoiding fumes, chemicals, radiation, and excessive heat;
- eating a healthy diet;
- taking prenatal vitamins—if possible, beginning before becoming pregnant;
- getting exercise (after discussing it with the doctor);
- getting plenty of rest;
- getting prenatal care—if possible, beginning with a preconception visit to the doctor to see if anything needs to change before you get pregnant.

Chapter 18

Immunization Issues for Pregnant Women

Ideally, women of childbearing age should be immunized before becoming pregnant to protect their babies against serious diseases. For instance, rubella causes serious damage to the unborn fetus and is preventable by rubella vaccine. Varicella (chickenpox) can cause birth defects in the fetus and fatal pneumonia in the mother; it is preventable by varicella vaccine. Tetanus in the newborn, often fatal, is prevented if the mother has been immunized, as is the case with many other vaccine-preventable diseases.

Although many medications, including some vaccines, are avoided during pregnancy because of potential harm to the mother or fetus, some vaccines are actually recommended for pregnant women. Certain immunizations during pregnancy will enhance the mother's health and others will protect the child by means of the mother's antibodies that remain in the child for the first 3–6 months of life.

While certain drugs may harm the developing fetus, the risk of a developing fetus being harmed by vaccination of the mother during pregnancy remains only theoretical. Currently, no evidence exists of risk from vaccinating pregnant women with any inactivated viral or bacterial vaccine or toxoid. Live attenuated vaccines, including MMR [measles, mumps, and rubella] and varicella, are of greater theoretical concern, so it is recommended that women avoid pregnancy as a precautionary measure for at least 28 days after administration of these vaccines. This 28-day rule is used even though there is no evidence in prior studies of damage to the fetus when the pregnant mother received one of these vaccines.

Pregnant women and health care providers should always consider the risks and benefits of the vaccine as well as the risks of the disease before administering or receiving the vaccine. Immunization before conception is always preferred to immunization during pregnancy to prevent disease in the child. After delivery, women susceptible to rubella or varicella should be immunized with MMR or varicella vaccine before discharge from the hospital.

Breast-feeding does not interfere with the response to the vaccines recommended for adults. Although rubella vaccine virus has been found in human milk, this and other vaccines provided to the mother during pregnancy or immediately postpartum have not been shown to interfere with the immune response of children to the vaccine. Also, no child has developed illness from a vaccine administered to their mother. Human milk contains antibodies and other factors that may help protect infants against many infectious diseases.

The Centers for Disease Control and Prevention (CDC) has published a recommended adult immunization schedule [http://www.cdc.gov/vaccines/recs/schedules/adult-schedule.htm], including for pregnant women.

Vaccines Recommended for All Pregnant Women

Influenza: Pregnant women who become infected with influenza viruses are at increased risk of hospitalization, serious medical complications, and adverse pregnancy outcomes. Immunization of the pregnant woman with inactivated influenza virus vaccine is effective at reducing febrile respiratory infections in pregnant woman. Immunizing the mother during pregnancy also protects her newborn because she passes immune antibodies across the placenta (influenza antibodies are actually higher in umbilical cord blood than in the mother's blood). Infants with influenza virus infection account for many hospitalizations and are predisposed to bacterial respiratory infections. Childhood deaths associated with influenza virus infection occur most frequently in infants less than 6 months of age. Unfortunately, during the first 6 months of life, there are no vaccines or anti-influenza virus drugs available. For these reasons, pregnant women should receive inactivated influenza virus vaccine and those who will be helping to care for the newborn should be vaccinated as well. Studies of influenza vaccination of more than 2,000 pregnant women have demonstrated no adverse effects to the fetus from the vaccine. However, the nasal influenza vaccine should not be given to pregnant women because it is a live virus vaccine.

Tetanus: Tetanus in newborn infants—once common throughout the Americas—is prevented if the mother has been immunized. This is because an immune mother passes antibodies to the baby across the placenta. The mother is immune if she has been immunized before becoming pregnant or during pregnancy. An expectant mother whose tetanus immunization status is uncertain or whose last immunization was more than 10 years ago should be immunized against tetanus. This is usually given combined with diphtheria toxoid vaccine (a product called Td). Recently a new Td vaccine that also contains vaccine for pertussis has been licensed for adults (Tdap) including for use for women in the child-bearing age group. Pregnancy is not a contraindication to Tdap immunization. However, at this time, CDC recommends that pregnant women who received the last tetanus toxoid-containing vaccine less than 10 years ago receive Tdap in the post-partum period according to the routine vaccination recommendations. If the last dose of tetanus toxoid-containing vaccine was more than 10 years before, they prefer that she be immunized with Td during the second and third trimester instead of Tdap.

Vaccines That Pregnant Women Should Not Receive

Generally, live-attenuated vaccines are contraindicated for pregnant women because of the theoretical risk of transmission of the vaccine virus to the fetus. The following live, attenuated vaccines should not be administered during pregnancy except in unusual circumstances:

- influenza live virus vaccine (nasal spray)
- oral poliovirus vaccine (no longer distributed in the United States)
- measles-containing vaccines
- mumps-containing vaccines
- rubella-containing vaccines
- smallpox (vaccinia) vaccine
- typhoid vaccine (Ty21a)

- varicella (chickenpox) live virus vaccine

- yellow fever vaccine

Varicella: Varicella (or, chickenpox) vaccine is universally recommended for all children and nonpregnant adults who are susceptible, but it is not given to pregnant women. Pregnant women who develop chickenpox (varicella) are at increased risk of having severe illness and a small proportion of their newborns may be born with congenital varicella syndrome. Susceptible women who are exposed to varicella (or shingles, which is caused by the same virus) should receive varicella-zoster immune globulin (VariZIG) within 96 hours, which may prevent or modify infection. Antiviral drugs usually are reserved for pregnant women with severe chickenpox illness. Infants born to mothers who had chickenpox within 5 days of delivery are also given VariZIG within 48 hours of delivery to prevent them from having serious illness. Vaccination with varicella live virus vaccine during pregnancy is not recommended, although inadvertent vaccinations have not been associated with adverse outcomes. A pregnant household member is not a contraindication for varicella immunization of a child within that household, however.

The varicella vaccine virus rarely spreads from a vaccinated person who develops rash to susceptible persons within households. The risk for a susceptible pregnant woman and her fetus should be very low after this type of exposure. However, the pregnant woman who believes that she is susceptible to chickenpox and who has a household exposure to someone who develops rash after varicella immunization should inform her physician.

Ideally, women should be immune to chickenpox before pregnancy, either from vaccine or chickenpox. At the completion of pregnancy, susceptible women should receive the first dose of chickenpox vaccine before discharge from the healthcare facility. A second dose should be administered four to eight weeks later.

Measles, mumps, and rubella: Measles, mumps, and rubella live virus vaccines—usually given together as MMR—should not be administered during pregnancy. However, because measles increases the risk for spontaneous abortion or premature delivery, pregnant susceptible women are given immune globulin within six days of exposure. The mumps virus has not been associated with problems during pregnancy. Wild rubella virus infection in early pregnancy has a high risk of causing congenital rubella syndrome (CRS) in fetuses. This is a devastating disease that is preventable by the use of vaccine prior to pregnancy. Pregnant women are screened early in pregnancy to be certain that they are immune. If susceptible and exposed, the pregnant woman and her physician together will need to consider her options. The rubella-susceptible woman should be immunized with MMR in the immediate post-partum period. However, CDC has followed the outcomes of inadvertent rubella vaccination of pregnant women and no cases of CRS have been detected.

Transmission of MMR vaccine viruses within households has not been demonstrated (except rubella virus from nursing mothers to their infants). Thus, susceptible children should be immunized whether or not there is a pregnant household contact.

Yellow fever: Live attenuated yellow fever vaccine is not known to cause developmental malformations. It is only administered to pregnant women if travel to an endemic area where she is going to be at risk of exposure to yellow fever is unavoidable.

Typhoid fever: Neither the live attenuated Ty21a nor the Vi polysaccharide typhoid fever vaccines have been tested in pregnant or breastfeeding women. Some experts might consider the polysaccharide vaccine for pregnant or lactating women if travel to an endemic area is unavoidable and she is likely to be at risk of exposure to Salmonella typhi (the cause of typhoid fever).

Vaccines for Some Pregnant Women

The following vaccines should be considered for pregnant women who are at risk for acquiring or being exposed to these diseases. Because spontaneous abortion occurs more commonly in the first trimester of pregnancy, some obstetricians prefer to avoid administering vaccines during this time, if possible, to avoid any temporal associations that might occur. Specific recommendations for travel by pregnant women (and others) can be obtained at www.cdc.gov/travel.

Hepatitis B virus: Hepatitis B (HBV) infection during pregnancy can result in severe disease for both the mother, the fetus, and ultimately for the neonate. Immunization is recommended universally in the United States for everyone under the age of 18 years and those older than that who have increased risk of exposure. Pregnancy is not a contraindication for HBV immunization and vaccine should be given to persons with occupational or lifestyle risks, special patients risk groups (such as those undergoing hemodialysis), those who have another sexually transmitted disease, household and sexual contacts of

HBV carriers, prison inmates, and for international travelers to endemic areas. All pregnant women should have early prenatal screening for immunity and, if susceptible and if they have a risk factor, should be immunized.

All pregnant women should be screened for active hepatitis B virus infection because most women who are infected do not know it and, if they have hepatitis B infection, the newborn infant will need to receive a birth dose of hepatitis B vaccine and hepatitis B immune globulin—giving both within hours of birth reduces the likelihood that the child will become infected with hepatitis B virus and, if infected, reduces the chances that the baby will be chronically infected.

Pneumococcal infection: Pneumococcal polysaccharide vaccine (PPV23) is indicated for specific medical conditions (such as asplenia [absence of the spleen], metabolic, renal, cardiac, and pulmonary diseases, and immunosuppression). Pregnant women with those conditions should also receive the vaccine, preferably prior to pregnancy—but it can be given to a pregnant woman if she has not previously been immunized.

Rabies exposure: The risk of rabies far exceeds the theoretical risk from the vaccine if the expectant mother has been exposed to the disease.

Meningococcal infection: Studies of pregnant women immunized with meningococcal polysaccharide vaccine and their newborns have not demonstrated any adverse effects. This means that that vaccine would likely be safe for a pregnant woman at high risk for meningococcal infection. Because the new meningococcal conjugate vaccine (MCV4) is the preferred vaccine for people 11–55 years of age, many experts would prefer to give MCV4 in this setting, although there are no data on the safety of MCV4 during pregnancy.

Hepatitis A: Pregnant women are at risk of acquiring hepatitis A virus infection if there is someone infected in the household, if they have occupational exposure, or if traveling to areas where hepatitis A is endemic. Although formal studies of hepatitis A vaccine in pregnant women have not been performed, the vaccine is produced from inactivated virus so the theoretical risk for the fetus should be low. The vaccine has been used in pregnant women without adverse events having been reported. Because international travel is now the most frequent source of exposure for Americans to hepatitis A, vaccination prior to travel to endemic areas is particularly important. For pregnant women who have been exposed to hepatitis A virus, testing for susceptibility may be warranted but should not delay the administration of immune globulin (gamma globulin).

Polio: Wild-type polioviruses have been eliminated in the United States and thus there is not usually an indication for immunization of the pregnant woman except for those women traveling to endemic areas. If polio vaccine is indicated, only the inactivated vaccine should be given to a pregnant woman and not the oral live virus vaccine.

Anthrax: Women vaccinated against anthrax earlier in life have had no problems with their pregnancies or babies. No studies have been published regarding use of anthrax vaccine among pregnant women, although an ongoing study by the Naval Health Research Center and the National Center for Birth Defects and Developmental Disabilities suggest that children born to women who were immunized with anthrax vaccine in the first trimester of pregnancy could have an increased risk of birth defects. The Advisory Committee for Immunization Practices recommends that pregnant women not be vaccinated against anthrax. However, in the circumstances of an exposure to aerosolized anthrax (such as might occur in a bioterror attack), the theoretical risks of the vaccine would likely be far less than the risk of disease; pregnant women should be vaccinated against anthrax only if the potential benefits of vaccination outweigh the potential risks to the fetus.

Human papillomavirus: Although the initial clinical trials of human papillomavirus (HPV) vaccine specifically excluded pregnant women, 1,244 pregnancies occurred in the vaccine group and 1,272 occurred among the women who received placebo. There were no differences in the rates of miscarriage, late pregnancy fetal deaths, or birth defects among their babies. Infants of 500 women who were breast feeding when they received vaccine had no more adverse events than did those who got placebo and none of the events was considered related to vaccine. The FDA [U.S. Food and Drug Administration] has established a registry to record the outcomes of pregnancy among women who are inadvertently given HPV vaccine while pregnant.

References

1. Gall, SA 2003. Maternal Immunization. *Obstetrics and Gynecology Clinics of North America,* 30(4):632–636.

2. CDC (2008). Guiding principles for development of ACIP recommendations for vaccination during pregnancy and breastfeeding. *MMWR* 57(21): 580.

3. CDC (2009). Recommended adult immunization schedule—United States, 2009. *MMWR* 57(53):Q1–4.

4. Zaman K, Roy E, Arifeen SE, et al. 2008. Effectiveness of maternal influenza immunization in mothers and infants. *N Engl J Med* 359: 1555–64.

5. CDC. 2008. Summary of ACIP recommendations for prevention of pertussis, tetanus and diphtheria among pregnant and postpartum women and their infants. *MMWR* 57(04):48–9.

6. CDC (2008). Prevention and control of influenza: Recommendations of the Advisory Committee on Immunization Practices (ACIP), 2008. *MMWR,* 57 (RR-07), 1–60.

7. AAP, Committee on Infectious Diseases (2006). Varicella-Zoster Infections. In: LK Pickering (Ed.), *Red Book: Report of the Committee on Infectious Diseases* (27th ed., pp. 711–25). Elk Grove Village, IL.

8. AAP, Committee on Infectious Diseases (2006). Rubella. In: LK Pickering (Ed.), *Red Book: Report of the Committee on Infectious Diseases* (27th ed., pp. 574–9). Elk Grove Village, IL.

9. American College of Obstetricians and Gynecologists (2003). Immunization during Pregnancy. ACOG Committee Opinion 282.

10. CDC (2006). General recommendations on immunization: recommendations of the Advisory Committee on Immunization Practices (ACIP). *MMWR* 55(RR15);1–48.

11. CDC (2002). Notice to Readers: Status of U.S. Department of Defense Preliminary Evaluation of the Association of Anthrax Vaccination and Congenital Anomalies. *MMWR* February 15, 2002 / 51(06);127.

Chapter 19

Taking Medicines during Pregnancy

Chapter Contents

Section 19.1

Is It Safe to Use Medicines during Pregnancy?

Excerpted from "Pregnancy and Medicines: Frequently Asked Questions," by the Office of Women's Health (www.4women.gov), part of the U.S. Department of Health and Human Services, May 1, 2007.

Is it safe to use medicine while I am pregnant?

There is no clear-cut answer to this question. Before you start or stop any medicine, it is always best to speak with the doctor who is caring for you while you are pregnant. Read on to learn about deciding to use medicine while pregnant.

How should I decide whether to use a medicine while I am pregnant?

When deciding whether to use a medicine in pregnancy, you and your doctor need to talk about the medicine's benefits and risks.

- **Benefits:** What are the good things the medicine can do for me and my growing baby (fetus)?

- **Risks:** What are the ways the medicine might harm me or my growing baby (fetus)?

There may be times during pregnancy when using medicine is a choice. Some of the medicine choices you and your doctor make while you are pregnant may differ from the choices you make when you are not pregnant. For example, if you get a cold, you may decide to "live with" your stuffy nose instead of using the "stuffy nose" medicine you use when you are not pregnant.

Other times, using medicine is not a choice—it is needed. Some women need to use medicines while they are pregnant. Sometimes, women need medicine for a few days or a couple of weeks to treat a problem like a bladder infection or strep throat. Other women need to use medicine every day to control long-term health problems like asthma, diabetes, depression, or seizures. Also, some women have a pregnancy problem that needs medicine treatment. These problems include severe nausea and vomiting, earlier pregnancy losses, or preterm labor.

How do prescription and over-the-counter (OTC) medicine labels help my doctor choose the right medicine for me when I am pregnant?

Doctors use information from many sources when they choose medicine for a patient, including medicine labels. To help doctors, the U.S. Food and Drug Administration (FDA) created pregnancy letter categories to help explain what is known about using medicine during pregnancy. This system assigns letter categories to all prescription medicines. The letter category is listed in the label of a prescription medicine. The label states whether studies were done in pregnant women or pregnant animals and if so, what happened. Over-the-counter (OTC) medicines do not have a pregnancy letter category. Some OTC medicines were prescription medicines first and used to have a letter category. Talk to your doctor and follow the instructions on the label before taking OTC medicines.

The FDA chooses a medicine's letter category based on what is known about the medicine when used in pregnant women and animals.

The FDA is working hard to gather more knowledge about using medicine during pregnancy. The FDA is also trying to make medicine labels more helpful to doctors. Medicine label information for prescription medicines is now changing, and the pregnancy part of the label will change over the next few years.

OTC medicines: All OTC medicines have a Drug Facts label. The Drug Facts label is arranged the same way on all OTC medicines. This makes information about using the medicine easier to find. One section of the Drug Facts label is for pregnant women. With OTC medicines, the label usually tells a pregnant woman to speak with her doctor before using the medicine. Some OTC medicines are known to cause certain problems in pregnancy. The labels for these medicines give pregnant women facts about why and when they should not use the medicine. Here are some examples:

- Nonsteroidal anti-inflammatory drugs (NSAIDs) like ibuprofen (Advil®, Motrin®), naproxen (Aleve®), and aspirin (acetylsalicylate), can cause serious blood flow problems in the baby if used

Table 19.1. Definition of Medicine Categories: Prescription Medicines

Pregnancy Category	Definition	Examples of Drugs
A	In human studies, pregnant women used the medicine and their babies did not have any problems related to using the medicine.	Folic acid; Levothyroxine (thyroid hormone medicine)
B	In humans, there are no good studies. But in animal studies, pregnant animals received the medicine, and the babies did not show any problems related to the medicine. Or in animal studies, pregnant animals received the medicine, and some babies had problems. But in human studies, pregnant women used the medicine and their babies did not have any problems related to using the medicine.	Some antibiotics like amoxicillin; Zofran® (ondansetron) for nausea; Glucophage® (metformin) for diabetes; some insulin used to treat diabetes such as regular and NPH [neutral protamine Hagedorn] insulin
C	In humans, there are no good studies. In animals, pregnant animals treated with the medicine had some babies with problems. However, sometimes the medicine may still help the human mothers and babies more than it might harm. Or no animal studies have been done, and there are no good studies in pregnant women.	Diflucan® (fluconazole) for yeast infections; Ventolin® (albuterol) for asthma; Zoloft® (sertraline) and Prozac® (fluoxetine) for depression
D	Studies in humans and other reports show that when pregnant women use the medicine, some babies are born with problems related to the medicine. However, in some serious situations, the medicine may still help the mother and the baby more than it might harm.	Paxil® (paroxetine) for depression; Lithium for bipolar disorder; Dilantin® (phenytoin) for epileptic seizures; some cancer chemotherapy
X	Studies or reports in humans or animals show that mothers using the medicine during pregnancy may have babies with problems related to the medicine. There are no situations where the medicine can help the mother or baby enough to make the risk of problems worth it. These medicines should never be used by pregnant women.	Accutane® (isotretinoin) for cystic acne; Thalomid® (thalidomide) for a type of skin disease

during the last third of pregnancy (after 28 weeks). Also, aspirin may increase the chance for bleeding problems in the mother and the baby during pregnancy or at delivery.

- The labels for nicotine therapy drugs, like the nicotine patch and lozenge, remind women that smoking can harm an unborn child. While the medicine is thought to be safer than smoking, the risks of the medicine are not fully known. Pregnant smokers are told to try quitting without the medicine first.

What if I'm thinking about getting pregnant?

If you are not pregnant yet, you can help your chances for having a healthy baby by planning ahead. Schedule a pre-pregnancy checkup. At this visit, you can talk to your doctor about the medicines, vitamins, and herbs you use. It is very important that you keep treating your health problems while you are pregnant. Your doctor can tell you if you need to switch your medicine. Ask about vitamins for women who are trying to get pregnant. All women who can get pregnant should take a daily vitamin with folic acid (a B vitamin) to prevent birth defects of the brain and spinal cord. You should begin taking these vitamins before you become pregnant or if you could become pregnant. It is also a good idea to discuss caffeine, alcohol, and smoking with your doctor at this time.

Is it safe to use medicine while I am trying to become pregnant?

It is hard to know exactly when you will get pregnant. Once you do get pregnant, you may not know you are pregnant for 10 to 14 days or longer. Before you start trying to get pregnant, it is wise to schedule a meeting with your doctor to discuss medicines that you use daily or every now and then. Sometimes, medicines should be changed, and sometimes they can be stopped before a woman gets pregnant. Each woman is different. So you should discuss your medicines with your doctor rather than making medicine changes on your own.

What if I get sick and need to use medicine while I am pregnant?

Whether or not you should use medicine during pregnancy is a serious question to discuss with your doctor. Some health problems need treatment. Not using a medicine that you need could harm you and your baby. For example, a urinary tract infection (UTI) that is not treated may become a kidney infection. Kidney infections can cause preterm labor and low birth weight. An antibiotic is needed to get rid of a UTI. Ask your doctor whether the benefits of taking a certain medicine outweigh the risks for you and your baby.

I have a health problem. Should I stop using my medicine while I am pregnant?

If you are pregnant or thinking about becoming pregnant, you should talk to your doctor about your medicines. Do not stop or change them on your own. This includes medicines for depression, asthma, diabetes, seizures (epilepsy), and other health problems. Not using medicine that you need may be more harmful to you and your baby than using the medicine.

For women living with HIV [human immunodeficiency virus], the Centers for Disease Control and Prevention (CDC) recommends using zidovudine (AZT) during pregnancy. Studies show that HIV positive women who use AZT during pregnancy greatly lower the risk of passing HIV to their babies. If a diabetic woman does not use her medicine during pregnancy, she raises her risk for miscarriage, stillbirth, and some birth defects. If asthma and high blood pressure are not controlled during pregnancy, problems with the fetus may result.

Are vitamins safe for me while I am pregnant?

Regular multivitamins and prenatal vitamins are safe to take during pregnancy and can be helpful. Women who are pregnant or trying to get pregnant should take a daily multivitamin or prenatal vitamin that contains at least 400 micrograms (mcg) of folic acid. It is best to start taking these vitamins before you become pregnant or if you could become pregnant. Folic acid reduces the chance of a baby having a neural tube defect, like spina bifida, where the spine or brain does not form the right way. Iron can help prevent a low blood count (anemia). It's important to take the vitamin dose prescribed by your doctor. Too many vitamins can harm your baby. For example, very high levels of vitamin A have been linked with severe birth defects.

Are herbal remedies, "natural" products, or dietary supplements safe for me while I am pregnant?

Except for some vitamins, little is known about using dietary supplements while pregnant. Some herbal remedy labels claim they

172

will help with pregnancy. But, most often there are no good studies to show if these claims are true or if the herb can cause harm to or your baby. Talk with your doctor before using any herbal product or dietary supplement. These products may contain things that could harm you or your growing baby during your pregnancy.

In the United States, there are different laws for medicines and for dietary supplements. The part of the FDA that controls dietary supplements is the same part that controls foods sold in the United States. Only dietary supplements containing new dietary ingredients that were not marketed before October 15, 1994, submit safety information for review by the FDA. However, unlike medicines, herbal remedies and "natural products" are not approved by the FDA for safety or for what they say they will do. Most have not even been evaluated for their potential to cause harm to you or the growing fetus, let alone shown to be safe for use in pregnancy. Before a company can sell a medicine, the company must complete many studies and send the results to the FDA. Many scientists and doctors at the FDA check the study results. The FDA allows the medicine to be sold only if the studies show that the medicine works and is safe to use.

Section 19.2

Aspirin and Pregnancy

Excerpted from "Aspirin," by the Center for the Evaluation of Risks to Human Reproduction (CERHR, cerhr.niehs.nih.gov), part of the National Institute of the Environmental Health Sciences, April 23, 2008.

Aspirin and Pregnancy

The Food and Drug Administration (FDA) has issued the following warning about aspirin use during pregnancy: "It is especially important not to use aspirin during the last three months of pregnancy, unless specifically directed to do so by a physician because it may cause problems in the unborn child or complications during delivery."

Aspirin is listed on the California Environmental Protection Agency (CAL/EPA) Proposition 65 list of developmental toxicants. A developmental toxicant is a substance that a group of expert scientists has determined can harm unborn children.

Aspirin and Breastfeeding

Aspirin is transferred to breast milk and it is estimated that a nursing baby receives about 4–8% of the mother's dose. Continued exposure to small doses of aspirin may be harmful to babies because aspirin tends to build up in their bodies. In some countries, nursing women are advised against aspirin use because of the possible development of Reye syndrome in their babies. Reye syndrome is a rare condition that affects the brain and liver and is most often observed in children given aspirin during a viral illness (National Reye's Syndrome Foundation). Because sufficient information is not available to accurately determine the extent of aspirin accumulation in babies and the resulting health outcomes, the World Health Organization (WHO) Working Group on Human Lactation considers aspirin intake by nursing mothers as unsafe.

The American Academy of Pediatrics Committee on Drugs listed aspirin as a drug that has been "associated with significant effects on some nursing infants and should be given to nursing mothers with caution." The report suggested that safer drugs such as acetaminophen should be used for pain relief during pregnancy.

Chapter 20

Folic Acid

Why can't I wait until I'm pregnant or planning to get pregnant to start taking folic acid?

Birth defects of the brain and spine (spina bifida and anencephaly) happen in the first few weeks of pregnancy; often before you find out you're pregnant. By the time you realize you're pregnant, it might be too late to prevent those birth defects. Also, half of all pregnancies in the United States are unplanned.

These are two reasons why it is important for all women who can get pregnant to be sure to get 400 mcg of folic acid every day, even if they aren't planning a pregnancy any time soon.

I'm planning to get pregnant this month. Is it too late to start taking folic acid?

The CDC recommends women to take 400 micrograms (mcg) of folic acid every day, starting at least three months before getting pregnant. If you are trying to get pregnant this month, or planning to get pregnant soon, start taking 400 mcg of folic acid today.

From "Folic Acid," by the Centers for Disease Control and Prevention (CDC, www.cdc.gov), National Center on Birth Defects and Developmental Disabilities, January 30, 2008.

I already have a child with spina bifida. Should I do anything different to prepare for my next pregnancy?

Women who had one pregnancy affected by a birth defect of the brain or spine might have another. Talk to your doctor about taking 4,000 micrograms (4.0 milligrams) of folic acid each day at least 1 month before getting pregnant and during the first few months of being pregnant. This is ten times the amount most people take. Your doctor will give you a prescription. You should not take more than one multivitamin each day. Taking more than one each day over time could be harmful to you and your baby.

Can't I get enough folic acid by eating a well-balanced healthy diet?

You might think that you can get all the folic acid and other vitamins you need from the food you eat each day. But it is hard to eat a diet that has all the nutrients you need every day. Even with careful planning, you might not get all the vitamins you need from your diet alone. That's why it's important to take a vitamin with folic acid every day.

I can't swallow large pills. How can I take a vitamin with folic acid?

These days, multivitamins with folic acid come in chewable chocolate or fruit flavors, liquids, and large oval or smaller round pills.

A single serving of many breakfast cereals also has the amount of folic acid that a woman needs each day. Check the label. Look for cereals that have 100% daily value (DV) of folic acid in a serving, which is 400 micrograms (mcg).

Vitamins cost too much. How can I get the vitamin with folic acid that I need?

Many stores offer a single folic acid supplement for just pennies a day. Another good choice is a store brand multivitamin, which includes more of the vitamins a woman needs each day. Unless your doctor suggests a special type, you do not have to choose among vitamins for women or active people. A basic multivitamin meets the needs of most women.

How can I remember to take a vitamin with folic acid every day?

Make it easy to remember by taking your vitamin at the same time every day. Try taking your vitamin when you:

- if you use a cell phone or PDA, program it to give you a daily reminder;
- brush your teeth;
- eat breakfast;
- finish your shower;
- brush your hair;
- if you have children, take your vitamin when they take theirs.

Seeing the vitamin bottle on the bathroom or kitchen counter can help you remember it, too.

Today's woman is busy. You know that you should exercise, eat right, and get enough sleep. You might wonder how you can fit another thing into your day. But it only takes a few seconds to take a vitamin to get all the folic acid you need.

Are there other health benefits of taking folic acid?

Folic acid might help to prevent some other birth defects, such as cleft lip and palate and some heart defects. There might also be other health benefits of taking folic acid for both women and men. More research is needed to confirm these other health benefits. All adults should take 400 micrograms (mcg) of folic acid every day.

Can women get too much folic acid?

Unless their doctor advises them to take more, most women should limit the amount they take to 1,000 mcg a day.

What is folate and how is it different from folic acid?

Folate is a form of the B vitamin folic acid. Folate is found naturally in some foods, such as leafy, dark green vegetables, citrus fruits and juices, and beans.

The body does not use folate as easily as folic acid. We cannot be sure that eating folate would have the same benefits as getting 400 micrograms of man-made (synthetic) folic acid. Women who can get pregnant should consume 400 micrograms of synthetic folic acid in addition to the natural food folate from a varied diet.

What is "synthetic" folic acid?

Synthetic folic acid is the simple, man-made form of the B vitamin folate. Folic acid is found in most multivitamins and has been added in U.S. foods labeled as "enriched" such as bread, pasta, rice, and breakfast cereals. The words, "folic acid" and "synthetic folic acid" mean the same thing.

Chapter 21

Nutrition and Pregnancy

Chapter Contents

Section 21.1

What to Eat: A Guide for Pregnant Women

Excerpted from "Staying Healthy and Safe," by the Office of
Women's Health (womenshealth.gov), part of the U.S. Department
of Health and Human Services, March 2009.

Eat this. Don't eat that. Do this. Don't do that. Pregnant women
are bombarded with dos and don'ts. Here's help to keep it all straight.

Eating for Two

Eating healthy foods is more important now than ever. You need
more protein, iron, calcium, and folic acid than you did before pregnancy. You also need more calories. But eating for two doesn't mean
eating twice as much. Rather, it means that the foods you eat are the
main source of nutrients for your baby. Sensible, balanced meals combined with regular physical fitness is still the best recipe for good
health during your pregnancy.

Calorie Needs

Your calorie needs will depend on your weight gain goals. Most
women need 300 calories a day more during at least the last 6 months
of pregnancy than they do prepregnancy. Keep in mind that not all
calories are equal. Your baby needs healthy foods that are packed with
nutrients—not empty calories such as those found in soft drinks, can-
dies, and desserts.

Although you want to be careful not to eat more than you need for
a healthy pregnancy, make sure not to restrict your diet during pregnancy either. If you don't get the calories you need, your baby might
not get the right amounts of protein, vitamins, and minerals. Low-
calorie diets can break down a pregnant woman's stored fat. This can
cause your body to make substances called ketones. Ketones can be
found in the mother's blood and urine and are a sign of starvation.
Constant production of ketones can result in a child with mental deficiencies.

Foods Good for Mom and Baby

A pregnant woman needs more of many important vitamins, minerals, and nutrients than she did before pregnancy. Making healthy food choices every day will help you give your baby what he or she needs to develop. Here are some foods to choose often:

- **Grains:** Fortified, cooked or ready-to-eat cereals; wheat germ

- **Vegetables:** Carrots, sweet potatoes, pumpkin, spinach, cooked greens, winter squash, tomatoes, red pepper

- **Fruits:** Cantaloupe, honeydew melon, mangoes, prunes or prune juice, bananas, apricots, oranges or orange juice, grapefruit, avocado

- **Dairy:** Nonfat or low-fat yogurt; nonfat milk (skim milk); low-fat milk (1% milk)

- **Meat and beans:** Cooked dried beans and peas; nuts and seeds; lean beef, lamb, and pork; shrimp, clams, oysters, and crab; cod, salmon, pollack, and catfish

Talk to your doctor if you have special diet needs for these reasons:

- **Diabetes:** Make sure you review your meal plan and insulin needs with your doctor. High blood glucose levels can be harmful to your baby.

- **Lactose intolerance:** Find out about low-lactose or reduced-lactose products and calcium supplements to ensure you are getting the calcium you need.

- **Vegetarian:** Ensure that you are eating enough protein, iron, vitamin B12, and vitamin D.

- **Phenylketonuria (PKU):** Keep good control of phenylalanine levels in your diet.

Food Safety

Most foods are safe for pregnant women and their babies. But you will need to use caution or avoid eating certain foods. Follow these guidelines:

- Clean, handle, cook, and chill food properly to prevent food-borne illness, including listeria and toxoplasmosis.

- Wash hands with soap after touching soil or raw meat.

- Keep raw meats, poultry, and seafood from touching other foods or surfaces.

- Cook meat completely.

- Wash produce before eating.

- Wash cooking utensils with hot, soapy water.

Do Not Eat

- Refrigerated smoked seafood like whitefish, salmon, and mackerel

- Hot dogs or deli meats unless steaming hot

- Refrigerated meat spreads

- Unpasteurized milk or juices

- Store-made salads, such as chicken, egg, or tuna salad

- Unpasteurized soft cheeses, such as unpasteurized feta, Brie, queso blanco, queso fresco, and blue cheeses

- Shark, swordfish, king mackerel, or tile fish (also called golden or white snapper)—these fish have high levels of mercury

- More than 6 ounces per week of white (albacore) tuna

- Herbs and plants used as medicines without your doctor's okay (The safety of herbal and plant therapies isn't always known. Some herbs and plants might be harmful during pregnancy, such as bitter melon [karela], noni juice, and unripe papaya)

- Raw sprouts of any kind (including alfalfa, clover, radish, and mung bean)

Vitamins and Minerals

In addition to making healthy food choices, ask your doctor about taking a prenatal vitamin and mineral supplement every day to be sure you are getting enough of the nutrients your baby needs. You also can check the label on the foods you buy to see how much of a certain nutrient the product contains. Women who are pregnant need more of these nutrients than women who are not pregnant.

Women who are pregnant also need to be sure to get enough vitamin D. The current recommendation for all adults under 50 (including pregnant women) is 5 micrograms (mcg) of vitamin D each day. But many health experts don't think this is enough. Ask your doctor how much vitamin D you need each day. Because vitamin D is important to your unborn baby's development, your doctor might want to measure your vitamin D levels to be sure you are getting enough.

Keep in mind that taking too much of a supplement can be harmful. For example, too much of the nutrient vitamin A can cause birth defects. For this reason, only take vitamins and mineral supplements that your doctor recommends.

Table 21.1. Nutrients and Pregnancy

Nutrient	How Much Pregnant Women Need Each Day
Folic acid*	400 micrograms (mcg)
Iron	27 milligrams (mg)
Calcium	1,000 milligrams (mg); 1,300 mg if 18 or younger
Vitamin A	770 micrograms (mcg); 750 mcg if 18 or younger
Vitamin B	122.6 micrograms (mcg)

*Note: Women who are sexually active also should take 400 micrograms of folic acid daily.

Don't Forget Fluids

All of your body's systems need water. When you are pregnant, your body needs even more water to stay hydrated and support the life inside you. Water also helps prevent constipation, hemorrhoids, excessive swelling, and urinary tract or bladder infections. Not getting enough water can lead to premature or early labor.

Your body gets the water it needs through the fluids you drink and the foods you eat. How much fluid you need to drink each day depends on many factors, such as your activity level, the weather, and your size. Your body needs more fluids when it is hot and when you are physically active. It also needs more water if you have a fever or if you are vomiting or have diarrhea.

The Institute of Medicine recommends that pregnant women drink about 10 cups of fluids daily. Water, juices, coffee, tea, and soft drinks all count toward your fluid needs. But keep in mind that some beverages are high in sugar and empty calories. A good way to tell if your fluid intake is okay is if your urine is pale yellow or colorless and you rarely feel thirsty. Thirst is a sign that your body is on its way to dehydration. Don't wait until you feel thirsty to drink.

Alcohol

There is no known safe amount of alcohol a woman can drink while pregnant. When you are pregnant and you drink beer, wine, hard liquor, or other alcoholic beverages, alcohol gets into your blood. The alcohol in your blood gets into your baby's body through the umbilical cord. Alcohol can slow down the baby's growth, affect the baby's brain, and cause birth defects.

Cravings

Many women have strong desires for specific foods during pregnancy. The desire for "pickles and ice cream" and other cravings might be caused by changes in nutritional needs during pregnancy. The fetus needs nourishment. And a woman's body absorbs and processes nutrients differently while pregnant. These changes help ensure normal development of the baby and fill the demands of breastfeeding once the baby is born.

Some women crave nonfood items such as clay, ice, laundry starch, or cornstarch. A desire to eat nonfood items is called pica. Eating nonfood items can be harmful to your pregnancy. Talk to your doctor if you have these urges.

Section 21.2

Vegetarian Diets and Pregnancy

"Staying Healthy on a Vegetarian Diet During Pregnancy," *Journal of Midwifery and Women's Health,* January/February 2008. © 2008 American College of Nurse-Midwives (www.midwife.org). Reprinted with permission.

Why choose a vegetarian diet?

You may choose a vegetarian diet for many reasons. You may not want to harm animals. You may have political reasons for not eating meat. You may feel that not eating meat is healthier. Or you may avoid meat for religious reasons.

Is it possible to stay healthy without eating meat?

The American Dietetic Association and many other health organizations say that vegetarian diets can be very healthy. Whatever your reason for choosing a vegetarian diet, you will need to learn a bit about nutrition in order to stay healthy—especially when you are pregnant.

What are the benefits of a vegetarian diet?

If you eat a well-balanced vegetarian diet, you will have a lower risk of:

- obesity;
- heart disease;
- diabetes;
- high blood pressure;
- colon cancer.

If you already have some of these health concerns, eating a vegetarian diet may improve your health.

Can I get enough protein without eating meat?

Yes, you can. Protein is made up of several amino acids. Animal products—like meat, fish, chicken, eggs, and milk—have all of the amino acids and are considered complete proteins. Plant foods—like grains, beans, and nuts—each have some of the amino acids, so they are usually incomplete proteins. By eating a wide range of plant foods, you can get all of the amino acids you need for complete protein. If you are not pregnant, you need about 46 grams of complete protein every day. That goes up to 71 grams per day when you are pregnant.

Are there other nutrients that I should pay attention to if I want to stay healthy on a vegetarian diet?

Other nutrients besides protein that you will want to make sure you get enough of are vitamin B12, vitamin D, calcium, iron, and essential fatty acids. The following text lists good food sources of these nutrients and some guidelines for how much to eat.

I've been a vegetarian for a while, but I just found out I am pregnant. What can I do to make sure my baby is as healthy as possible?

Most of us slip into habits and lose sight of exactly what we are eating every day. If you are newly pregnant, you might want to do something you probably did when you first became a vegetarian—keep a list of everything you eat every day for a while. Check your list against the recommendations to see if you are getting all the nutrients you need.

You can grow a healthy baby while eating a vegetarian diet.

What are diet guidelines for a healthy vegetarian diet during pregnancy?

In general, your daily diet should include:

- one to two servings of dark green vegetables;
- four to five servings of other vegetables and fruit;
- three to four servings of bean and soy products;
- six or more servings of whole-grain products;
- one to two servings of nuts, seeds, and wheat germ.

If you are pregnant or breastfeeding, you should add:

- four servings of vitamin B12-fortified foods;
- 15 minutes of sunshine on your arms and face or 200 IU [international units] of vitamin D;
- eight servings (1200–1500 mg) of calcium-rich foods;
- iron-rich foods;
- 1 tablespoon of ground flax seed or other N-3 fatty acid-rich food.

Vitamin B12: Vitamin B12 is important for the growth of nerve and blood cells. It is only found naturally in animal foods like meat, fish, and milk. Plant-based foods that are fortified with vitamin B12 include soymilk, tofu, cereal, and nutritional yeast.

Vitamin D: Vitamin D is important for growth of the bones and the teeth. It is found in animal foods, but can also be absorbed through the skin from sunlight. Vitamin D-fortified foods include cow's milk, some soymilk, and some breakfast cereals.

Calcium: Calcium is very important for bone growth and strength. Calcium is found in milk products. Plant-based food sources include broccoli, collards, kale, sesame seeds, almonds, and soy products.

Iron: Iron is used in making blood. It is most commonly found in meat and eggs. Plant-based iron-rich foods include soy, bean, lentils, spinach, molasses, dried apricots, prunes, and raisins. To make the most of your iron, eat it with a high vitamin C food like oranges or strawberries.

Essential fatty acids: Essential fatty acids are important to the function of cells and the development of the brain. There are two types of fatty acids: N-3 and N-6. Vegetarian diets tend to have a lot of N-6 fatty acids but be low in N-3. Sources of N-3 fatty acids include eggs, flaxseed, and canola and soybean oils.

Section 21.3

Anemia and Pregnancy

"Anemia and Pregnancy," © 2003 University of Pittsburgh Medical Center (www.upmc.com). Reprinted with permission. The text that follows this document under the heading "*Health Reference Series* Medical Advisor's Notes and Updates" was provided to Omnigraphics, Inc. by David A. Cooke, MD, FACP, March 31, 2009. Dr. Cooke is not affiliated with the University of Pittsburgh Medical Center.

What is anemia?

Anemia means you have low iron in your blood or "low blood."[1] Iron helps your red blood cells carry oxygen to all parts of your body.

What are the symptoms of anemia?

Anemia can make you feel very tired and have no energy. You may feel light-headed or dizzy and may "black out."

How does anemia affect my baby?

Your baby depends on you for oxygen. If you have severe anemia, your baby may not get enough oxygen to grow well. The baby may be small at birth. Anemia may increase the chance that you will give birth early. If you have anemia and bleed heavily after the birth, you may need a blood transfusion.

What treatment is available?

To treat anemia, you need to replace the iron in your body. It is important that you and your doctor work together to treat anemia.
Here are some tips for treating anemia:

- Take vitamins and iron pills every day as your doctor tells you to.

- Do not take iron pills with milk. The calcium in the milk does not let the iron work well in your body.

- Take your iron pill with juices that have vitamin C in them. Some examples are orange juice and tomato juice. This helps the iron get into your blood better.

- Do not take antacids like Tums or Maalox at the same time you take iron pills. These can affect how your body uses the iron pills.

- Iron pills can cause problems having a bowel movement. Eat more foods with fiber, like fruits, vegetables, and cereals.

- Drink 6 to 8 glasses of water or juice daily.

- Your bowel movements may turn dark black. This is normal.

- Eating foods that are high in iron is very important. Foods that help increase your iron level are:
  - red meats, like beef and pork;
  - liver;
  - black molasses;
  - peanut butter;
  - nuts, like almonds and cashews;
  - beans;
  - dried fruits, like prunes, apricots, figs, raisins, peaches, and dates;
  - egg yolks;
  - sweet potatoes;
  - dark green or yellow vegetables, like collard greens, kale, spinach, turnips, and mustard greens;
  - raisin bran cereal and wheat germ.

Eating right and taking iron and vitamins will help keep you and your baby healthy.

Health Reference Series *Medical Advisor's Notes and Updates*

1. Most cases of anemia in pregnancy are due to iron deficiency, and the advice in this article is directed toward this. However, not all anemia is due to iron deficiency. A variety of other conditions including kidney disease, bone marrow disease, drug

effects, and other vitamin deficiencies can also cause anemia. Check with your doctor that your anemia is due to iron deficiency, because treatment might be quite different with other conditions.

Section 21.4

What You Need to Know about Mercury in Fish and Shellfish

Excerpted from "What You Need to Know about Mercury in Fish and Shellfish," by the Environmental Protection Agency (EPA, www.epa.gov), August 14, 2008.

Fish and shellfish are an important part of a healthy diet. Fish and shellfish contain high-quality protein and other essential nutrients, are low in saturated fat, and contain omega-3 fatty acids. A well-balanced diet that includes a variety of fish and shellfish can contribute to heart health and children's proper growth and development. So, women and young children in particular should include fish or shellfish in their diets due to the many nutritional benefits.

However, nearly all fish and shellfish contain traces of mercury. For most people, the risk from mercury by eating fish and shellfish is not a health concern. Yet, some fish and shellfish contain higher levels of mercury that may harm an unborn baby or young child's developing nervous system. The risks from mercury in fish and shellfish depend on the amount of fish and shellfish eaten and the levels of mercury in the fish and shellfish. Therefore, the Food and Drug Administration (FDA) and the Environmental Protection Agency (EPA) are advising women who may become pregnant, pregnant women, nursing mothers, and young children to avoid some types of fish and eat fish and shellfish that are lower in mercury.

By following these three recommendations for selecting and eating fish or shellfish, women and young children will receive the benefits of eating fish and shellfish and be confident that they have reduced their exposure to the harmful effects of mercury.

1. Do not eat shark, swordfish, king mackerel, or tilefish because they contain high levels of mercury.

2. Eat up to 12 ounces (2 average meals) a week of a variety of fish and shellfish that are lower in mercury. Five of the most commonly eaten fish that are low in mercury are shrimp, canned light tuna, salmon, pollack, and catfish. Another commonly eaten fish, albacore ("white") tuna has more mercury than canned light tuna. So, when choosing your two meals of fish and shellfish, you may eat up to 6 ounces (one average meal) of albacore tuna per week.

3. Check local advisories about the safety of fish caught by family and friends in your local lakes, rivers, and coastal areas. If no advice is available, eat up to 6 ounces (one average meal) per week of fish you catch from local waters, but don't consume any other fish during that week.

Follow these same recommendations when feeding fish and shellfish to your young child, but serve smaller portions.

Section 21.5

Caffeine Use during Pregnancy

From "Caffeine," by the Center for the Evaluation of Risks to Human Reproduction (CERHR, cerhr.niehs.nih.gov), part of the National Institute of Environmental Health Sciences (NIEHS), April 23, 2008.

Numerous studies have examined the effects of caffeine intake on fertility and pregnancy. Most studies found that moderate caffeine intake does not affect fertility or increase the chance of having a miscarriage or a baby with birth defects; some studies did find a relationship between caffeine intake and fertility or miscarriages. However, most of those studies were judged to be inadequate because they did not consider other lifestyle factors that could contribute to infertility or miscarriages. The Organization of Teratology Information Services (OTIS) stated that there is no evidence that caffeine causes birth defects in humans. Groups such as OTIS and Motherisk agree that low caffeine intake (<150 mg/day or 1 1/2 cups of coffee) will not likely increase a woman's chance of having a miscarriage or a low birth weight baby. Motherisk recommends that caffeine intake by pregnant women not exceed 150 mg/day whereas OTIS stated that moderate caffeine intake of 300 mg/day (equivalent to about 3 cups of coffee) does not seem to reduce fertility in women or increase the chances of having a child with birth defects or other problems. Caffeine can enter breast milk, and high amounts can cause the baby to become wakeful and agitated. The American Academy of Pediatrics recommends that nursing women limit caffeine intake, but states that no harm is likely to occur in a nursing child whose mother drinks one cup of coffee a day. OTIS recommends that pregnant and nursing women drink plenty of water, milk, and juice and not substitute those fluids with caffeinated beverages.

Caffeine and Fertility

Numerous studies have been conducted to determine the effects of caffeine intake on fertility in women. The International Food Information Council (IFIC) has described and made conclusions about the following studies.

One small study in 1988 suggested that caffeine, equivalent to the amount consumed in 1 to 2 cups of coffee daily, might decrease female fertility. However, the researchers acknowledged that delayed conception could be due to other factors they did not consider, such as exercise, stress, or other dietary habits. Since then, larger, well-designed studies have failed to support the 1988 findings.

In 1990, researchers at the Centers for Disease Control and Prevention and Harvard University examined the association between the length of time to conceive and consumption of caffeinated beverages. The study involved more than 2,800 women who had recently given birth and 1,800 women with the medical diagnosis of primary infertility. Each group was interviewed concerning caffeine consumption, medical history, and lifestyle habits. The researchers found that caffeine consumption had little or no effect on the reported time to conceive in those women who had given birth. Caffeine consumption also was not a risk factor for infertility.

Supporting those findings, a 1991 study of 11,000 Danish women examined the relationship among number of months to conceive, cigarette smoking, and coffee and tea consumption. Although smokers who consumed eight or more cups of coffee per day experienced delayed conception, nonsmokers did not, regardless of caffeine consumption.

A study of 210 women, published in the *American Journal of Public Health* in 1998, examined the differences in fertility associated with consumption of different caffeinated beverages. This study, prompted by an inconsistency in previously reported findings, did not find a significant association between total caffeine consumption and reduced fertility. In fact, the researchers found that women who drank more than one-half cup of tea per day had a significant increase in fertility. This was particularly true with caffeine consumption in the early stages of a woman's attempt at conception. The caffeinated tea and fertility correlation was supported by a 1994 study; however, those women had significantly higher consumption levels. OTIS reviewed the studies examining caffeine effects on fertility and concluded that, "Low to moderate caffeine consumption (<300 mg/day) does not seem to reduce a woman's chance of becoming pregnant."

Caffeine and Pregnancy

The March of Dimes notes that during pregnancy, caffeine easily passes from the mother to her unborn child through the placenta. Because the systems for breaking down and eliminating chemicals are not fully developed in the unborn child, blood levels of caffeine may remain elevated for longer periods in the unborn child compared to the mother. OTIS notes that, "higher amounts of caffeine could affect babies in the same way as it does adults. Some reports have stated that children born to mothers who consumed >500 mg/day were more likely to have faster heart rates, tremors, increased breathing rate, and spend more time awake in the days following birth." The effects of caffeine intake on miscarriages, birth defects, and low birth weight have been studied, and different results were obtained in the various studies. The International Food Information Council (IFIC) has described and made conclusions about the following studies.

Recently, researchers from McGill University in Montreal published a study showing a relationship between caffeine intake and miscarriage. While caffeine intake before and during pregnancy appeared to be associated with increased fetal loss, the authors failed to account for a number of factors that could result in a false association, including effects of morning sickness or nausea, the number of cigarettes smoked, and amount of alcohol consumed.

Just prior to the McGill study, a research team from the U.S. National Institute of Child Health and Human Development conducted a study of 431 women. The researchers monitored the women and the amount of caffeine they consumed from conception to birth. After accounting for nausea, smoking, alcohol use, and maternal age, the researchers found no relationship between caffeine consumption of up to 300 mg per day and adverse pregnancy outcomes, including miscarriage.

Earlier, in 1992, researchers analyzed the effects of cigarettes, alcohol, and coffee consumption on pregnancy outcome in more than 40,000 Canadian women. Although alcohol consumption and smoking tended to have adverse effects on pregnancy outcome, moderate caffeine consumption was not associated with low birth weight or miscarriages. Further, the relationship of caffeine consumption to spontaneous abortion was investigated in a study of 5,342 pregnant women in 1997 in which researchers concluded that there was no increased risk for spontaneous abortion associated with moderate caffeine consumption. Another very comprehensive study, done in Uppsala, Sweden, and reported in December 2000, concluded reducing caffeine intake during early pregnancy may be prudent.

Studies published during the 1980s also support the conclusion that moderate caffeine consumption during pregnancy does not cause early birth or low birth-weight babies. A review of more than 20 studies conducted since 1980 found no evidence that caffeine consumption at moderate levels has any discernible adverse effect on pregnancy outcome.

A seven-year study of 1,500 women examined caffeine use during pregnancy and subsequent child development. Caffeine consumption, equivalent to about 1 1/2–2 cups of coffee per day had no effect on birth weight, birth length, or head circumference. Follow-up examinations at ages 8 months, 4 years, and 7 years also revealed no effects of caffeine consumption on a child's motor development or intelligence.

In the early 1980s, the U.S. Food and Drug Administration (FDA) conducted a study where rats were force-fed very high doses of caffeine through a stomach tube. While the results prompted an advisory to pregnant women to avoid caffeine, the study was criticized as not being representative of the way humans consume caffeine.

In 1986, FDA researchers carried out another study, in which rats consumed high doses of caffeine in their drinking water. At the conclusion of the second study, the FDA found no adverse effects in the offspring, contradicting the agency's earlier findings.

A recent study published in 2001 examined the effect of maternal caffeine consumption throughout pregnancy on fetal growth and found evidence that caffeine consumption during pregnancy has no adverse effect on fetal growth. Additionally, a 2002 study entitled "Effect of caffeine exposure during pregnancy on birthweight and gestational age," in the *American Journal of Epidemiology* found no association between moderate caffeine consumption and reduced birthweight, gestational age, or fetal growth.

Major studies over the last decade have shown no association between birth defects and caffeine consumption. FDA has evaluated this scientific evidence and concluded that caffeine does not adversely affect reproduction in humans. However, as with other dietary habits, the agency continues to advise pregnant women to consume caffeine in moderation.

Groups such as OTIS, March of Dimes, and Motherisk reviewed studies examining caffeine intake during pregnancy and are in agreement that high caffeine intake (>300 mg/day, equivalent to more than 3 cups of coffee/day) should be avoided during pregnancy. There is also general agreement that low caffeine intake (<150 mg/day, about 1½ cups of coffee) during pregnancy is not likely to harm the unborn child. However, there is some disagreement regarding moderate caffeine intake.

Following a statistical analysis of studies examining caffeine intake in pregnant woman, Motherisk stated, "Our results suggest a small but statistically significant increase in risk of spontaneous abortion and low birth weight babies in pregnant women consuming more than 150 mg of caffeine per day. Pregnant women should be encouraged to be aware of dietary caffeine intake and to consume less than 150 mg of caffeine a day from all sources throughout pregnancy."

Subsequent to their review of caffeine studies, OTIS stated that "Recent reports suggest that low to moderate consumption of caffeine does not increase the risk for miscarriage. A few studies have shown that there may be an increased risk for miscarriage with high caffeine consumption (>300 mg/day), particularly in combination with smoking or alcohol, or with very high levels of caffeine consumption (>800 mg/day)." OTIS goes on to say that, "In humans, even large amounts of caffeine have not been shown to cause an increased chance for birth defects." OTIS concluded that, "Most experts agree that moderation and common sense are the keys for consuming caffeinated items during pregnancy." Moderate caffeine consumption is approximately 300 mg/day, which is similar to 3 cups of coffee. It is also important for pregnant women to drink sufficient quantities of water, milk, and juice. These fluids should not be replaced with caffeinated beverages."

Chapter 22

Exercise during Pregnancy

Fitness goes hand in hand with eating right to maintain your physical health and well-being during pregnancy. Pregnant or not, physical fitness helps keep the heart, bones, and mind healthy. Healthy pregnant women should get at least 2 hours and 30 minutes of moderate-intensity aerobic activity a week. It's best to spread your workouts throughout the week. If you regularly engage in vigorous-intensity aerobic activity or high amounts of activity, you can keep up your activity level as long as your health doesn't change and you talk to your doctor about your activity level throughout your pregnancy.

Special benefits of physical activity during pregnancy:

- Exercise can ease and prevent aches and pains of pregnancy including constipation, varicose veins, backaches, and exhaustion.

- Active women seem to be better prepared for labor and delivery and recover more quickly.

- Exercise may lower the risk of preeclampsia and gestational diabetes during pregnancy.

- Fit women have an easier time getting back to a healthy weight after delivery.

- Regular exercise may improve sleep during pregnancy.

Excerpted from "Staying Healthy and Safe," by the Office of Women's Health (www.womenshealth.gov), March 2009.

- Staying active can protect your emotional health. Pregnant women who exercise seem to have better self-esteem and a lower risk of depression and anxiety.

- Results from a recent, large study suggest that women who are physically active during pregnancy may lower their chances of preterm delivery.

Getting Started

For most healthy moms-to-be who do not have any pregnancy-related problems, exercise is a safe and valuable habit. Even so, talk to your doctor or midwife before exercising during pregnancy. She or he will be able to suggest a fitness plan that is safe for you. Getting a doctor's advice before starting a fitness routine is important for both inactive women and women who exercised before pregnancy.

If you have one of these conditions, your doctor will advise you not to exercise:

- Risk factors for preterm labor

- Vaginal bleeding

- Premature rupture of membranes (when your water breaks early, before labor)

Best Activities for Moms-to-Be

Low-impact activities at a moderate level of effort are comfortable and enjoyable for many pregnant women. Walking, swimming, dancing, cycling, and low-impact aerobics are some examples. These sports also are easy to take up, even if you are new to physical fitness.

Some higher intensity sports are safe for some pregnant women who were already doing them before becoming pregnant. If you jog, play racquet sports, or lift weights, you may continue with your doctor's okay.

Keep these points in mind when choosing a fitness plan:

- Avoid activities in which you can get hit in the abdomen like kickboxing, soccer, basketball, or ice hockey.

- Steer clear of activities in which you can fall like horseback riding, downhill skiing, and gymnastics.

- Do not scuba dive during pregnancy. Scuba diving can create gas bubbles in your baby's blood that can cause many health problems.

Tips for Safe and Healthy Physical Activity

Follow these tips for safe and healthy fitness:

- When you exercise, start slowly, progress gradually, and cool down slowly.

- You should be able to talk while exercising. If not, you may be overdoing it. Take frequent breaks.

- Don't exercise on your back after the first trimester. This can put too much pressure on an important vein and limit blood flow to the baby.

- Avoid jerky, bouncing, and high-impact movements. Connective tissues stretch much more easily during pregnancy. So these types of movements put you at risk of joint injury.

- Be careful not to lose your balance. As your baby grows, your center of gravity shifts making you more prone to falls. For this reason, activities like jogging, using a bicycle, or playing racquet sports might be riskier as you near the third trimester.

- Don't exercise at high altitudes (more than 6,000 feet). It can prevent your baby from getting enough oxygen.

- Make sure you drink lots of fluids before, during, and after exercising.

- Do not workout in extreme heat or humidity.

- If you feel uncomfortable, short of breath, or tired, take a break and take it easier when you exercise again.

Stop exercising and call your doctor as soon as possible if you have any of the following:

- Dizziness
- Headache
- Chest pain
- Calf pain or swelling
- Abdominal pain
- Blurred vision
- Fluid leaking from the vagina
- Vaginal bleeding

- Less fetal movement
- Contractions

Work out Your Pelvic Floor (Kegel Exercises)

Your pelvic floor muscles support the rectum, vagina, and urethra in the pelvis. Toning these muscles with Kegel exercises will help you push during delivery and recover from birth. It also will help control bladder leakage and lower your chance of getting hemorrhoids.

- Pelvic muscles are the same ones used to stop the flow of urine. Still, it can be hard to find the right muscles to squeeze. You can be sure you are exercising the right muscles if when you squeeze them you stop urinating. Or you can put a finger into the vagina and squeeze. If you feel pressure around the finger, you've found the pelvic floor muscles. Try not to tighten your stomach, legs, or other muscles.

- Tighten the pelvic floor muscles for a count of three, then relax for a count of three.

- Repeat 10 to 15 times, three times a day.

- Start Kegel exercises lying down. This is the easiest position. When your muscles get stronger, you can do Kegel exercises sitting or standing as you like.

Chapter 23

Weight Gain during Pregnancy

Chapter Contents

Section 23.1

How Much Weight Should You Gain?

Excerpted from "Managing Gestational Diabetes: A Patient's Guide to a Healthy Pregnancy," by the National Institute of Child Health and Human Development (NICHD, www.nichd.nih.gov), part of the National Institutes of Health, September 2006.

Healthy weight gain can mean either your overall weight gain, or your weekly rate of weight gain. Some health care providers focus only on overall gain or only on weekly gain, but some keep track of both types of weight gain. First, let's look at overall weight gain.

The amount of weight gain that is healthy for you depends on how much you weighed before you were pregnant. Find your prepregnancy weight and height in Table 23.1. Then look at the bottom row of the table to find your overall healthy weight gain goal.

If you are expecting twins, an overall weight gain of 35 to 45 pounds is considered healthy.

Remember that these goals are only a general range for overall weight gain. Your health care provider will let you know if you're gaining too much or too little weight for a healthy pregnancy. Weight loss can be dangerous during any part of your pregnancy. Report any weight loss to your health care provider right away.

How do I do it?

To maintain a healthy weight gain, eat a healthy diet as outlined by your health care provider, and get regular, moderate physical activity.

If you think your weight gain is out-of-control, but you are following a recommended diet and physical activity program, tell your health care provider. He or she will adjust your treatment plan to get your weight gain back into healthy range.

When do I do it?

It's a good idea to keep track of how much weight you gain from the time you learn you are pregnant to the time you have the baby.

Knowing your weight status can help your health care provider detect possible problems before they become dangerous.

It's also a good idea to weigh yourself on the same day of the week and at the same time of day. Your health care provider can make a schedule for you so you know how often to weigh yourself and at what time of day. You will also be weighed at your prenatal appointments.

How do I know that I'm doing it right?

One way to determine if your overall weight gain is within the healthy range is to follow your weekly rate of weight gain. The information below gives some general guidelines for weekly rate of weight gain.

Table 23.1. Overall Weight Gain Goals by Prepregnancy Height and Weight

Height (Without Shoes)		Weight Status Category (Weight in pounds, in light, indoor clothing)			
ft.	in.	A*	B	C	D
4	9	92 or less	93-113	114–134	135 or more
4	10	94 or less	95–117	118–138	139 or more
4	11	97 or less	98–120	121–142	143 or more
5	0	100 or less	101–123	124–146	147 or more
5	1	103 or less	104–127	128–150	151 or more
5	2	106 or less	107–131	132–155	156 or more
5	3	109 or less	110–134	135–159	160 or more
5	4	113 or less	114–140	141–165	166 or more
5	5	117 or less	118–144	145–170	171 or more
5	6	121 or less	122–149	150–176	177 or more
5	7	124 or less	125–153	154–181	182 or more
5	8	128 or less	129–157	158–186	187 or more
5	9	131 or less	132–162	163–191	192 or more
5	10	135 or less	136–166	167–196	197 or more
5	11	139 or less	140–171	172–202	203 or more
6	0	142 or less	143–175	176–207	208 or more
Your overall weight gain goal is:		35–40*	30–35	22–27	15–20

*The weight gain goal for women in this category may range from 40 to 45 pounds.

If your weekly rate of gain is low, you might need to adjust your diet to get more calories. If your weekly rate of gain is high, you may be developing a condition called preeclampsia, which can be dangerous.

What is a good weekly rate of weight gain?

Aim to keep your weekly rate of weight gain within these healthy ranges:

- In the first trimester of pregnancy (the first 3 months): 3 to 6 pounds for the entire 3 months.

- During the second and third trimesters (the last 6 months): between 1/2 and 1 pound each week.

- If you gained too much weight early in the pregnancy: limit weight gain to 3/4 of a pound each week (3 pounds each month).

A weight gain of 2 pounds or more each week is considered high.

Keep in mind that your weekly rate of weight gain may go up and down throughout the course of your pregnancy. Some weeks you may gain weight, other weeks you won't; as a result, your weekly rate of gain may not match your overall weight gain goal exactly. Your health care provider will let you know if you're gaining too much or too little weight for a healthy pregnancy. Weight loss can be dangerous during any part of your pregnancy. Report any weight loss to your health care provider right away.

You may also notice that your weight gain slows down or stops for a time. It should start going up again after 1 to 2 weeks. If not, tell your health care provider immediately. He or she may need to adjust your treatment plan.

Are there any other ways I can maintain a healthy weight gain?

Some general guidelines that might help you reach your target weekly rate of gain include:

- Try to get more light or moderate physical activity, if your health care provider says it's safe.

- Use the Nutrition Facts labels on food packages to make lower-calorie food choices that fit into your meal plan.

- Eat fewer fried foods and fast foods.

- Eat healthy foods that fit into your meal plan, such as salads with low-fat dressings and broiled or grilled chicken.

- Use less butter and margarine on food, or don't use them at all.

- Use spices and herbs (such as curry, garlic, and parsley) and low-fat or lower calorie sauces to flavor rice and pasta.

- Eat smaller meals and have low-calorie snacks more often, to ensure that your body has a constant glucose supply, and to prevent yourself from getting very hungry.

- Avoid skipping meals or cutting back too much on breakfast or lunch. Eating less food or skipping meals could make you overly hungry at the next meal, causing you to overeat.

Section 23.2

Gestational Weight Gain Warnings

"Researcher Warns about Gestational Weight Gain," by Eddy Ball, in *Environmental Factor*, by the National Institute of Environmental Health Sciences (NIEHS, www.niehs.nih.gov), part of the National Institutes of Health, March 2008.

Nutritional epidemiologist Anna Maria Siega-Riz, Ph.D., had good reason to sound alarmed when she talked about pregnancy and weight gain in February 2008.

According to the University of North Carolina at Chapel Hill professor, overweight and obese women, as well as women who gain too much weight during their pregnancies, may be endangering their own health and the health of their children.

In her talk, "Maternal Obesity: The Number One Problem Facing Prenatal Care Providers in the New Millennium," Siega-Riz presented a preponderance of evidence that these women have a significantly greater risk of suffering from metabolic syndrome-related diseases, of bearing children with birth defects, such as spina bifida, and of giving birth to babies who will experience problems with their own health.

More women are overweight and obese worldwide, and more of them are gaining excessive weight during pregnancy. Compounding the problem, Siega-Riz added, is the complacency of many pregnant women and, even more disturbing, their health care providers.

"Maternal obesity is not unique to the United States," Siega-Riz said as she began her lecture. "It is occurring globally." Many developing countries are facing the same problems as the United States, with obesity rates between 20 and 30 percent. Not only are rates increasing, Siega-Riz noted, but obesity is also emerging as a health disparity issue due to its greater prevalence among minority women.

According to Siega-Riz, in the United States about a third of women are overweight and 10 to 15 percent are obese. The majority of pregnant women are gaining 21 to 40 pounds during pregnancy, and since the 1990s, there has been a 30 percent increase in the number of women who gain 40 or more pounds. "Only about a third of women are gaining weight within the targeted weight-gain recommendations," she said. In addition to the significant health problems that obesity contributes to on its own, such as diabetes and cardiovascular disease, Siega-Riz pointed to studies suggesting that about 25 percent of problems with fecundity and fertility are due to obesity.

Maternal overweight and obesity have been associated with a dramatic increase in risk for gestational diabetes, gestational hypertension, preeclampsia, cesarean delivery, fetal death, and birth defects. The effects of overweight and obesity persist beyond childbirth and include postpartum weight retention, postpartum anemia related to the higher rate of cesarean sections, shorter duration of breastfeeding, and persistent glucose intolerance. Moreover, with excessive weight gain, a woman is also more likely to find herself in a higher weight classification at 12 months postpartum than she was at conception, putting her at even greater risk for complications in a subsequent pregnancy.

Because of these trends, physicians are seeing a growing number of pregnant women weighing as much as 300 pounds. "Quite frankly, they don't know how to manage them," Siega-Riz observed. One study found that 33 percent of subjects reported receiving no advice on gestational weight gain from their providers. The few intervention studies thus far have failed to show promising results and have found poor rates of compliance with interventions on the part of physicians and pregnant women.

As she and her colleagues strive to close the gaps in research on gestational weight gain, Siega-Riz continues to push for translation of this research through education and policy change. She currently serves a member of the Institute of Medicine's (IOM) Committee to Reexamine IOM Pregnancy Weight Guidelines. In 2004, she served on the IOM's Committee to Review the WIC [Women, Infants, and Children] Food Packages. As result of the recommendations from this committee, the United States Department of Agriculture made the first major changes to the food packages since WIC's inception 30 years ago.

Chapter 24

Sleep during Pregnancy

Women from adolescence to postmenopause are underrepresented in studies of sleep and its disorders. Although sleep complaints are twice as prevalent in women, 75% of sleep research has been conducted in men. More sleep studies in the past five years have included women, but small sample sizes prohibit meaningful sex comparisons. Thus, sex differences in sleep and sleep disorder characteristics, in responses to sleep deprivation, and in sleep-related physiology remain unappreciated. Furthermore, findings from studies based primarily in men are often considered to be representative of 'normal' even when it is recognized that there are important sleep-related physiological differences in women, including timing of nocturnal growth hormone secretion and differential time course of delta activity across the night.

Hormonal changes and physical discomfort are common during pregnancy and both can affect sleep. Although nearly all pregnant women will experience disturbed sleep by the third trimester, there have been only two longitudinal sleep studies of subjective and objective sleep measures during pregnancy. There have been no reports of intervention studies to improve sleep quality during pregnancy. Some have assumed that disturbed sleep is a 'natural' consequence of pregnancy, labor, delivery, and postpartum that resolves over time

Excerpted from "Sleep, Sex Differences, and Women's Health: National Sleep Disorders Research Plan," by the National Heart, Lung and Blood Institute (NHLBI, www.nhlbi.nih.gov), part of the National Institutes of Health, July 2003. Revised by David A. Cooke, MD, FACP, April 29, 2009.

since few women seek assistance to improve sleep. Research has not shown a relationship between sleep quality and quantity and any perinatal adverse outcome, length of labor, or type of delivery.

More studies are needed, however, to clarify the extent to which sleep-related problems during pregnancy may have adverse fetal, perinatal, or infant-related consequences.

Very little is known about the effects of late stage pregnancy sleep disturbances on labor and delivery, emotional distress, or postpartum depression. However, nighttime labor and a history of sleep disruption in late stage pregnancy are related to a higher incidence of postpartum blues. Certain sleep disorders such as restless legs syndrome (RLS), periodic limb movement disorder (PLMS), sleep-disordered breathing (SDB), or insomnia may emerge during pregnancy and the extent to which these disorders resolve or place women at higher risk for sleep disorders later in life is not clear. Pregnancy induces changes in the upper airway and in functional residual capacity that predispose women to snoring, SDB, and reduced oxygen stores.

Pregnant women who snore may be at risk for preeclampsia and/or SDB. The number of pregnant women with SDB may be substantial, but the prevalence has not been defined in either uncomplicated or complicated pregnancy. Women with preeclampsia and excessive weight gain during pregnancy are at greater risk for the development of SDB and pregnancy-induced hypertension, which have been associated with adverse perinatal outcomes, but few polysomnographic studies have been done in these women.

Sleep in Pregnancy and Postpartum

- Longitudinal studies indicate that age combined with anemia is related to first trimester fatigue and that reduced sleep time is related to fatigue during the third trimester. Both reduced sleep time and anemia are related to fatigue postpartum. Significant changes in sleep are evident in the first trimester of pregnancy with increased total sleep time coupled with more awakenings, but postpartum sleep efficiency is lower than prepregnancy. Slow wave sleep percentage is reduced throughout pregnancy compared to prepregnancy and postpartum. REM sleep was reduced during pregnancy in one study, but was reduced in another longitudinal study, most notably during the third trimester.

- Restless legs syndrome (RLS) occurs in about 15%–25% of pregnant women and becomes more common in later pregnancy. RLS is known to be associated with iron deficiency in non-pregnant patients, and some data suggest this is true in pregnant women as well. There is also some evidence that RLS in pregnancy may be associated with reduced levels of folate. It is unclear whether taking iron or folic acid supplements (both of which are usually recommended in pregnancy for other reasons) affects the risk of pregnancy-related RLS.

- Thirty percent of pregnant women begin snoring for the first time during the second trimester. However, there continues to be very limited information regarding whether pregnancy increases the risk for sleep apnea.

- Preeclamptic women show evidence of SDB associated with increased blood pressure. Pregnant women who snore have a two-fold greater incidence of hypertension, preeclampsia, and fetal growth restriction compared to nonsnorers.

- Self-reported sleep quality derived from sleep diaries shows considerable sleep disturbances in the early postpartum period. Sleep efficiency improves during the first year postpartum, but it is unclear whether sleep quantity and quality return to pre-pregnancy levels.

- There is a relationship between sleep and mood during pregnancy and through the first three to four months postpartum. Increased disturbances in self-reported sleep and decreased reported total sleep time are associated with depressed mood postpartum.

Chapter 25

Sex during Pregnancy

If you're pregnant or even planning a pregnancy, you've probably found an abundance of information about sex before pregnancy (that is, having sex in order to conceive) and sex after childbirth (general consensus: expect a less active sex life when there's a newborn in the house).

But there's less talk about the topic of sex during pregnancy, perhaps because of our culture's tendency to dissociate expectant mothers from sexuality. Like many parents-to-be, you may have questions about the safety of sex and what's normal for most couples.

Well, what's normal tends to vary widely, but you can count on the fact that there will be changes in your sex life. Open communication will be the key to a satisfying and safe sexual relationship during pregnancy.

Is It Safe to Have Sex during Pregnancy?

If you're having a normal pregnancy, sex is considered safe during all stages of the pregnancy.

So what's a "normal pregnancy"? It's one that's considered low-risk for complications such as miscarriage or pre-term labor. Talk to your doctor, nurse-midwife, or other pregnancy health care provider if

"Sex During Pregnancy," October 2007, reprinted with permission from www.kidshealth.org. Copyright © 2007 The Nemours Foundation. This information was provided by KidsHealth, one of the largest resources online for medically reviewed health information written for parents, kids, and teens. For more articles like this one, visit www.KidsHealth.org, or www.TeensHealth.org.

you're uncertain about whether you fall into this category. (The next section of this text may help, too.)

Of course, just because sex is safe during pregnancy doesn't mean you'll necessarily want to have it! Many expectant mothers find that their desire for sex fluctuates during certain stages in the pregnancy. Also, many women find that sex becomes uncomfortable as their bodies get larger.

You and your partner need to keep the lines of communication open regarding your sexual relationship. Talk about other ways to satisfy your need for intimacy, such as kissing, caressing, and holding each other. You also may need to experiment with other positions for sex to find those that are the most comfortable.

Many women find that they lose their desire and motivation for sex late in the pregnancy—not only because of their size but also because they're preoccupied with the impending delivery and the excitement of becoming a new parent.

When It's Not Safe

There are two types of sexual behavior that aren't safe for any pregnant woman:

- If you engage in oral sex, your partner should not blow air into your vagina. Blowing air can cause an air embolism (a blockage of a blood vessel by an air bubble), which can be potentially fatal for mother and child.

- You should not have sex with a partner whose sexual history is unknown to you or who may have a sexually transmitted disease, such as herpes, genital warts, chlamydia, or HIV [human immunodeficiency virus]. If you become infected, the disease may be transmitted to your baby, with potentially dangerous consequences.

If your doctor, nurse-midwife, or other pregnancy health care provider anticipates or detects certain significant complications with your pregnancy, he or she is likely to advise against sexual intercourse. The most common risk factors include:

- a history or threat of miscarriage

- a history of pre-term labor (you've previously delivered a baby before 37 weeks) or signs indicating the risk of pre-term labor (such as premature uterine contractions)

- unexplained vaginal bleeding, discharge, or cramping

- leakage of amniotic fluid (the fluid that surrounds the baby)

- placenta previa, a condition in which the placenta (the blood-rich structure that nourishes the baby) is situated down so low that it covers the cervix (the opening of the uterus)

- incompetent cervix, a condition in which the cervix is weakened and dilates (opens) prematurely, raising the risk for miscarriage or premature delivery

- multiple fetuses (you're having twins, triplets, etc.)

Common Questions and Concerns

The following are some of the most frequently asked questions about sex during pregnancy.

Can sex harm my baby?

No, not directly. Your baby is fully protected by the amniotic sac (a thin-walled bag that holds the fetus and surrounding fluid) and the strong muscles of the uterus. There's also a thick mucus plug that seals the cervix and helps guard against infection. The penis does not come into contact with the fetus during sex.

Can intercourse or orgasm cause miscarriage or contractions?

In cases of normal, low-risk pregnancies, the answer is no. The contractions that you may feel during and just after orgasm are entirely different from the contractions associated with labor. However, you should check with your health care provider to make sure that your pregnancy falls into the low-risk category. Some doctors recommend that all women stop having sex during the final weeks of pregnancy, just as a safety precaution, because semen contains a chemical that may actually stimulate contractions. Check with your health care provider to see what he or she thinks is best.

Is it normal for my sex drive to increase or decrease during pregnancy?

Actually, both of these possibilities are normal (and so is everything in between). Many pregnant women find that symptoms such as fatigue,

215

nausea, breast tenderness, and the increased need to urinate make sex too bothersome, especially during the first trimester. Generally, fatigue and nausea subside during the second trimester, and some women find that their desire for sex increases. Also, some women find that freedom from worries about contraception, combined with a renewed sense of closeness with their partner, makes sex more fulfilling. Desire generally subsides again during the third trimester as the uterus grows even larger and the reality of what's about to happen sets in.

Your partner's desire for sex is likely to increase or decrease as well. Some men feel even closer to their pregnant partner and enjoy the changes in their bodies. Others may experience decreased desire because of anxiety about the burdens of parenthood, or because of concerns about the health of both the mother and their unborn child.

Your partner may have trouble reconciling your identity as a sexual partner with your new (and increasingly visible) identity as an expectant mother. Again, remember that communication with your partner can be a great help in dealing with these issues.

When to Call Your Doctor

Call your health care provider if you're unsure whether sex is safe for you. Also, call if you notice any unusual symptoms after intercourse, such as pain, bleeding, or discharge, or if you experience contractions that seem to continue after sex.

Remember, "normal" is a relative term when it comes to sex during pregnancy. You and your partner need to discuss what feels right for both of you.

Chapter 26

Working and Traveling during Pregnancy

Chapter Contents

Section 26.1

Work and Travel Considerations for Pregnant Women

"Work and Travel During Pregnancy,"
© 2009 A.D.A.M., Inc. Reprinted with permission.

Generally, women who are pregnant may continue to work during their pregnancy. Some women are able to work right up until they are ready to deliver, while others may need to cut back on their work schedule or stop completely before their due date. Whether you can work during your pregnancy or not depends on your health, the health of the baby, and the type of job that you have. Here are some factors to consider:

- **Heavy lifting:** If your job requires heavy lifting, standing, or walking, your doctor may recommend that you work fewer hours a day. This is especially true as you get closer to your delivery date.

- **Exposure to environmental hazards:** If you work in a job where you are exposed to hazardous or poisonous agents, you may need to temporarily change positions until after the baby is born. Some agents that may pose a threat to the health of the baby include:
  - chemotherapy medications (may impact health care workers such as nurses and pharmacists);
  - lead (workers in lead smelting, paint manufacturing, printing, ceramics, glass manufacturing, pottery glazing and battery manufacturing; toll booth attendants; and people working on heavily traveled roads);
  - ionizing radiation (X-ray technicians, some physicists and researchers).

Get information on possible toxic substances present at your workplace. Find out if these are at toxic levels and if the workplace is adequately ventilated and workers adequately equipped with protective devices. Radiation from computers, color TVs, and microwaves is called non-ionizing radiation and is not harmful.

- **Stress:** All people experience mental and physical stress as part of life. Too much stress, however, may cause various symptoms such as headaches, depression, and weight gain. Stress may have an impact on how well your body can fight off infection or disease. While you are pregnant, stress should be minimized to the best of your ability. Depending on how much stress your pregnancy adds to your existing load, you may need to get extra help from your spouse or someone else so you can get the rest you need.

Travel

Traveling is generally considered safe during pregnancy. The key to traveling while pregnant is to make sure you are going to be comfortable and as safe as possible. It is best to notify your doctor of your travel plans and ask for any recommendations specific to your pregnancy.

Whether you are traveling by plane, car, or train it is important to do the following:

- Continue to eat regularly.
- Drink plenty of fluids to avoid dehydration.
- Get up and walk around every hour or so to help your circulation and to keep swelling down.
- Wear comfortable shoes and clothing that doesn't bind.
- Take crackers and juice with you to prevent nausea.

Do not take over the counter medicines or any non-prescribed medications without checking with your doctor. This includes medication for motion sickness or bowel problems related to traveling.

Foreign travel: If you are planning a trip out of the country, discuss your trip with your doctor. Plan ahead to allow time for any shots or medications you may need, and be prepared to take a copy of your prenatal record with you.

Traveling to high altitudes may cause problems during pregnancy, as your body and your fetus adjust to the lower air pressure and lower levels of oxygen. It's generally best to let your body adjust to moderate altitudes—6,000–8,000 feet—for a few days before going above 8,000 feet. Women with complicated pregnancies may want to avoid mountain-top excursions altogether.

The American College of Obstetricians and Gynecologists (ACOG) recommends the following when traveling by land, air, or sea:

- **Land:** Travel no more than 5–6 hours a day. Always wear your seatbelt. Place the lap belt under your abdomen and across your hips so that it fits snugly and comfortably. Put the shoulder strap between your breasts and across your shoulder. Always wear the lap shoulder strap when traveling while pregnant. The fluid-filled sac inside the uterus, which is further protected by muscles, organs, and bones, cushions the baby. Unless the mother has a serious injury in an accident, the baby will likely not be harmed. However, if you are in an accident you should always check with your doctor to make sure you and your baby are fine.

- **Air:** Flying during pregnancy is generally safe. In the United States, pregnant women are allowed to fly up to 36 weeks of pregnancy. You should consider getting an aisle seat for more room and to make it easier to walk around and get to the bathroom. Wear layered clothing so you can have some control when there are temperature changes. Be sure to get up and walk at least once an hour, and drink plenty of fluids, to reduce the risk of blood clots forming in your legs. Women with complicated pregnancies—those with high risk of preterm delivery, pre-eclampsia, or signs of poor fetal growth—may need supplemental oxygen when flying. Talk to your health care provider before you travel to see if you need additional oxygen. Air travel also exposes passengers to small amounts of cosmic radiation. This is rarely an issue for passengers, but flight attendants and pilots may be exposed to inappropriate levels of radiation.

- **Sea:** If you have never been on a cruise it may not be the best time to take one. Travel by sea may upset your stomach even if you're not pregnant, and may be more uncomfortable if you are. If you do decide to go on a cruise, check what medical care will be available to you and what emergency measures your cruise is prepared to employ.

Section 26.2

International Travel during Pregnancy

Excerpted from "Planning for a Healthy Pregnancy and Traveling While Pregnant," Chapter 9, Travelers' Health–*Yellow Book*, by the Centers for Disease Control and Prevention (CDC, www.cdc.gov), June 18, 2007.

Factors Affecting the Decision to Travel before and during Pregnancy

Reproductive-aged women who may be planning both pregnancy and international travel should consider preconceptional immunization, when practical, to prevent disease in the offspring. Since as many as 50% of pregnancies are unplanned, reproductive-aged women should consider maintaining current immunizations during routine checkups in case an unplanned pregnancy coincides with a need to travel. Preconceptional immunizations are preferred to vaccination during pregnancy, because they decrease risk to the unborn child. A woman should defer pregnancy for at least 28 days after receiving live vaccines (e.g., MMR [measles, mumps, rubella], yellow fever), because of theoretical risk of transmission to the fetus. However, no harm to the fetus has been reported from the unintentional administration of these vaccines during pregnancy, and pregnancy termination is not recommended after an inadvertent exposure. Vaccination of susceptible women during the postpartum period, especially for rubella and varicella, is another opportunity for prevention, and these vaccines should be encouraged and administered (even for breastfeeding mothers) before discharge from the hospital.

According to the American College of Obstetrics and Gynecology, the safest time for a pregnant woman to travel is during the second trimester (18-24 weeks), when she usually feels best and is in least danger of spontaneous abortion or premature labor. A woman in the third trimester should be advised to stay within 300 miles of home because of concerns about access to medical care in case of problems such as hypertension, phlebitis, or premature labor. Pregnant women should be advised to consult with their health-care providers before making any travel decisions. Collaboration between travel health experts and obstetricians is helpful in weighing benefits and risks based on destination and recommended preventive and treatment measures. In general, pregnant women with serious underlying illnesses should be advised not to travel to developing countries.

Preparation for Travel during Pregnancy

Once a pregnant woman has decided to travel, a number of issues need to be considered before her departure.

- An intrauterine pregnancy should be confirmed by a clinician and ectopic pregnancy excluded before beginning any travel.

- Health insurance should provide coverage while abroad and during pregnancy. In addition, a supplemental travel insurance policy and a prepaid medical evacuation insurance policy should be obtained, although most may not cover pregnancy-related problems.

- Check medical facilities at the destination. For a woman in the last trimester, medical facilities should be able to manage complications of pregnancy, toxemia, and cesarean sections.

- Determine beforehand whether prenatal care will be required abroad and, if so, who will provide it. The pregnant traveler should also make sure prenatal visits requiring specific timing are not missed.

- Determine, before traveling, whether blood is screened for HIV [human immunodeficiency virus] and hepatitis B at the destination. The pregnant traveler should also be advised to know her blood type, and Rh-negative pregnant women should receive the anti-D immune globulin (a plasma-derived product) prophylactically at about 28 weeks' gestation. The immune globulin dose should be repeated after delivery if the infant is Rh positive.

General Recommendations for Travel

A pregnant woman should be advised to travel with at least one companion; she should also be advised that, during her pregnancy, her level of comfort may be adversely affected by traveling. Typical problems of pregnant travelers are the same as those experienced by any pregnant woman: fatigue, heartburn, indigestion, constipation, vaginal discharge, leg cramps, increased frequency of urination, and hemorrhoids. During travel, pregnant women can take preventive measures including avoidance of gas-producing food or drinks before scheduled flights (entrapped gases can expand at higher altitudes) and periodic movement of the legs (to decrease venous stasis). Pregnant women should always use seatbelts while seated, as air turbulence is not predictable and may cause significant trauma.

Signs and symptoms that indicate the need for immediate medical attention are vaginal bleeding, passing tissue or clots, abdominal pain or cramps, contractions, ruptured membranes, excessive leg swelling or pain, headaches, or visual problems.

Greatest Risks for Pregnant Travelers

Motor vehicle accidents are a major cause of morbidity and mortality for pregnant women. When available, safety belts should be fastened at the pelvic area. Lap and shoulder restraints are best; in most accidents, the fetus recovers quickly from the safety belt pressure. However, even after seemingly mild blunt trauma, a physician should be consulted.

Hepatitis E, which is not vaccine preventable, can be especially dangerous for pregnant women, for whom the case-fatality rate is 17%–33%. Therefore, pregnant women should be advised that the best preventive measures are to avoid potentially contaminated water and food, as with other enteric infections.

Scuba diving should be avoided in pregnancy because of the risk of decompression syndrome in the fetus.

Chapter 27

Nicotine, Alcohol, and Drug Use during Pregnancy

Chapter Contents

Section 27.1

Smoking and Pregnancy

Excerpted from "Staying Healthy and Safe," by the Office
of Women's Health (www.womenshealth.gov), part of the U.S.
Department of Health and Human Services, March 2009.

Smoking cigarettes is very harmful to your health and could also affect the health of your baby. Not only does smoking cause cancer and heart disease in people who smoke, a recent large study confirmed that smoking during pregnancy increases the risk of low birth weight. Low-birth-weight babies are at higher risk of health problems shortly after birth. Also, some studies have linked low birth weight with a higher risk of health problems later in life, such as high blood pressure and diabetes. Women who smoke during pregnancy are more likely than other women to have a miscarriage and to have a baby born with cleft lip or palate, types of birth defects. Also, mothers who smoke during or after pregnancy put their babies at greater risk of sudden infant death syndrome (SIDS).

Mothers who smoke have many reasons to quit smoking. Take care of your health and your unborn baby's health by asking your doctor for help quitting smoking. Quitting smoking is hard, but you can do it with help.

Section 27.2

Alcohol Use and Pregnancy

This section includes text from "Alcohol Use and Pregnancy," by the National Center on Birth Defects and Developmental Disabilities (NCBDDD, www.cdc.gov/ncbddd), part of the Centers for Disease Control and Prevention (CDC), September 15, 2005, and "When You Are Pregnant Drinking Can Hurt Your Baby," by the National Institute of Alcohol Abuse and Alcoholism (NIAAA, www.niaaa.nih.gov), part of the National Institutes of Health, 2006.

Alcohol Use and Pregnancy

A mother's alcohol use during pregnancy is one of the top preventable causes of birth defects and developmental disabilities. There is no known amount of alcohol that is safe to drink while pregnant. There is no time during pregnancy when it is safe to drink. When a pregnant woman drinks alcohol, her baby does, too.

- Drinking alcohol during pregnancy can cause many birth defects and developmental disabilities. These are known as fetal alcohol spectrum disorders (FASDs) and include fetal alcohol syndrome.

- FASDs can cause problems in how a person looks, grows, thinks, and acts. FASDs can also cause birth defects of the heart, brain, and other major organs.

- About 1 in 12 pregnant women in the United States reports alcohol use. And about 1 in 30 pregnant women in the United States reports binge drinking (having five or more drinks at one time).

- Alcohol can harm a baby at any time during pregnancy. It can cause problems in the early weeks of pregnancy, before a woman even knows she is pregnant.

- The good news is that FASDs are 100% preventable—if a woman does not drink alcohol while she is pregnant.

227

- Health professionals should ask all of their female patients of childbearing age about alcohol use. They should tell women about the risks of using alcohol during pregnancy and advise them not to drink alcohol during pregnancy.

The U.S. Surgeon General wants women to know they should not drink alcohol during pregnancy. In a 2005 advisory on alcohol use in pregnancy, he stated:

- A pregnant woman should not drink alcohol.

- A pregnant woman who has already used alcohol during her pregnancy should stop right away.

- A woman who is thinking about getting pregnant should stop using alcohol.

- Nearly half of all births in the United States are unplanned. Therefore, any woman who could become pregnant should talk to her doctor and take steps to lower the chance of exposing her baby to alcohol.

When You Are Pregnant Drinking Can Hurt Your Baby

When you are pregnant, your baby grows inside you. Everything you eat and drink while you are pregnant affects your baby. If you drink alcohol, it can hurt your baby's growth. Your baby may have physical and behavioral problems that can last for the rest of his or her life. Children born with the most serious problems caused by alcohol have fetal alcohol syndrome.

Children with fetal alcohol syndrome may:

- be born small;
- have problems eating and sleeping;
- have problems seeing and hearing;
- have trouble following directions and learning how to do simple things;
- have trouble paying attention and learning in school;
- need special teachers and schools;
- have trouble getting along with others and controlling their behavior; and
- need medical care all their lives.

Can I drink alcohol if I am pregnant?

No. Do not drink alcohol when you are pregnant. Why? Because when you drink alcohol, so does your baby. Think about it. Everything you drink, your baby also drinks.

Is any kind of alcohol safe to drink during pregnancy?

No. Drinking any kind of alcohol when you are pregnant can hurt your baby. Alcoholic drinks are beer, wine, wine coolers, liquor, or mixed drinks. A glass of wine, a can of beer, and a mixed drink all have about the same amount of alcohol.

What if I drank during my last pregnancy and my baby was fine?

Every pregnancy is different. Drinking alcohol may hurt one baby more than another. You could have one child that is born healthy and another child that is born with problems.

Will these problems go away?

No. These problems will last for a child's whole life. People with severe problems may not be able to take care of themselves as adults. They may never be able to work.

What if I am pregnant and have been drinking?

If you drank alcohol before you knew you were pregnant, stop drinking now. You will feel better, and your baby will have a good chance to be born healthy. If you want to get pregnant, do not drink alcohol. You may not know you are pregnant right away. Alcohol can hurt a baby even when you are only 1 or 2 months pregnant.

How can I stop drinking?

There are many ways to help yourself stop drinking. You do not have to drink when other people drink. If someone gives you a drink, it is OK say no. Stay away from people or places that make you drink. Do not keep alcohol at home.

If you cannot stop drinking, get help. You may have a disease called alcoholism. There are programs that can help you stop drinking. They are called alcohol treatment programs. Your doctor or nurse can find a program to help you. Even if you have been through a treatment program before, try it again. There are programs just for women.

Section 27.3

Fetal Alcohol Spectrum Disorders

Excerpted from "Fetal Alcohol Spectrum Disorders," by the National Center on Birth Defects and Developmental Disabilities (NCBDDD, www.cdc.gov/ncbddd), part of the Centers for Disease Control and Prevention (CDC), May 2, 2006.

What is FAS?

FAS stands for fetal alcohol syndrome. It is one of the leading known preventable causes of mental retardation and birth defects. FAS represents the severe end of a spectrum of effects that can occur when a woman drinks alcohol during pregnancy. Fetal death is the most extreme outcome. FAS is characterized by abnormal facial features, growth deficiency, and central nervous system (CNS) problems.

People with FAS can have problems with learning, memory, attention span, communication, vision, hearing, or a combination of these things. These problems often lead to difficulties in school and problems getting along with others. FAS is a permanent condition. It affects every aspect of an individual's life and the lives of his or her family. However, FAS is 100% preventable—if a woman does not drink alcohol while she is pregnant.

What are FAE, ARND, and ARBD?

Prenatal exposure to alcohol can cause a spectrum of disorders. Many terms have been used to describe children who have some, but not all, of the clinical signs of FAS. Three terms are fetal alcohol effects (FAE), alcohol-related neurodevelopmental disorder (ARND), and alcohol-related birth defects (ARBD). The term FAE has been used to describe behavioral and cognitive problems in children who were prenatally exposed to alcohol, but who do not have all of the typical diagnostic features of FAS. In 1996, the Institute of Medicine (IOM)

230

replaced FAE with the terms ARND and ARBD. People with ARND can have functional or mental problems linked to prenatal alcohol exposure. These include behavioral or cognitive deficits, or both. Examples are learning difficulties, poor school performance, and poor impulse control. They can have difficulties with mathematical skills, memory, attention, judgment, or a combination of these. People with ARBD can have problems with the heart, kidneys, bones, hearing, or a combination of these.

What are FASDs?

The term fetal alcohol spectrum disorders (FASDs) has emerged to address the need to describe the spectrum of disorders related to fetal alcohol exposure. It is an umbrella term describing the range of effects that can occur in an individual whose mother drank alcohol during pregnancy. These effects can include physical, mental, behavioral, learning disabilities, or a combination of these, with possible lifelong implications. The term FASDs is not intended for use as a clinical diagnosis. Unlike people with FAS, those with other prenatal alcohol-related conditions under the umbrella of FASDs do not show the identifying physical characteristics of FAS and, as a result, they often go undiagnosed.

How common are fetal alcohol syndrome (FAS) and other prenatal alcohol-related conditions (known collectively as FASDs)?

The reported rates of FAS vary widely. These different rates depend on the population studied and the surveillance methods used. CDC studies show FAS rates ranging from 0.2 to 1.5 cases per 1,000 live births in different areas of the United States. Other prenatal alcohol-related conditions, such as ARND and ARBD, are believed to occur about three times as often as FAS.

How do I know if my child has been affected by maternal alcohol use?

Children with FAS have evidence of growth deficiency, CNS (central nervous system) problems, and a distinct pattern of facial characteristics such as a thin upper lip, smooth philtrum (the groove running vertically between the nose and lips), and small eye openings. Children with different FASDs have CNS problems like children with FAS and/or a pattern of behavior or cognitive abnormalities such as learning difficulties and poor school performance. People with FASDs can have poor

coordination or hyperactive behavior. They can have developmental disabilities such as speech and language delays, learning disabilities, mental retardation, or low IQ (intelligence quotient). They can have problems
with self-care such as tying shoes or organizing one's day. People with
FASDs can have poor reasoning and judgment skills. Infants with
FASDs have sleep and sucking disturbances. People with FASDs often
have problems as they get older. These might include mental health
problems, disrupted school experiences, trouble with the law, unemploy-
ment, inappropriate sexual behavior, or a combination of these.

Can FASDs be treated?

FASDs are permanent conditions. They last a lifetime and affect
every aspect of a child's life and the lives of his or her family members.
There is no cure for these conditions. However, FASDs can be completely
prevented—if a woman does not drink alcohol while she is pregnant.
With early identification and diagnosis, a child with an FASD can get
services that can help him or her lead a more productive life.

If a woman has an FASD, but does not drink during preg-nancy, can her child have an FASD? Are FASDs hereditary?

FASDs are not genetic or hereditary. If a woman drinks alcohol
during her pregnancy, her baby can be born with an FASD. But if a
woman has an FASD, her own child cannot have an FASD, unless she
drinks alcohol during pregnancy.

Is there any safe amount of alcohol to drink during preg-nancy? Is there a safe time during pregnancy to drink al-cohol?

When a pregnant woman drinks alcohol, so does her unborn baby.
There is no known safe amount of alcohol that a woman can drink
during pregnancy. There is also no safe time during pregnancy to drink
alcohol. Alcohol can have negative effects on a fetus in every trimester of pregnancy. Therefore, women should not drink if they are pregnant, planning to become pregnant, or could become pregnant (that
is, sexually active and not using an effective form of birth control).

What is a drink? What if I drink only beer or wine coolers?

All drinks containing alcohol can hurt an unborn baby. A standard
drink is defined as .60 ounces of pure alcohol. This is equivalent to

one 12-ounce beer or wine cooler, one 5-ounce glass of wine, or 1.5 ounces of 80 proof distilled spirits (hard liquor). Some alcoholic drinks have high alcohol concentrations and come in larger containers (22–45 ounce containers). There is no safe kind of alcohol. If you have any questions about your alcohol use and its risks to your health, talk to your health care provider.

How does alcohol cause these problems?

Alcohol in the mother's blood crosses the placenta freely and enters the embryo or fetus through the umbilical cord. Alcohol exposure in the first 3 months of pregnancy can cause structural defects (e.g., facial changes). Growth and CNS problems can occur from drinking alcohol any time during pregnancy. The brain is developing throughout pregnancy. It can be damaged at any time. It is unlikely that one mechanism can explain the harmful effects of alcohol on the developing fetus. For example, brain images of some people with FAS show that certain areas have not developed normally. The images show that certain cells are not in their proper place and tissues have died in some areas.

Is there anything I can do now to decrease the chances of having a child with an FASD?

If a woman is drinking during pregnancy, it is never too late for her to stop. The sooner a woman stops drinking, the better it will be for her baby. A woman should use an effective form of birth control until her drinking is under control. If a woman is not able to stop drinking, she should contact her physician, local Alcoholics Anonymous, or local alcohol treatment center, if needed. The Substance Abuse and Mental Health Services Administration has a Substance Abuse Treatment Facility locator. This locator helps people find drug and alcohol treatment programs in their area.

If a woman is sexually active and not using an effective form of birth control, she should not drink alcohol. She could be pregnant and not know it for several weeks or more.

Mothers are not the only ones who can prevent FASDs. Spouses, partners, family members, friends, schools, health and social service organizations, and communities can help prevent FASDs through education and support.

I just found out I am pregnant. I have stopped drinking now, but I was drinking in the first few weeks of my pregnancy, before I knew I was pregnant. Could my baby have an FASD? What should I do now?

The most important thing is that you have completely stopped drinking after learning of your pregnancy. It is never too late to stop drinking. The sooner you stop, the better the chances for your baby's health. It is not possible to know what harm might have been done already. Some women can drink heavily during pregnancy and their babies do not seem to have any problems. Others drink less and their babies show various signs of alcohol exposure. Many body parts and organs are developing in the embryonic stage (weeks 3 to 8 of the pregnancy). This is the time when most women do not know they are pregnant. There is no known safe amount of alcohol or safe time to drink alcohol during pregnancy. It is recommended not to drink at all if one is pregnant or planning to become pregnant. Also, if a woman is sexually active and not using an effective form of birth control, she should avoid alcohol. The best advice is to try not to be alarmed, talk to your doctor about this, and be sure to receive routine prenatal care throughout your pregnancy.

Can a father's drinking cause FASDs?

How alcohol affects the male sperm is currently being studied. Whatever the effects are found to be, they are not FASDs. FASDs are caused specifically by the mother's alcohol use during pregnancy. However, the father's role is important. He can help the woman avoid drinking alcohol during pregnancy. He can encourage her abstinence from alcohol by avoiding social situations that involve drinking. He can also help her by avoiding alcohol himself.

Section 27.4

Drug Use during Pregnancy

Excerpted from "Drugs," by the Center for the Evaluation of the
Risks for Human Reproduction (CERHR, cerhr.niehs.gov), part of the
National Institute of Environmental Health Sciences, April 23, 2008.

Drugs use by pregnant women can result in harm to unborn children. The March of Dimes provides information about pregnancy and the use of legal drugs such as tobacco and alcohol and illegal drugs such as cocaine, PCP [phencyclidine], and heroin. Because some prescription and over-the-counter drugs can also harm unborn children, the March of Dimes recommends that pregnant women speak to their doctors before taking any medication.

Cocaine Use during Pregnancy

The March of Dimes offers the following information about cocaine use during pregnancy.

What are the risks with use of cocaine during pregnancy?

Cocaine use during pregnancy can affect a pregnant woman and her unborn baby in many ways. During the early months of pregnancy, it may increase the risk of miscarriage. Later in pregnancy, it can trigger preterm labor (labor that occurs before 37 weeks of pregnancy) or cause the baby to grow poorly. As a result, cocaine-exposed babies are more likely than unexposed babies to be born with low birthweight (less than 5 1/2 pounds). Low-birthweight babies are 20 times more likely to die in their first month of life than normal-weight babies, and face an increased risk of lifelong disabilities such as mental retardation and cerebral palsy. Cocaine-exposed babies also tend to have smaller heads, which generally reflect smaller brains.

Some studies suggest that cocaine-exposed babies are at increased risk of birth defects, including urinary tract defects and, possibly, heart defects. Cocaine also may cause an unborn baby to have a stroke, which

235

can result in irreversible brain damage or a heart attack, and sometimes death.

Cocaine use also may cause the placenta to pull away from the wall of the uterus before labor begins. This condition, called placental abruption, can lead to extensive bleeding and can be fatal for both mother and baby. (Prompt cesarean delivery, however, can prevent most deaths.)

Babies who were regularly exposed to cocaine before birth may score lower than unexposed babies on tests given at birth to assess the newborn's physical condition and overall responsiveness. They may not do as well as unexposed babies on measures of motor ability, reflexes, attention and mood control, and they appear less likely to respond to a human face or voice.

Babies who are regularly exposed to cocaine before birth sometimes have feeding difficulties and sleep disturbances. As newborns, some are jittery and irritable, and they may startle and cry at the gentlest touch or sound. Therefore, these babies may be difficult to comfort and may be described as withdrawn or unresponsive. Other cocaine-exposed babies "turn off" surrounding stimuli by going into a deep sleep for most of the day. Generally, these behavioral disturbances are temporary and resolve over the first few months of life. Some studies suggest that cocaine-exposed babies have a greater chance of dying of sudden infant death syndrome (SIDS). However, other studies suggest that poor health practices that often accompany maternal cocaine use (such as use of other drugs) also may play a major role in these deaths.

What is the long-term outlook for babies who were exposed to cocaine before birth?

Some studies suggest that most children who are exposed to cocaine before birth have normal intelligence. This is encouraging, in light of earlier predictions that many of these children would be severely brain damaged. A 2002 study at Harvard Medical School and Boston University found that children up to age 2 who were heavily exposed to cocaine before birth scored just as well on tests of infant development as lightly exposed or unexposed children. However, other studies suggest that cocaine may sometimes affect mental development, possibly lowering IQ [intelligence quotient] levels.

A 2002 study at Case Western Reserve University found that cocaine-exposed 2-year-olds were twice as likely as unexposed children from similar low socioeconomic backgrounds to have significant delays in mental development (14 percent and 7 percent, respectively).

It is not known whether these children will continue to have learning problems when they reach school age.

Studies are inconclusive regarding the risk of learning and behavioral problems. Studies from the National Institute on Drug Abuse suggest that most adolescents who were exposed to cocaine before birth seem to function normally. However, some may have subtle impairments in the ability to control emotions and focus attention that could put them at risk of behavioral and learning problems. Other studies suggest that cocaine exposure may adversely affect language abilities. Researchers continue to follow cocaine-exposed children through their teen years to clarify their long-term outlook.

Marijuana Use and Pregnancy

Marijuana is often mistakenly viewed as a "safe" drug. However, a study funded by the National Institute on Drug Abuse (NIDA) and the National Institute on Child Health and Human Development (NICHD) suggests that exposure to cannabinoids, psychoactive chemicals present in marijuana, can affect early embryonic development.

What are the risks with use of marijuana during pregnancy?

Some studies suggest that use of marijuana during pregnancy may slow fetal growth and slightly decrease the length of pregnancy (possibly increasing the risk of premature delivery). Both of these factors can increase a woman's chance of having a low-birthweight baby. These effects are seen mainly in women who use marijuana regularly (six or more times a week).

After delivery, some babies who were regularly exposed to marijuana in the womb appear to undergo withdrawal-like symptoms including excessive crying and trembling.

Couples who are planning pregnancy also should keep in mind that marijuana can reduce fertility in both men and women, making it more difficult to conceive.

What is the long-term outlook for babies exposed to marijuana before birth?

There have been a limited number of studies following marijuana-exposed babies through childhood. Some did not find any increased risk of learning or behavioral problems. However, others found that

237

children who are exposed to marijuana before birth are more likely to have subtle problems that affect their ability to pay attention and to solve visual problems. Exposed children do not appear to have a decrease in IQ.

Chapter 28

Prenatal Radiation Exposures and Home Monitoring

Chapter Contents

Section 28.1

X-Rays, Pregnancy, and You

From "X-Rays, Pregnancy, and You," by the Centers for Devices and Radiological Health (CDRH, www.fda.gov/cdrh), part of the U.S. Food and Drug Administration, May 11, 2001. Reviewed by David A. Cooke, MD, FACP, April 12, 2009.

Pregnancy is a time to take good care of yourself and your unborn child. Many things are especially important during pregnancy, such as eating right, cutting out cigarettes and alcohol, and being careful about the prescription and over-the-counter drugs you take.

Diagnostic x-rays and other medical radiation procedures of the abdominal area also deserve extra attention during pregnancy. This information is to help you understand the issues concerning x-ray exposure during pregnancy. Diagnostic x-rays can give the doctor important and even life-saving information about a person's medical condition. But like many things, diagnostic x-rays have risks as well as benefits. They should be used only when they will give the doctor information needed to treat you.

You'll probably never need an abdominal x-ray during pregnancy. But sometimes, because of a particular medical condition, your physician may feel that a diagnostic x-ray of your abdomen or lower torso is needed. If this should happen—don't be upset. The risk to you and your unborn child is very small, and the benefit of finding out about your medical condition is far greater. In fact, the risk of not having a needed x-ray could be much greater than the risk from the radiation. But even small risks should not be taken if they're unnecessary.

You can reduce those risks by telling your doctor if you are, or think you might be, pregnant whenever an abdominal x-ray is prescribed. If you are pregnant, the doctor may decide that it would be best to cancel the x-ray examination, to postpone it, or to modify it to reduce the amount of radiation. Or, depending on your medical needs, and realizing that the risk is very small, the doctor may feel that it is best to proceed with the x-ray as planned. In any case, you should feel free to discuss the decision with your doctor.

What Kind of X-Rays Can Affect the Unborn Child?

During most x-ray examinations—like those of the arms, legs, head, teeth, or chest—your reproductive organs are not exposed to the direct x-ray beam. So these kinds of procedures, when properly done, do not involve any risk to the unborn child. However, x-rays of the mother's lower torso—abdomen, stomach, pelvis, lower back, or kidneys—may expose the unborn child to the direct x-ray beam. They are of more concern.

What Are the Possible Effects of X-Rays?

There is scientific disagreement about whether the small amounts of radiation used in diagnostic radiology can actually harm the unborn child, but it is known that the unborn child is very sensitive to the effects of things like radiation, certain drugs, excess alcohol, and infection. This is true, in part, because the cells are rapidly dividing and growing into specialized cells and tissues. If radiation or other agents were to cause changes in these cells, there could be a slightly increased chance of birth defects or certain illnesses, such as leukemia, later in life.

It should be pointed out, however, that the majority of birth defects and childhood diseases occur even if the mother is not exposed to any known harmful agent during pregnancy. Scientists believe that heredity and random errors in the developmental process are responsible for most of these problems.

What If I'm X-Rayed before I Know I'm Pregnant?

Don't be alarmed. Remember that the possibility of any harm to you and your unborn child from an x-ray is very small. There are, however, rare situations in which a woman who is unaware of her pregnancy may receive a very large number of abdominal x-rays over a short period. Or she may receive radiation treatment of the lower torso. Under these circumstances, the woman should discuss the possible risks with her doctor.

How You Can Help Minimize the Risks

- Most important, tell your physician if you are pregnant or think you might be. This is important for many medical decisions, such as drug prescriptions and nuclear medicine procedures, as well

241

as x-rays. And remember, this is true even in the very early weeks of pregnancy.

- Occasionally, a woman may mistake the symptoms of pregnancy for the symptoms of a disease. If you have any of the symptoms of pregnancy—nausea, vomiting, breast tenderness, fatigue—consider whether you might be pregnant and tell your doctor or x-ray technologist (the person doing the examination) before having an x-ray of the lower torso. A pregnancy test may be called for.

- If you are pregnant, or think you might be, do not hold a child who is being x-rayed. If you are not pregnant and you are asked to hold a child during an x-ray, be sure to ask for a lead apron to protect your reproductive organs. This is to prevent damage to your genes that could be passed on and cause harmful effects in your future descendants.

- Whenever an x-ray is requested, tell your doctor about any similar x-rays you have had recently. It may not be necessary to do another. It is a good idea to keep a record of the x-ray examinations you and your family have had taken so you can provide this kind of information accurately.

- Feel free to talk with your doctor about the need for an x-ray examination. You should understand the reason x-rays are requested in your particular case.

Section 28.2

Pregnant Women Should Avoid Fetal Keepsake Images and Heartbeat Monitors

From "Avoid Fetal Keepsake Images, Heartbeat Monitors,"
by the U.S. Food and Drug Administration (FDA, www.fda.gov),
March 24, 2008.

While ultrasonic fetal scanning is generally considered a safe medical procedure, the use of it for unapproved and unintended purposes raises concerns.

The use of ultrasound imaging devices for producing fetal keepsake videos is viewed as an unapproved use by the Food and Drug Administration (FDA). Doppler ultrasound heartbeat monitors are not intended for over-the-counter (OTC) use. Both products are approved for use only with a prescription.

"Although there are no known risks of ultrasound imaging and heartbeat monitors, the radiation associated with them can produce effects on the body," says Robert Phillips, Ph.D., a physicist with FDA's Center for Devices and Radiological Health (CDRH). "When ultrasound enters the body, it heats the tissues slightly. In some cases, it can also produce small pockets of gas in body fluids or tissues."

Phillips says the long-term effects of tissue heating and of the formation of partial vacuums in a liquid by high-intensity sound waves (cavitation) are not known.

Using ultrasound equipment only through a prescription ensures that pregnant women will receive professional care that contributes to their health and to the health of their babies, and that ultrasound will be used when medically indicated.

Fetal Keepsake Videos

"Performing prenatal ultrasounds without medical oversight may put a mother and her unborn baby at risk," says Phillips. "The bottom line is: Why take a chance with your baby's health for the sake of a video?"

Fetal keepsake videos are viewed as a problem because there is no medical benefit derived from the exposure. Further, there is no control on how long a single imaging session will take or how many sessions will occur.

FDA is aware of entrepreneurs that are commercializing ultrasonic imaging of fetuses by making keepsake videos. In some cases, the ultrasound machine may be used for as long as an hour to get a video of the fetus.

Doppler Ultrasound Heartbeat Monitors

Similar concerns surround the OTC sale of Doppler ultrasound heartbeat monitors. These devices, which people use to listen to the heartbeat of a fetus, are currently marketed legally as "prescription devices" that should only be used by or under the supervision of a health care professional.

"When the product is purchased over the counter and used without prior consultation with a health care professional, there is no oversight of how the device is used and little or no medical benefit derived from the exposure," Phillips says. "The number of sessions or the length of a session to which a fetus is exposed is uncontrolled, thus raising the potential for harm to the fetus."

Section 28.3

Home Uterine Monitors Not Useful for Predicting Premature Birth

From "Home Uterine Monitors Not Useful For Predicting Premature Birth," by the National Institute of Child Health and Human Development (NICHD, www.nichd.nih.gov), updated July 25, 2006.

Portable monitors that detect contractions of the uterus do not appear to be useful for identifying women likely to have a preterm delivery, according to a study by the National Institute of Child Health and Human Development (NICHD).

Although they are widely prescribed for women at risk of giving birth prematurely, the NICHD study confirms earlier findings that the monitors are not useful for predicting or preventing preterm birth. The study also confirmed that several other methods being assessed as ways to predict preterm labor were of little value.

"The study found that while women who gave birth prematurely did have slightly more contractions throughout pregnancy than did women who gave birth at term, there was no detectable pattern that would predict premature birth," said Duane Alexander, MD, Director of the NICHD.

The study was conducted at the 11 centers participating in the NICHD Network of Maternal-Fetal Medicine Units and appears in the January 25 [2002] *New England Journal of Medicine*. The study was led by Jay Iams, MD, director of the Division of Maternal-Fetal Medicine at the Ohio State University Medical Center.

The portable, or ambulatory, monitors cost up to $100 a day and may be worn for up to 10 weeks. The monitors relay information to a central monitoring office, where any potential signs of early labor can be passed on to a physician.

The researchers analyzed 34,908 hours of recordings from 306 women. When the women began the study, they were in their 22nd through 24th week of pregnancy. The authors wrote that the women who gave birth before the 35th week of pregnancy had a slightly greater frequency of contractions than did the women who gave birth after the 35th week, but this information did not allow them to predict impending premature labor. A pregnancy is considered full term at 37 weeks.

"We could identify no threshold frequency that effectively identified women who delivered preterm infants," the study authors wrote in the *New England Journal of Medicine* article.

The researchers also found little value of some other techniques in predicting preterm labor, including measuring the cervix and collecting a substance known as fetal fibronectin from the cervix.

"Our data indicate that ambulatory monitoring of uterine contractions does not identify women destined to have preterm delivery," the authors wrote.

Preterm birth complicates from 8 to 10 percent of all births, said Catherine Spong, MD, Chief of NICHD's Pregnancy and Perinatology Branch and coordinator of the Maternal-Fetal Medicine Units. Premature infants are at greater risk for life-threatening infections, for a serious lung condition known as respiratory distress syndrome, and for serious damage to the intestines (necrotizing enterocolitis). Most deaths of premature infants occur among those born before the 32nd week of pregnancy. In addition, the cost of caring for premature infants in the United States exceeds $4 billion each year.

Chapter 29

Common Safety
Concerns during Pregnancy

Chapter Contents

Section 29.1

Hot Tubs, High Temperatures, and Pregnancy Risks

"Hyperthermia and Pregnancy," © 2006 Organization of Teratology Information Services (OTIS). Reprinted with permission. Member programs of OTIS are located throughout the U.S. and Canada. To find the Teratogen Information Service in your area, call OTIS toll-free 866-626-OTIS (866-626-6847), or visit www.otispregnancy.org.

This information talks about the risks that hyperthermia can have during pregnancy. With each pregnancy, all women have a 3% to 5% chance of having a baby with a birth defect. This information should not take the place of medical care and advice from your health care provider.

What is hyperthermia?

Hyperthermia refers to an abnormally high body temperature. A person's normal body temperature averages about 98.6 degrees Fahrenheit (37 degrees Celsius). In pregnancy, a body temperature of at least 101 degrees Fahrenheit (38.3 degrees Celsius) can be of concern. However, most studies have not shown a concern until your temperature reaches 102 degrees Fahrenheit (38.9 degrees Celsius) or higher for an extended period of time.

What can cause hyperthermia?

Hyperthermia most often occurs from a fever due to illness. Extremely heavy exercise or prolonged exposure (longer than 10 minutes) to heat sources such as hot tubs, very hot baths, or saunas can also raise body temperature.

What effect does hyperthermia in early pregnancy have?

Some studies have shown an increased risk for birth defects called neural tube defects (NTD) in babies of women who had high temperatures early in pregnancy.

Studies have suggested there may also be an increased risk for miscarriage. Possible associations between high fever and birth defects such as heart defects and abdominal wall defects have been suggested. However, most studies did not find these results. The potential risk for these problems is small.

It is important to know what caused your fever during pregnancy. Risks may be associated with the cause of the fever, such as rubella infection, rather than from the fever itself. Please discuss any concerns you may have with your health care provider.

What is a neural tube defect?

Neural tube defects occur when the spine or skull does not close properly. About 1 to 2 out of every 1,000 births has a neural tube defect. An opening in the spinal column is called spina bifida. The majority of babies with spina bifida grow to adulthood. The most severe open skull defect is called anencephaly. Infants with anencephaly have a severely underdeveloped brain and usually die at or shortly after birth.

Babies with spina bifida may need surgery to close the opening. While spina bifida can be of varying severity, most children will have some degree of paralysis and may have problems with walking and with bowel and bladder control. Some children with spina bifida may also develop hydrocephalus or "water on the brain." The very mildest form of spina bifida is covered by skin and causes no major problems.

When does the neural tube close?

The neural tube (which forms the spinal cord) is completely closed by the beginning of your 6th week of pregnancy (dating from the first day of your last menstrual period). After the neural tube has closed, a neural tube defect cannot occur. Therefore, if your high temperature occurs after the 6th week of pregnancy, the neural tube has already closed. Then, your pregnancy is not at an increased risk for this birth defect due to the hyperthermia.

I am 5 weeks pregnant and have a high fever. Can this hurt my baby?

There may be an increased risk for a neural tube defect if a woman has a fever of 101 degrees Fahrenheit (38.3 degrees Celsius) or higher for an extended period of time during the first 6 weeks of pregnancy. It is not possible to determine the exact risk. With an illness like the flu, it is often hard to separate the effects of a high temperature from

249

the other effects of an illness. You should contact your health care provider if you have a fever during pregnancy.

What testing is available for neural tube defects during my pregnancy?

Neural tube defects are detectable during pregnancy through a combination of ultrasound and alpha-fetoprotein (AFP) screening at approximately 15–20 weeks. AFP screening is a blood test that measures the level of AFP in the mother's blood. This screen can detect 80–90% of fetuses with open neural tube defects. Skin-covered neural tube defects are hard to detect during pregnancy.

Elevated levels of AFP in maternal blood indicate an increased risk for neural tube defects and suggest a need for further diagnostic testing, such as amniocentesis or a targeted ultrasound exam. Please talk to your health care provider if you have questions about these prenatal tests.

I have a fever of less than 101 degrees Fahrenheit (38.3 degrees Celsius) and am pregnant. Is there a risk to my baby?

A temperature below 101 degrees Fahrenheit (38.3 degrees Celsius) does not appear to increase the risk for birth defects above that seen in any pregnancy. However, you should discuss with your health care provider whether the illness causing your fever poses a risk.

I have been using the hot tub and sauna. Is this a risk during my pregnancy?

Hot tub or sauna use during pregnancy should be limited to less than 10 minutes. This is because it may take only 10 to 20 minutes in a hot tub or sauna to raise your body temperature to 102 degrees Fahrenheit (38.9 degrees Celsius). You may not even feel uncomfortable at this temperature.

Although sauna use alone has not been as strongly associated with an increased risk for neural tube defects, the same safety measures are recommended. If you were in a hot tub or sauna for a long period of time early in pregnancy, you may want to talk with your health care provider about ways to detect neural tube defects during pregnancy.

After 6 weeks of pregnancy, normal hot tub and sauna use does not appear to increase the risk for birth defects. However, you should still be careful to limit your use to 10 minutes or less and not get overheated or dehydrated.

250

Will using my electric blanket or heated waterbed during pregnancy increase the risk for hyperthermia?

Electric blankets and heated waterbeds are not likely to raise your body temperature enough to increase the risk for neural tube defects. Although one recent study showed no increased risk, concerns have been raised, but not confirmed, that use during pregnancy may increase the risk for pregnancy loss or low birth weight.

Can ultrasound hurt my baby?

The use of ultrasound has not been associated with adverse pregnancy outcomes. Ultrasound uses sound waves to create an image of a fetus on a screen. Although this procedure can slightly increase body temperature, even a lengthy ultrasound exposure is unlikely to increase your body temperature significantly.

References

Chambers CD, et al. 1998. Maternal fever and birth outcome: a prospective study. *Teratology*. 58:251–257.

Edwards MJ, et al. 1995. Hyperthermia and birth defects. *Reprod Toxicol* 9(5):411.

Harvey MAS, et al. 1981. Suggested limits to the use of hot tub and sauna by pregnant women. *CMAJ* 125:50.

Layde PM, et al. 1980. Maternal fever and neural tube defects. *Teratology* 21:105.

Lipson A, et al. 1985. Saunas and birth defects. *Teratology* 32:147.

Lyndberg MC, et al. 1994. Maternal flu, fever, and the risk of neural tube defects: A population based case-control study. *Am J Epidemiol* 140(3):244.

Milunsky A, et al. 1992. Maternal heat exposure and neural tube defects. *JAMA* 268(7):882.

Morctti ME, et al. 2005. Maternal hyperthermia and the risk for neural tube defects in offspring: Systematic review and meta-analysis. *Epidemiol* 16:216–219.

NCRP. 1983. National Council on Radiation Protection and Measurements Report No 74, Bethesda, MD, p. 72.

Ridge BR and Budd GM. 1990. How long is too long in a spa pool? *NEJM* 323(12):835.

Sandford MK, et al. 1992. Neural tube defect etiology: Evidence concerning maternal hyperthermia, health and diet. *Dev Med Child Neurol* 34:661.

Warkany J. 1986. Teratogen Update. Hyperthermia. *Teratology* 33:365.

Wertheimer N and Leeper E. 1986. Possible effects of electric blankets and heated waterbeds on fetal development. *Bioelectromagnetics* 7:13.

If you have questions about the information here or other exposures during pregnancy, call OTIS at 1-866-626-6847.

Section 29.2

Pregnancy and Chiropractic Care

Chiropractic care is health maintenance of the spinal column, disks, related nerves and bone geometry without drugs or surgery. It involves the art and science of adjusting misaligned joints of the body, especially of the spine, which reduces spinal nerve stress and therefore promotes health throughout the body.

Is chiropractic care safe during pregnancy?

There are no known contraindications to chiropractic care throughout pregnancy. All chiropractors are trained to work with women who are pregnant. Investing in the fertility and pregnancy wellness of women who are pregnant or trying to conceive is a routine treatment for most chiropractors.

Some chiropractors take a specific interest in prenatal and perinatal care and seek additional training. Below represents designations of chiropractors who have taken advanced steps in working with infertility and pregnancy wellness.

- DACCP—Diplomate with ICPA reflecting highest level of advanced training

- CACCP—Certified with the ICPA reflecting advanced training

- Member of ICPA reflecting special interest

- Webster Certified—trained to specifically work with breech positions

Chiropractors that have been trained to work with pregnant women may use tables that adjust for a pregnant woman's body, and they will use techniques that avoid unneeded pressure on the abdomen.

A chiropractor who is versed in the needs of women who are pregnant will also provide you with exercises and stretches that are safe to use during pregnancy and complement any adjustments made to your spine.

Why should I have chiropractic care during pregnancy?

During pregnancy, there are several physiological and endocrinological changes that occur in preparation for creating the environment for the developing baby. The following changes could result in a misaligned spine or joint:

- protruding abdomen and increased back curve

- pelvic changes

- postural adaptations

Establishing pelvic balance and alignment is another reason to obtain chiropractic care during pregnancy. When the pelvis is misaligned it may reduce the amount of room available for the developing baby. This restriction is called intrauterine constraint. A misaligned pelvis may also make it difficult for the baby to get into the best possible position for delivery.

The nervous system is the master communication system to all the body systems including the reproductive system. Keeping the spine aligned helps the entire body work more effectively.

What are the benefits of chiropractic care during pregnancy?

Chiropractic care during pregnancy may provide benefits for women who are pregnant. Potential benefits of chiropractic care during pregnancy include:

- maintaining a healthier pregnancy;
- controlling symptoms of nausea;
- reducing the time of labor and delivery;
- relieving back, neck or joint pain; and
- prevent a potential cesarean section.

What about chiropractic care and breech deliveries?

The late Larry Webster, D.C., Founder of the International Chiropractic Pediatric Association, developed a specific chiropractic analysis and adjustment which enables chiropractors to establish balance in the pregnant woman's pelvis and reduce undue stress to her uterus and supporting ligaments. This balanced state in the pelvis makes it easier for a breech baby to turn naturally. The technique is known as the Webster Technique.

It is considered normal by some for a baby to present breech until the third trimester. Most birth practitioners are not concerned with breech presentations until a patient is 37 weeks along. Approximately 4% of all pregnancies result in a breech presentation.

The *Journal of Manipulative and Physiological Therapeutics* reported in the July/August 2002 issue an 82% success rate of babies turning vertex when doctors of chiropractic used the Webster Technique. Further, the results from the study suggest that it may be beneficial to perform the Webster Technique as soon as the 8th month of pregnancy when a woman has a breech presentation.

Currently, the International Chiropractic Pediatric Association recommends that women receive chiropractic care throughout pregnancy to establish pelvic balance and optimize the room a baby has for development throughout pregnancy. With a balanced pelvis, babies have a greater chance of moving into the correct position for birth, and the crisis and worry associated with breech and posterior presentations may be avoided altogether. Optimal baby positioning at the time of birth also eliminates the potential for dystocia (difficult labor) and therefore results in easier and safer deliveries for both the mother and baby.

Talk to Your Health Care Provider

As more women are seeking the benefits of chiropractic care throughout pregnancy, more health care providers are seeking trained doctors of chiropractic in their communities to refer their pregnant patients to. Discuss these options with your health care provider. If they are not yet familiar with chiropractic care in pregnancy, ask them to find out more about its many benefits. Most importantly, seek options that support your body's natural abilities to function and find a team of providers who are respectful of your choices.

Your Next Steps

- Find a chiropractor [http://www.americanpregnancy.org/members/chiropractors] in your area.

- Talk to your health care provider regarding chiropractic care or other alternative interventions.

- Need help covering the cost of chiropractic care? Receive free info from the Maternity Card discount program [http://www.americanpregnancy.org/insuranceform.html].

Section 29.3

Hair Treatment during Pregnancy

"Hair Treatments and Pregnancy," © 2006 Organization of Teratology Information Services (OTIS). Reprinted with permission. Member programs of OTIS are located throughout the U.S. and Canada. To find the Teratogen Information Service in your area, call OTIS toll-free at 866-626-OTIS (866-626-6847), or visit www.otispregnancy.org.

This text talks about the risks that exposure to hair treatments can have during pregnancy. With each pregnancy, all women have a 3% to 5% chance of having a baby with a birth defect. This information should not take the place of medical care and advice from your health care provider.

What are the different types of hair treatments?

Hair treatments include hair coloring, hair curling (permanents), hair bleaching, and hair straightening (relaxers) agents. Hair coloring procedures are divided into several groups determined by the length of time the color stays in the hair. These categories include temporary dyes, semi-permanent dyes, and permanent dyes. Permanent dyes have received the most attention, and they include a variety of chemicals. Hair curling or permanent waves are produced by placing two solutions in the hair. The first solution is a waving fluid and the second is a fixation or neutralization solution. Hair bleaching involves the use of hydrogen peroxide, and hair straighteners or hair relaxers involve a variety of chemicals.

The amount of an exposure, the timing during the pregnancy, and frequency of use may be important factors when thinking about hair treatments in pregnancy. Since many different chemicals are used and manufacturers frequently change formulations, these general guidelines are offered based upon small doses, animal data, and limited data in pregnant women. Cosmetic products are frequently used, but are not generally evaluated for effects on pregnancy.

Do I absorb hair coloring/dye through my skin?

Low levels of hair dye can be absorbed through the skin after application, and the dye is excreted into the urine. This minimal amount is not thought to be enough to cause a problem for the baby.

Before I was pregnant, I had my hair dyed every couple of months. Is this safe now that I am pregnant?

There are very few studies of hair dye use during human pregnancy. In animal studies, at doses 100 times higher than what would normally be used in human application, no significant changes were seen in fetal development. We know that only a small amount of any product applied to your scalp is actually absorbed into your system and therefore, little would be available to get to the developing baby. In addition, many women have dyed their hair during pregnancy with no known reports of negative outcomes. This information, in combination with the minimal absorption through the skin makes hair treatment in pregnancy unlikely to be of concern.

I would like to have my hair permed and am currently in the first trimester of my pregnancy. Is there any risk for birth defects or miscarriage?

Similar to hair dyes, there is limited information available for the safety of hair permanents in pregnancy. The fixation solution used during the application of the permanent may irritate the scalp, but this has not been associated with any other effects in the body. Very little absorption is likely to occur and it does not seem to cause effects in other parts of the body.

I have my hair straightened every two months. Can I continue this into pregnancy?

A study in humans examined the use of hair straighteners during pregnancy. The use of these products was not found to increase the chance of low birth weight or preterm delivery. The study did not address the chance of other abnormal outcomes (such as birth defects). Again, it is likely that only a small amount of hair straightening products are actually absorbed into your system, so the developing baby would only be exposed to small amounts.

I work full time as a cosmetologist and recently became pregnant. Should I stop working until the baby is born?

A large study looked at the risk of miscarriage in cosmetologists. A slightly increased risk of miscarriage was found for cosmetologists who had specific work activities. Activities that seemed to contribute to the slightly increased risk included working more than 40 hours per week, standing more than 8 hours per day, higher numbers of bleaches and permanents applied per week, and working in salons where nail sculpturing was performed. Part time cosmetologists (less than 35 hours per week) did not seem to have an increased risk of miscarriage during pregnancy.

In another study, miscarriage rates among hairdressers were reviewed, and newer data was compared to older data. The older data (from 1986–1988) showed an increased risk of miscarriage, an extended time trying to get pregnant, and low birth weight. The newer data (from 1991–1993) did not find increased risks. The authors suggest that newer restrictions on some dye formulas and better working conditions have contributed to the better outcomes.

Both studies support the importance of proper working conditions. Working in a well ventilated area, wearing protective gloves, taking frequent breaks, and avoiding eating or drinking in the workplace are all important factors that can decrease chemical exposures.

Is it safe to have hair treatments while I am breastfeeding?

There is no information on having hair treatments during breastfeeding. It is highly unlikely that a significant amount would enter the breast milk because so little enters the mom's bloodstream. Many women receive hair treatments while breastfeeding, and there are no known reports of negative outcomes.

References

Blackmore-Prince C, et al 1999. Chemical hair treatments and adverse pregnancy outcome among Black women in central North Carolina. *Am J Epidemiol* 149:712–716.

Burnett C, et al. 1976. Teratology and percutaneous toxicity studies on hair dyes. *J Toxicol Environ Health* 1:1027–1040.

DiNardo JC, et al. 1985. Teratological assessment of five oxidative hair dyes in the rat. *Toxicology and Applied Pharmacology* 78:163–166.

Inouye M. and Murakami U. 1976. Teratogenicity of 2,5-diaminotoluene, a hair dye component, in mice. *Teratology* 14:241–242.

John EM, et al. 1994. Spontaneous abortions among cosmetologists. *Epidemiol* 5:147–155.

Kersemaekers WM, et al. 1996. Reproductive disorders among hairdressers. *Epidemiol* 8:396–401.

Koren G (ed.) 1994. *Maternal-Fetal Toxicology: A Clinician's Guide.* New York: Marcel Dekker, Inc.

Koren G. 1996. Hair care during pregnancy. *Can Fam Physician* 42:625–626.

Kramer S, et al. 1987. Medical and drug risk factors associated with neuroblastoma: A case-control study. *J Natl Cancer Inst* 78:797–803.

Maibach HI, et al. 1975. Percutaneous penetration following use of hair dyes. *Arch Dermatol* 111:1444–1445.

Marks TA, et al. 1979. Teratogenicity of 4-nitro-1,2-diaminobenzene (4NDB) and 2-nitro-1,4-diaminobenzene (2NDB) in the mouse. *Teratology* 19:37A–38A.

Marks TA, et al. 1981. Teratogenic evaluation of 2-nitro-p-phenylenediamine, 4-nitro-o-phenylenediamine, and 2,5-toluenediamine sulfate in the mouse. *Teratology* 24:253–265.

Paul M (ed.) 1993. *Occupational and Environmental Reproductive Hazards: A Guide for Clinicians.* Baltimore: Williams and Wilkins.

Rylander L, et al. 2002. Reproductive outcome among female hairdressers. *Occup Environ Med* 59:517–522.

Section 29.4

Tanning during Pregnancy

"Self-Tanners, Tanning Pills, Tanning Booths and Pregnancy," © 2007 Organization of Teratology Information Services (OTIS). Reprinted with permission. Member programs of OTIS are located throughout the U.S. and Canada. To find the Teratogen Information Service in your area, call OTIS toll-free at 866-626-OTIS (866-626-6847), or visit www.otispregnancy.org.

This text talks about the risks that exposure to self-tanners, tanning pills, and tanning booths can have during pregnancy. With each pregnancy, all women have a 3% to 5% chance of having a baby with a birth defect. This information should not take the place of medical care and advice from your health care provider.

What are self-tanners?

Self-tanners are lotions, gels, and sprays that are applied to the skin to darken it, making the skin look "tan" without sun exposure. The active ingredient in self-tanners that makes your skin darker is dihydroxyacetone (DHA). DHA often comes from plant sources such as sugar beets and sugar cane, and is considered a safe skin-coloring agent. The Food and Drug Administration (FDA) has approved DHA as a tanning product in the United States since the 1970s. Most self-tanning products that you can buy in stores contain 3–5% DHA, while the products used by professionals contain 5–15% DHA.

The tan color will last about a week, and eventually disappears as new skin replaces old skin. Self-tanning products do not provide protection from the harmful effects of the sun. You should still use sunscreen and protective clothing to shield yourself from the sun when using these products.

Are self-tanners absorbed into my bloodstream if I'm using them on my skin?

Although not well-studied, it is estimated that only one-half of one percent (0.5%) of DHA is absorbed into the bloodstream when self-tanners are applied on the skin. There is no information available as to whether this very small amount is able to cross the placenta and get into the baby's circulation.

What about using booths which spray self-tanner on me?

The FDA limits the use of DHA to external application only. It is not approved for use on the eyes, lips, or mucous membranes, or for internal use. This may be hard to avoid when using a "spray tanning" booth, so it is a good idea to protect your mouth, nose, lungs, and eyes when using one. You should request protective measures to cover your eyes and nose, to prevent inhaling the chemical.

Can using self-tanners during my pregnancy cause birth defects?

There is no published information suggesting that using self-tanners during pregnancy causes birth defects. When self-tanners are used, it is thought that only very small amounts of DHA are absorbed into the bloodstream through the skin. Therefore, very little DHA would be available to get to the baby if it does cross the placenta. It is possible that if you are inhaling the self-tanning spray fumes in tanning booths, or applying the product to mucous membranes, more of the DHA could get into your system and result in higher blood levels. Unfortunately, there is no information to prove the safety of using self-tanners while pregnant.

Can I use self-tanners while breastfeeding?

If you decide to use self-tanners while breastfeeding, it is a good idea to avoid putting the self-tanner on areas that the baby's mouth comes in contact with, such as the nipple and areola. There is no evidence suggesting that using self-tanners while breastfeeding is unsafe for a baby.

Can I use tanning pills when I am pregnant or breastfeeding?

Tanning pills are tablets containing a chemical called canthaxanthin as the main active agent. A person has to ingest a very large amount of canthaxanthin in order for his or her skin to change color. Although canthaxanthin, when used in small amounts, is approved by the FDA as a color additive in food, tanning pills are not approved by the FDA. There are no studies examining the use of canthaxanthin during pregnancy or breastfeeding. Be aware that harmful effects in adults have been reported, including eye damage, liver damage, nausea, cramping, diarrhea, severe itching, and welts. Therefore, it may be best to avoid the use of tanning pills during pregnancy or while breastfeeding.

What about using tanning booths while pregnant?

Ultraviolet rays do not penetrate the uterus, so the baby is protected while you are pregnant. However, if your body becomes overheated, your body temperature will rise, causing the baby's body temperature to increase. This condition is called hyperthermia, which may increase the risk for miscarriage or spina bifida. It is recommended that you spend as little as 10–15 minutes at a time in a tanning booth while pregnant.

Can using self-tanners, tanning pills, or tanning booths make it more difficult for me to become pregnant?

There is no evidence to suggest that using self-tanners makes it more difficult to become pregnant, as very little of the DHA is absorbed into the bloodstream. Tanning pills are taken orally, so there is a greater chance that a person could ingest a very large amount of canthaxanthin. There are no studies regarding the safety of using tanning pills while trying to become pregnant. Using tanning booths is not expected to make it more difficult to become pregnant.

Is it a problem if the baby's father is using self-tanners, tanning pills, or tanning booths while I am trying to become pregnant?

For males, there is no evidence that using any of the self-tanning products or tanning pills will cause birth defects. However, constant spikes in body temperature can decrease sperm production, so a male should be careful not to become overheated in a tanning booth.

References

Lapunzina P. 1996. Ultraviolet light-related neural tube defects? *Am J Med Genet* 67:106.

Merck Index, 12th Edition, p. 3225.

Meadows M. 2003. Don't Be in the Dark about Tanning. *FDA Consumer Magazine* 37:6.

United States Food and Drug Administration. 2000. Tanning Pills: Office of Cosmetics and Colors Fact Sheet. Available at: http:// www.cfsan.fda.giv/~dms/cos-tan2.html.

United States Food and Drug Administration. 2003. DHA-Spray Sunless 'Tanning' Booths: Office of Cosmetics and Colors Fact Sheet. Available at: http://www.cfsan.fda.giv/~dms/cos-tan4.html

Yourick JJ, et al. 2004. Fate of chemicals in skin after dermal application: Does the in vitro skin reservoir affect the estimate of systemic absorption? *Toxicol Appl Pharmacol* 195:309–320.

Part Four

High-Risk Pregnancies

Chapter 30

What Is a High-Risk Pregnancy?

Chapter Contents

Section 30.1

Understanding Pregnancy Risk

From "High-Risk Pregnancy," by the National Institute of Child
Health and Human Development (NICHD, www.nichd.nih.gov), part
of the National Institutes of Health, December 4, 2006.

What causes a high-risk pregnancy?

Before a woman becomes pregnant, it is important for her to have
good nutrition and a healthy lifestyle. Good prenatal care and medical treatment during pregnancy can help prevent complications.

But there are factors that can be present before a woman becomes
pregnant that can cause a high-risk pregnancy. Risk factors for a high-
risk pregnancy can include:

- young or old maternal age;

- being overweight or underweight;

- having had problems in previous pregnancies;

- pre-existing health conditions, such as high blood pressure, diabetes, or HIV (human immunodeficiency virus).

Health problems can also develop during a pregnancy that can
make it high-risk. Such problems may occur even in a woman who
was previously healthy.

What are some conditions that may cause a high-risk preg-nancy?

- **Preeclampsia** is a syndrome that includes high blood pressure,
  urinary protein, and changes in blood levels of liver enzymes during pregnancy. It can affect the mother's kidneys, liver, and brain.
  With treatment, many women will have healthy babies. If left untreated, the condition can be fatal for the mother and/or the baby
  and can lead to long-term health problems. **Eclampsia** is a more
  severe form of preeclampsia that can cause seizures and coma in
  the mother.

- **Gestational diabetes mellitus** (or gestational diabetes) is a type of diabetes that only pregnant women get. If a woman gets diabetes when she is pregnant, but never had it before, then she has gestational diabetes. Many women with gestational diabetes have healthy pregnancies and healthy babies because they follow a treatment plan from their health care provider.

- **HIV/AIDS** (acquired immunodeficiency syndrome) kills or damages cells of the body's immune system, progressively destroying the body's ability to fight infections and certain cancers. The term AIDS applies to the most advanced stages of HIV infection. Women can give HIV to their babies during pregnancy, while giving birth, or through breastfeeding. But, there are effective ways to prevent the spread of mother-to-infant transmission of HIV.

- **Preterm labor** is labor that begins before 37 weeks of pregnancy. Because the baby is not fully grown at this time, it may not be able to survive outside the womb. Health care providers will often take steps to try to stop labor if it occurs before this time. Although there is no way to know which women will experience preterm labor or birth, there are factors that place women at higher risk, such as certain infections, a shortened cervix, or previous preterm birth.

- **Other medical conditions** like high blood pressure, diabetes, or heart, breathing, or kidney problems can become more serious during a woman's pregnancy. Regular prenatal care can help ensure a healthier pregnancy for a woman and her baby.

What can a woman do to promote a healthy pregnancy?

Many health care providers recommend that a woman who is thinking about becoming pregnant see a health care provider to ensure she is in good preconception health.

During pregnancy, there are also steps a woman can take to reduce the risk of certain problems, such as:

- getting at least 400 micrograms of folic acid every day if she thinks she could become pregnant, and continuing folic acid when she does get pregnant;

- getting proper immunizations;

- maintaining a healthy weight and diet, getting regular physical activity, and avoiding smoking, alcohol, or drug use; and

- starting prenatal care appointments early in pregnancy.

267

Section 30.2

Teen Pregnancy

"Teen Pregnancy and Other Health Issues,"
© 2009 National Campaign to Prevent Teen and Unplanned Pregnancy
(www.thenationalcampaign.org). Reprinted with permission.

Teen pregnancy can have negative health implications for both the mother and child. Of course, the health and health-related behavior of teen mothers before, during, and after pregnancy affects the health of the baby. Evidence suggests that babies born to teen mothers are at increased risk for specific health problems compared to babies born to older mothers. In addition to these personal costs, there are considerable costs to taxpayers associated with the public health care expenses of teen childbearing. Reducing teen pregnancy will not only improve the health of teens and their future children, it will also reduce some of the costs of public health services.

- Infants born to teen mothers are at increased risk of being born prematurely and at a low birthweight. This puts newborns at greater risk for infant death, respiratory distress syndrome, bleeding in the brain, vision loss, and serious intestinal problems.[1,2]

- Teen mothers are also more likely than mothers over the age of 25 to smoke during pregnancy, and often teen mothers are not at adequate pre-pregnancy weight and/or do not gain the appropriate amount of weight while pregnant.[1]

- Compared to older pregnant women, pregnant teens are far less likely to receive timely and consistent prenatal care.[1]

- Recent research indicates that while there is little difference in their child's health status as reported by teen mothers or by older mothers, the children of teen mothers are less likely to visit a medical care provider.[3] Teen mothers are also slightly more likely than similarly situated older mothers to report that their child has a chronic health condition.[3]

- The children of teen mothers are more likely to depend on publicly provided health care than the children of older mothers. In fact, 84 percent of health care expenses for children (ages 0–1) of teen mothers aged 18–19 are provided through public programs. Three quarters of health care expenses for pre-school children of teen mothers 17 and younger are provided through public programs. This is compared to about half of the expenses for children born to mothers who were aged 20 or 21.[3]

- Despite their lower utilization of health care resources, the costs associated with providing health and medical care (primarily Medicaid and SCHIP [State Children's Health Insurance Program]) to the children of teen mothers is nearly $2 billion each year.[3]

- Furthermore, approximately 72 percent of teen births in the United States are financed by Medicaid.[4]

Early pregnancy not only has health implications for the children of young mothers, it has implications for the teens as well. Helping more teens to avoid or reduce risky sexual behavior (by either delaying sex or using contraception effectively) will help prevent teen pregnancy and sexually transmitted diseases (STDs) including HIV/AIDS (human immunodeficiency virus/acquired immunodeficiency syndrome).

- Even though young people aged 15–24 represent 25 percent of the sexually active population, they account for about half of all new cases of STDs.[5]

- The rate of reported chlamydia cases among teens age 15–19 increased 20 percent between 2000 and 2004—the second highest rate among all age groups and nearly five times the overall rate.[6]

- Although the rate of reported gonorrhea cases decreased slightly between 2000 and 2004, the rate among teens remains second only to young adults aged 20–24 years and is almost four times the overall rate.[6]

- Between 2001 and 2005, the estimated number of HIV/AIDS cases increased among teens aged 15–19. By the end of 2005, there were more than 6,300 reported AIDS cases among teens aged 13–19 in the United States.[7] In addition, in the 33 areas with confidential HIV infection reporting, an estimated 5,300 teenagers were reported to be living with HIV/AIDS in 2005.

- Approximately half of all new HIV infections occur among young people aged 15–24 annually.[8]

269

Sources

1. March of Dimes, Teenage Pregnancy, in Quick Reference and Fact Sheets. 2004.

2. Martin, J.A., Hamilton, B.E., Ventura, S.J., Menacker, F. and Kirmeyer, S., *Births: Final Data for 2004.* National Vital Statistics Reports, 2006. 55(1).

3. Hoffman, S.D., *By the Numbers: The Public Costs of Adolescent Childbearing.* 2006, The National Campaign to Prevent Teen Pregnancy Washington, DC.

4. National Campaign analysis of, *National Survey of Family Growth, 2002.* 2005, National Campaign to Prevent Teen Pregnancy: Washington, DC.

5. Weinstock, H., Berman, S., and Cates, W., Sexually Transmitted Diseases Among American Youth: Incidence and Prevalence Estimates. *Perspectives on Sexual and Reproductive Health,* 2004. 36(1): p. 6–10.

6. Centers for Disease Control and Prevention, *Sexually Transmitted Disease Surveillance, 2004.* 2005, U.S. Department of Health and Human Services: Atlanta, GA.

7. Centers for Disease Control and Prevention, *HIV/AIDS Surveillance Report,* 2005. 2006, U.S. Department of Health and Human Services, Centers for Disease Control and Prevention: Atlanta, GA.

8. Guttmacher Institute, Facts on American Teens' Sexual and Reproductive Health in *In Brief.* 2006, Guttmacher Institute: New York, NY.

Section 30.3

Pregnancy after Age 35

Today, many women are waiting until their mid-30s or later before having their first child.

Women over age 35 can have normal pregnancies and deliver healthy babies. But 35 is the age often used to measure an increased risk of problems with pregnancy.

A woman's chance of having problems during pregnancy goes up a little each year after a woman is in her early 20s. These problems usually fall into 2 categories: a decrease in fertility (a woman's ability to become pregnant) and genetic conditions that may affect the baby.

Decline in Fertility

As you get older, it is harder to become pregnant. This is because your body does not release eggs (ovulate) as often. Even though you may have regular menstrual periods, your body may not be releasing eggs every month. There is less chance that your partner's sperm will fertilize the eggs that are released. Fertilized eggs are less likely to attach to your uterus.

Some physical conditions, such as a blocked fallopian tube or endometriosis, also may decrease your chance of becoming pregnant. These problems are more common in women over age 35.

Also, if you and your partner have been together for a long time, chances are you may be having sex less often. Any of these factors may make it difficult for you to become pregnant. If you and your partner have sex without using birth control for 6 months without your getting pregnant, you should make an appointment with your doctor for a fertility test.

Genetic Conditions

The most common genetic problem in babies born to women older than 35 is Down syndrome. Down syndrome causes birth defects such as mental retardation and heart problems, among others. Children born to women of any age can have Down syndrome. But the older the mother is, the greater the risk.

Prenatal testing can detect a pregnancy with Down syndrome. Two tests—chorionic villi sampling and amniocentesis are invasive and have some risk. The most serious risk is losing the baby (miscarriage). At age 35, the risk of having a child with a birth defect is about the same as the risk from the test. For this reason, prenatal testing is routinely offered to pregnant women who are 35 or older.

Another test is the multiple marker screen. It is a simple blood test that measures the amount of a certain substance in the mother's blood. This test can tell if there is a greater risk of having a baby with Down syndrome or other birth defects like spina bifida and anencephaly. It is important to remember that these are screening tests and are not 100 percent accurate. Also, they cannot identify all birth defects or genetic conditions.

Genetic counseling can help you and your partner estimate your chances of having a child with a birth defect. If you or your partner has a family history of birth defects or genetic problems, you should have genetic counseling before you become pregnant.

Other Considerations

If you are over 35 and planning to become pregnant, you also need to consider that chronic health problems, such as diabetes or high blood pressure, often develop with age. Miscarriage and stillbirth (the birth of a baby who has died before delivery) rates also are higher in women over age 35. By staying in good physical health, you can avoid many of these possible problems.

Preparing for Pregnancy

One of the best things you and your partner can do is prepare for pregnancy, both physically and emotionally. Even though you may feel your "biological clock" speeding up, you should not become pregnant unless you and your partner are ready for the responsibilities and changes that come with having a baby.

When you and your partner decide you are ready to have a child, you should make an appointment with your doctor to discuss your pre-pregnancy care. The father-to-be may want to come to this appointment.

Early and regular care is important to having a healthy pregnancy. Your doctor may recommend that you take prenatal vitamins, especially folic acid (also known as folate), before getting pregnant to help reduce the risks of some birth defects. Always check with your doctor before you take any medicine or vitamins.

Section 30.4

Multiple Pregnancy: Twins, Triplets, and Beyond

When a woman is carrying two or more babies (fetuses), it is called a multiple pregnancy. In the past two decades, the number of multiple births in the United States has jumped dramatically. Between 1980 and 2003, the number of twin births increased by two-thirds (66 percent), and the number of higher-order multiples (triplets or more) increased four-fold, according to the National Center for Health Statistics.[1] Today, more than 3 percent of babies in this country are born in sets of two, three or more, and about 94 percent of these multiple births are twins.[1]

The rising number of multiple pregnancies is a concern because women who are expecting more than one baby are at increased risk of certain pregnancy complications, including preterm delivery (before 37 completed weeks of pregnancy). Premature babies are at risk of serious health problems during the newborn period, as well as lasting disabilities and death.

Some of the complications associated with multiple pregnancy can be minimized or prevented when they are diagnosed early. There are a number of steps a pregnant woman and her health care provider can take to help improve the chances that her babies will be born healthy.

Why are multiple pregnancies increasing?

About one-third of the increase in multiple pregnancies is due to the fact that more women over age 30 are having babies.[2] Women in this age group are more likely than younger women to conceive multiples.

The remainder of the increase is due to the use of fertility-stimulating drugs and assisted reproductive techniques (ART), such as in vitro fertilization (IVF). In IVF, eggs are removed from the mother, fertilized in a laboratory dish and then transferred to the uterus. About 45 percent of ART pregnancies result in twins and about 7 percent in triplets or more.[3]

Doctors now monitor fertility treatments carefully so that women will have fewer, but healthier, babies. This involves limiting the number of embryos transferred during IVF.

In 2004, the American Society for Reproductive Medicine and the Society for Assisted Reproductive Technology issued guidelines on the best number of embryos to transfer, depending on a woman's age and other factors.[4] For example, the guidelines recommend that doctors transfer no more than two embryos for women under age 35, and consider transferring only one embryo for women in this age group who are considered most likely to become pregnant.

Doctors monitor women taking certain fertility drugs with ultrasound. If ultrasound shows that a large number of eggs could be released during that treatment cycle, the doctor will stop the treatment. In fact, the rate of higher-order multiple births has remained stable since 1999.[1]

A woman has a higher-than-average chance of conceiving twins if she has a personal or family history of fraternal (non-identical) twins or if she is obese or tall.[2,5] African-American women are more likely to have twins than Caucasian women, and Asian women are the least likely to have twins.[5]

What is the difference between identical and fraternal twins?

Identical twins (also called monozygotic twins) occur when one fertilized egg splits and develops into two (or occasionally more) fetuses. The fetuses usually share one placenta. Identical twins have the same chromosomes, so they generally look alike and are the same sex.

Fraternal twins (also called dizygotic twins) develop when two separate eggs are fertilized by two different sperm. Each twin usually has its own placenta. Fraternal twins (like other siblings) share about 50 percent of their chromosomes, so they can be different sexes. They generally do not look any more alike than brothers or sisters born from different pregnancies. Fraternal twins are more common than identical twins.

Triplets and other higher-order multiples can result from three or more eggs being fertilized, one egg splitting twice (or more) or a combination of both. A set of higher-order multiples may contain all fraternal siblings or a combination of identical and fraternal siblings.

How are multiple pregnancies diagnosed?

Although previous generations often were surprised by the delivery of twins (or other multiples), today most parents-to-be learn the news fairly early. An ultrasound examination can detect most multiples by the beginning of the second trimester.

(Sometimes a twin pregnancy that is identified very early is later found to have only one fetus. This is called "vanishing twin syndrome," and its cause is not well understood. The surviving twin generally is not harmed.)

Other factors can alert a health care provider that a woman may be expecting twins or more. These include:

- abnormal results on a blood test done around 16 weeks of pregnancy to screen for certain birth defects;

- more than one heartbeat heard by a provider using a hand-held ultrasound device (Doppler);

- rapid weight gain during the first trimester;

- larger uterus than expected;

- severe pregnancy-related nausea and vomiting (morning sickness);

- more fetal movement than experienced by the woman in a previous singleton pregnancy.

When a health care provider suspects a multiple pregnancy, he will likely recommend an ultrasound examination to find out for sure.

What complications occur more frequently in a multiple pregnancy?

Women who are expecting more than one baby are at increased risk of a number of pregnancy complications. The more babies a woman is carrying at once, the greater her risk. Common complications include:

- **Premature birth:** More than 50 percent of twins, more than 90 percent of triplets, and virtually all quadruplets and higher

275

multiples are born preterm.[6] The length of pregnancy decreases with each additional baby. On average, most singleton pregnancies last 39 weeks; for twins, 35 weeks; for triplets, 33 weeks; and for quadruplets, 29 weeks.[5]

- **Low birthweight (LBW):** About half of twins and almost all higher order multiples are born with low birthweight (less than 5 1/2 pounds or 2,500 grams).[3] LBW can result from preterm birth and/or poor fetal growth. Both are common in multiple pregnancies. Low-birthweight babies, especially those born before about 32 weeks gestation and/or weighing less than 3 1/3 pounds (1,500 grams), are at increased risk of health problems in the newborn period as well as lasting disabilities, such as mental retardation, cerebral palsy and vision and hearing loss. While advances in health care have brightened the outlook for these tiny babies, chances remain slim that all infants in a set of sextuplets or more will survive and thrive.

- **Twin-twin transfusion syndrome:** About 20 percent of identical twins who share a placenta develop this complication.[7] It occurs when a connection between the two babies' blood vessels in the placenta results in one baby getting too much blood flow and the other too little. Until recently, severe cases often resulted in the loss of both babies. Recent studies, though, suggest that the use of amniocentesis to drain off excess fluid can save up to 64 percent of affected babies.[7] Removing the excess fluid appears to improve blood flow in the placenta and reduces the risk of preterm labor. Studies also suggest that using laser surgery to seal off the connection between the blood vessels may save a similar number of babies.[7] An advantage of laser surgery is that only one treatment is needed, while amniocentesis generally must be repeated more than once.

- **Preeclampsia:** Women expecting twins are more than twice as likely as women with a singleton pregnancy to develop this complication, characterized by high blood pressure and protein in the urine.[8] Severe cases can be dangerous for mother and baby. In some cases, the baby must be delivered early to prevent serious complications.

- **Gestational diabetes:** Women carrying multiples are at increased risk of this pregnancy-related form of diabetes (high blood sugar).[8] This condition can cause the baby to grow especially large, increasing the risk of injuries during vaginal delivery. Babies born to women with gestational diabetes also may have breathing and other problems during the newborn period.

Early diagnosis and management of these complications can help protect mother and babies.

What special care is needed in a multiple gestation?

Women who are expecting multiples generally need to visit their health care providers more frequently than women expecting one baby to help prevent, detect, and treat the complications that develop more often in a multiple pregnancy. Health care providers may recommend twice-monthly visits during the second trimester and weekly (or more frequent) visits during the third trimester.

Starting around the 20th week of pregnancy, a health care provider will monitor the pregnant woman carefully for signs of preterm labor. She may do an internal exam or recommend a vaginal ultrasound examination to see if the woman's cervix is shortening (a possible sign that labor may begin soon).

If a woman develops preterm labor, her provider may recommend bed rest in the hospital and, possibly, treatment with drugs that may postpone labor. If the provider believes the babies are likely to be born before 34 weeks gestation, she will probably recommend that the pregnant woman be treated with drugs called corticosteroids. These drugs help speed fetal lung development and reduce the likelihood and severity of breathing and other problems during the newborn period.

Even if a woman pregnant with multiples has no signs of preterm labor, her provider may recommend cutting back on activities sometime between the 20th and 24th weeks of pregnancy. She may be advised to cut back on activities even sooner and to rest several times a day if she is expecting more than two babies.

As a multiple gestation progresses, the health care provider will regularly check the pregnant woman's blood pressure for preeclampsia. The provider also may recommend regular ultrasound examinations starting around 20 weeks of pregnancy to check that all babies are growing at about the same rate.

During the third trimester, the provider may recommend tests of fetal well-being. These include the non-stress test, which measures fetal heart rate when the baby is moving, and the biophysical profile, which combines the non-stress test with a special ultrasound examination.

Should a woman expecting multiples gain extra weight?

Eating right and gaining the recommended amount of weight reduces the risk of having a premature or low-birthweight baby in singleton, as well as multiple, gestations. A healthy weight gain is especially important if a woman is pregnant with twins or more, as multiples have a higher risk of preterm birth and low birthweight than singletons.

Women who begin pregnancy at a normal weight and who are expecting one baby usually should gain 25 to 35 pounds over 9 months. Women pregnant with multiples should discuss their weight-gain goals with their health care provider. Women of normal weight who are expecting twins usually should gain 35 to 45 pounds.[9] This breaks down to about 1 pound per week in the first half of pregnancy, and a little more than a pound a week for the remainder of pregnancy. Women pregnant with triplets or more may need to gain more.

The American College of Obstetricians and Gynecologists recommends that women with multiple pregnancies consume about 500 more calories a day than usual (a total of about 2,700 calories a day).[9] Women pregnant with multiples should discuss with their health care providers the number of extra calories they should eat.

Women who are carrying more than one baby should take a prenatal vitamin that is recommended by their health care provider and that contains at least 30 milligrams of iron. Iron-deficiency anemia is common in multiple gestations, and it can increase the risk of preterm delivery.

Can a woman expecting multiples deliver vaginally?

The chance of a cesarean delivery is higher in twin than in singleton births. However, a pregnant woman has a good chance of having a normal vaginal delivery if both babies are in a head-down position and there are no other complications. When a woman is carrying three or more babies, a cesarean delivery is usually recommended because it is safer for the babies.

Does the March of Dimes support research relevant to multiple gestation?

The March of Dimes supports a number of grants aimed at improving understanding of the causes of preterm delivery. Although these studies generally focus on singleton pregnancies, the largely unknown mechanisms leading to preterm delivery of singletons and of multiples may be much the same. One grantee is studying the causes of conjoined ("Siamese") twinning, with the ultimate goal of learning how to prevent this severe complication of twinning.

For More Information

The Fetal Hope Foundation [http://www.fetalhope.org] provides support and information about twin-to-twin transfusion syndrome.

References

1. Martin, J.A., et al. Births: Final Data for 2003. National Vital Statistics Reports, volume 54, number 2, September 8, 2005.

2. Reddy, U.M., et al. Relationship of Maternal Body Mass Index and Height to Twinning. *Obstetrics and Gynecology,* volume 105, number 3, March 2005, pages 593–597.

3. Wright, V.C., et al. Assisted Reproductive Technology Surveillance—2003. *Morbidity and Mortality Weekly Report,* volume 55 (SS04), May 26, 2006.

4. Practice Committee of the Society for Assisted Reproductive Technology and the American Society for Reproductive Medicine. *Fertility and Sterility,* volume 82, number 3, September 2004, pages 773–774.

5. American Society for Reproductive Medicine. Multiple Pregnancy and Birth: Twins, Triplets, and Higher Order Multiples: A Guide for Patients. Birmingham AL, 2004, accessed 6/8/06.

6. Hoyert, D.L., et al. Annual Summary of Vital Statistics: 2004. *Pediatrics,* volume 117, number 1, January 2006, pages 168–183.

7. Fox, C., et al. Contemporary Treatments for Twin-Twin Transfusion Syndrome. *Obstetrics and Gynecology,* 2005, volume 105, number 6, pages 1469–1477.

8. American College of Obstetricians and Gynecologists (ACOG). Multiple Gestation: Complicated Twin, Triplet, and Higher-Order Multifetal Pregnancy. *ACOG Practice Bulletin*, number 56, October 2004.

9. American College of Obstetricians and Gynecologists (ACOG). *Your Pregnancy and Birth, 4th Edition.* ACOG, Washington, DC, 2004.

Chapter 31

Allergies, Asthma, and Pregnancy

Asthma is the most common potentially serious medical condition to complicate pregnancy. In fact, asthma affects approximately 8 percent of women in their childbearing years. Well-controlled asthma is not associated with significant risk to mother or fetus. Uncontrolled asthma can cause serious complications to the mother, including high blood pressure, toxemia, premature delivery and rarely death. For the baby, complications of uncontrolled asthma include increased risk of stillbirth, fetal growth retardation, premature birth, low birth weight and a low APGAR score at birth.

Asthma can be controlled by careful medical management and avoidance of known triggers, so asthma need not be a reason for avoiding pregnancy. Most measures used to control asthma are not harmful to the developing fetus and do not appear to contribute to either miscarriage or birth defects.

Although the outcome of any pregnancy can never be guaranteed, most women with asthma and allergies do well with proper medical management by physicians familiar with these disorders and the changes that occur during pregnancy.

What is asthma and what are its symptoms?

Asthma is a condition characterized by obstruction in the airways of the lungs caused by spasm of surrounding muscles, accumulation of mucus, and swelling of the airway walls due to the gathering of inflammatory cells. Unlike individuals with emphysema who have irreversible destruction of their lung cells, asthmatic patients usually have a condition that can be reversed with vigorous treatment.

Individuals with asthma most often describe what they feel in their airways as a "tightness." They also describe wheezing, shortness of breath, chest pain, and cough. Symptoms of asthma can be triggered by allergens (including pollen, mold, animals, feathers, house dust mites, and cockroaches), other environmental factors, exercise, infections, and stress.

What are the effects of pregnancy on asthma?

When women with asthma become pregnant, one-third of the patients improve, one-third worsen, and the last third remain unchanged. Although studies vary widely on the overall effect of pregnancy on asthma, several reviews find the following similar trends:

- Women with severe asthma are more likely to worsen, while those with mild asthma are more likely to improve or remain unchanged.

- The change in the course of asthma in an individual woman during pregnancy tends to be similar on successive pregnancies.

- Asthma exacerbations are most likely to appear during the weeks 24 to 36 of gestation, with only occasional patients (10 percent or fewer) becoming symptomatic during labor and delivery.

- The changes in asthma noted during pregnancy usually return to pre-pregnancy status within three months of delivery.

Pregnancy may affect asthmatic patients in several ways. Hormonal changes that occur during pregnancy may affect both the nose and sinuses, as well as the lungs. An increase in the hormone estrogen contributes to congestion of the capillaries (tiny blood vessels) in the lining of the nose, which in turn leads to a "stuffy" nose in pregnancy (especially during the third trimester). A rise in progesterone causes increased respiratory drive, and a feeling of shortness of breath may be experienced as a result of this hormonal increase. These events may be confused with or add to allergic or other triggers of asthma. Spirometry and peak flow are measurements of airflow obstruction (a marker of asthma) that help your physician determine if asthma is the cause of shortness of breath during pregnancy.

Fetal monitoring: For pregnant women with asthma, the type and frequency of fetal evaluation is based on gestational age and maternal risk factors. Ultrasound can be performed before 12 weeks if there is concern about the accuracy of an estimated due date and repeated later if a slowing of fetal growth is suspected. Electronic heart rate monitoring, called "non-stress testing" or "contraction stress testing," and ultrasonic determinations in the third trimester may be used to assess fetal well being. For third trimester patients with significant asthma symptoms, the frequency of fetal assessment should be increased if problems are suspected. Asthma patients should record fetal activity or kick counts daily to help monitor their baby according to their physician's instructions.

During a severe asthma attack in which symptoms do not quickly improve, there is risk for significant maternal hypoxemia, a low oxygen state. This is an important time for fetal assessment; continuous electronic fetal heart rate monitoring may be necessary along with measurements of the mother's lung function.

Fortunately during labor and delivery, the majority of asthma patients do well, although careful fetal monitoring remains very important. In low risk patients whose asthma is well-controlled, fetal assessment can be accomplished by 20 minutes of electronic monitoring (the admission test). Intensive fetal monitoring with careful observation is recommended for patients who enter labor and delivery with severe asthma, have a non-reassuring admission test, or other risk factors.

Avoidance and control: The connection between asthma and allergies is common. Most asthmatic patients (75 percent to 85 percent) will be allergic to one or more substances such as pollens, molds, animals, house dust mites, and cockroaches. Pet allergies are caused by protein found in animal dander, urine, and saliva. These allergens may trigger asthma symptoms or make existing symptoms worse.

Other non-allergic substances may also worsen asthma and allergies. These include tobacco smoke, paint and chemical fumes, strong odors, environmental pollutants (including ozone and smog), and drugs, such as aspirin or beta-blockers (used to treat high blood pressure, migraine headache, and heart disorders).

Avoidance of specific triggers should lessen the frequency and intensity of asthmatic and allergic symptoms. Allergist-immunologists recommend the following methods:

- Remove allergy causing pets from the house, or at the least keep them out of the bedroom at all times.

- Seal pillows, mattresses, and box springs in special dust mite-proof casings (your allergist should be able to give you information regarding comfortable cases).

- If possible, wash bedding weekly in 130-degree Fahrenheit water (comforters may be dry-cleaned periodically) to kill dust mites.

- However, keeping the hot water tank at this temperature may not be advisable if there are small children or others at risk of scalding at home.

- Keep home humidity under 50 percent to control dust mite and mold growth.

- Use filtering vacuums or "filter vacuum bags" to control airborne dust when cleaning.

- Close windows, use air conditioning, and limit outdoor activity between 5 a.m. and 10 a.m., when pollen and pollution are at their highest.

- Limit exposure to chemical fumes and, most importantly, tobacco smoke.

Can asthma medications safely be used during pregnancy?

Though no medication has been proven entirely safe for use during pregnancy, your doctor will carefully balance medication use and symptom control. Your treatment plan will be individualized so that potential benefits of medications outweigh the potential risks of these medications or of uncontrolled asthma.

Asthma is a disease in which intensity of symptoms can vary from day to day, month to month, or season to season regardless of pregnancy. Therefore, a treatment plan should be chosen based both on asthma severity and experience during pregnancy with those medications. Remember that the use of medications should not replace avoidance of allergens or irritants, as avoidance will potentially reduce medication needs.

In general, asthma medications used in pregnancy are chosen based on the following criteria:

- Inhaled medications are generally preferred because they have a more localized effect with only small amounts entering the bloodstream.

- When appropriate, time-tested older medications are preferred since there is more experience with their use during pregnancy.

- Medication use is limited in the first trimester as much as possible when the fetus is forming. Birth defects from medications are rare (no more than 1 percent of all birth defects are attributable to all medications.)

In general, the same medications used during pregnancy are appropriate during labor and delivery and when nursing.

Bronchodilator medication: Short-acting inhaled beta2-agonists, often called "asthma relievers" or "rescue medications," are used as necessary to control acute symptoms. Albuterol is the preferred short-acting inhaled beta2-agonist for use during pregnancy since there are more available reassuring human gestational safety data.

Two long-acting inhaled beta agonists, salmeterol (Serevent®) and formoterol (Foradil®), are available. No large-scale trials of these medications in pregnancy have been performed. However, because of their inhaled route, chemical relation to albuterol, and efficacy data, long-acting beta agonists are recommended during pregnancy for patients not controlled on inhaled corticosteroids.

Theophylline has extensive human experience without evidence of significant abnormalities. Newborns can have jitteriness, vomiting, and fast pulse if the maternal blood level is too high. Therefore, patients who receive theophylline should have blood levels checked during pregnancy.

Ipratropium (Atrovent®), an anticholinergic bronchodilator medication, does not cause problems in animals; however, there is no published experience in humans. Ipratropium is absorbed less than similar medications in this class, such as atropine.

Anti-inflammatory medication: The anti-inflammatory medications are preventive, or "asthma controllers," and include inhaled cromolyn (Intal®), corticosteroids, and leukotriene modifiers. Patients requiring the use of beta2-agonists more often than three times a week, or who have reduced peak flow readings or spirometry (lung function studies), usually need daily anti-inflammatory medication. Inhaled cromolyn sodium is virtually devoid of side effects but is less effective than inhaled corticosteroids.

Budesonide (Pulmicort®): Budesonide is recommended as the inhaled corticosteroid of choice for use during pregnancy due to a large amount of reassuring human gestational safety data. However, other inhaled corticosteroids (such as beclomethasone [Qvar®], fluticasone [Flovent®], flunisolide [AeroBid®], mometasone [Asmanex®], and triamcinolone [Azmacort®] have not been proven to be unsafe during pregnancy and can be continued in patients well-controlled by them prior to pregnancy.

In some cases oral or injectable corticosteroids, such as prednisone, prednisolone, or methylprednisolone may be necessary for a few days in patients with severe asthma exacerbations or throughout pregnancy in women with severe asthma. Some studies have demonstrated a slight increase in the incidence of pre-eclampsia, premature deliveries or low-birth-weight infants with chronic use of corticosteroids. However, they are the most effective drugs for the treatment of patients with more severe asthma and other allergic disorders. Therefore, their significant benefit usually far exceeds their minimal risk.

Three leukotriene modifiers, montelukast (Singulair®), zafirlukast (Accolate®), and zileuton (Zyflo®) are available. Results of animal studies are reassuring for montelukast and zafirlukast , but there are minimal data in human pregnancy with this new class of anti-inflammatory drugs.

Can allergy medications safely be used during pregnancy?

Antihistamines may be useful during pregnancy to treat the nasal and eye symptoms of seasonal or perennial allergic rhinitis, allergic conjunctivitis, the itching of urticaria (hives) or eczema, and as an adjunct to the treatment of serious allergic reactions, including anaphylaxis (allergic shock). With the exception of life-threatening anaphylaxis, the benefits from their use must be weighed against any risk to the fetus. Because symptoms may be of such severity to affect maternal eating, sleeping, or emotional well-being, and because uncontrolled rhinitis may pre-dispose to sinusitis or may worsen asthma, antihistamines may provide definite benefit during pregnancy.

Chlorpheniramine (Chlor-Trimeton®) and diphenhydramine (Benadryl®) have been used for many years during pregnancy with reassuring animal studies. Generally, chlorpheniramine would be the preferred choice, but a major drawback of these medications is drowsiness and performance impairment in some patients.. Two of the newer less sedating antihistamines—loratadine (Claritin®) and cetirizine (Zyrtec®)—have reassuring animal and human study data and are currently recommended when indicated for use during pregnancy.

The use of decongestants is more problematic. The nasal spray oxymetazoline (Afrin®, Neo-Synephrine® Long-Acting, etc.) appears to be the safest product because there is minimal, if any, absorption into the bloodstream. However, these and other over-the-counter nasal sprays can cause rebound congestion and actually worsen the condition for which they are used. Their use is generally limited to very intermittent use or regular use for only 3 consecutive days.

Although pseudoephedrine (Sudafed®) has been used for years, and studies have been reassuring, there have been recent reports of a slight increase in abdominal wall defects in newborns. Use of decongestants during the first trimester should only be entertained after consideration of the severity of maternal symptoms unrelieved by other medications. Phenylephrine and phenylpropanolamine are less desirable than pseudoephedrine based on the information available.

A corticosteroid nasal spray should be considered in any patient whose allergic nasal symptoms are more than mild and last for more than a few days. These medications prevent symptoms and lessen the need for oral medications. There are few specific data regarding the safety of intranasal corticosteroids during pregnancy. However, based on the data for the same medications used in an inhaled form (for asthma), budesonide (Rhinocort®) would be considered the intranasal corticosteroid of choice, but other intranasal corticosteroids could be continued if they were providing effective control prior to pregnancy.

Immunotherapy and influenza vaccine: Allergen immunotherapy (allergy shots) is often effective for those patients in whom symptoms persist despite optimal environmental control and proper drug therapy. Allergen immunotherapy can be carefully continued during pregnancy in patients who are benefiting and not experiencing adverse reactions. Due to the greater risk of anaphylaxis with increasing doses of immunotherapy and a delay of several months before it becomes effective, it is generally recommended that this therapy not be started during pregnancy.

Patients receiving immunotherapy during pregnancy should be carefully evaluated. It may be appropriate to lower the dosage in order to further reduce the chance of an allergic reaction to the injections.

Influenza (flu) vaccine is recommended for all patients with moderate and severe asthma. There is no evidence of associated risk to the mother or fetus.

Can asthma medications safely be used while nursing?

Nearly all medications enter breast milk, though infants are generally exposed to very low concentrations of the drugs. Hence, the medications described above rarely present problems for the infant during breastfeeding. Specifically, very little of the inhaled beta agonists, inhaled or oral steroids, and theophylline will appear in mother's milk.

Some infants can have irritability and insomnia if exposed to higher doses of medication or to theophylline. In general, the lowest drug concentration in mother's milk can be obtained by taking theophylline 15 minutes after nursing or 3 to 4 hours before the next feeding.

Summary

It is important to remember that the risks of asthma medications are lower than the risks of uncontrolled asthma, which can be harmful to both mother and child. The use of asthma or allergy medication needs to be discussed with your doctor, ideally before pregnancy. Therefore, the doctor should be notified whenever you are planning to discontinue birth control methods or as soon as you know that you are pregnant. Regular follow up for evaluation of asthma symptoms and medications is necessary throughout the pregnancy to maximize asthma control and to minimize medication risks.

This information has been prepared by members of the Pregnancy Committee of the American College of Allergy, Asthma and Immunology, an organization whose members are dedicated to providing optimal care to all patients with asthma, including those who are pregnant.

Chapter 32

Cancer and Pregnancy

Chapter Contents

Section 32.1

Breast Cancer and Pregnancy

Excerpted from "Pregnancy and Breast Cancer Risk," by
the National Cancer Institute (NCI, www.cancer.gov), part of
the National Institutes of Health, April 30, 2008.

Every woman's hormone levels change throughout her life for a variety of reasons, and hormone changes can lead to changes in the breasts. Hormone changes that occur during pregnancy may influence a woman's chances of developing breast cancer later in life. Research continues to help us understand reproductive events and breast cancer risk.

Pregnancy-Related Factors That Protect against Breast Cancer

Some factors associated with pregnancy are known to reduce a woman's chance of developing breast cancer later in life:

- The younger a woman has her first child, the lower her risk of developing breast cancer during her lifetime.

- A woman who has her first child after the age of 35 has approximately twice the risk of developing breast cancer as a woman who has a child before age 20.

- A woman who has her first child around age 30 has approximately the same lifetime risk of developing breast cancer as a woman who has never given birth.

Having more than one child decreases a woman's chances of developing breast cancer. In particular, having more than one child at a younger age decreases a woman's chances of developing breast cancer during her lifetime.

Although not fully understood, research suggests that preeclampsia, a pathologic condition that sometimes develops during pregnancy, is associated with a decrease in breast cancer risk in the offspring, and there is some evidence of a protective effect for the mother.

After pregnancy, breastfeeding for a long period of time (for example, a year or longer) further reduces breast cancer risk by a small amount.

Pregnancy-Related Factors That Increase Breast Cancer Risk

Some factors associated with pregnancy are known to increase a woman's chances of developing breast cancer:

- After a woman gives birth, her risk of breast cancer is temporarily increased. This temporary increase lasts only for a few years.

- A woman who during pregnancy took DES (diethylstilbestrol), a synthetic form of estrogen that was used between the early 1940s and 1971, has a slightly higher risk of developing breast cancer. (So far, research does not show an increased breast cancer risk for their female offspring who were exposed to DES before birth. Those women are sometimes referred to as DES daughters.)

Other Breast Cancer Risk Factors Not Related to Pregnancy

At present, other factors known to increase a woman's chance of developing breast cancer include age (a woman's chances of getting breast cancer increase as she gets older), a family history of breast cancer in a first degree relative (mother, sister, or daughter), an early age at first menstrual period (before age 12), a late age at menopause (after age 55), use of menopausal hormone replacement drugs, and certain breast conditions. Obesity is also a risk factor for breast cancer in postmenopausal women.

Misunderstandings about Breast Cancer Risk Factors

There are a number of misconceptions about what can cause breast cancer. These include, but are not limited to, using deodorants or antiperspirants, wearing an underwire bra, having a miscarriage or induced abortion, or bumping or bruising breast tissue. However, none of these factors has been shown to increase a woman's risk of breast cancer. In addition, cancer is not contagious; no one can "catch" cancer from another person.

Preventing Breast Cancer

There are some things women can do to reduce their breast cancer risk. Because some studies suggest that the more alcoholic beverages a woman drinks the greater her risk of breast cancer, it is important to limit alcohol intake. Maintaining a healthy body weight is important because being overweight increases risk of postmenopausal breast cancer. New evidence suggests that being physically active may also reduce risk. Physical activity that is sustained throughout lifetime or, at a minimum, performed after menopause, may be particularly beneficial in reducing breast cancer risk. Eating a diet high in fruits and vegetables, and energy and fat intake balanced to energy expended in exercise are useful approaches to avoiding weight gain in adult life.

Detecting Breast Cancer

A woman can be an active participant in improving her chances for early detection of breast cancer. NCI recommends that, beginning in their 40s, women have a mammogram every year or two. Women who have a higher than average risk of breast cancer (for example, women with a family history of breast cancer) should seek expert medical advice about whether they should be screened before age 40, and how frequently they should be screened.

Section 32.2

Gestational Trophoblastic Tumors

From "Gestational Trophoblastic Tumors," by the National Cancer Institute (NCI, www.cancer.gov), part of the National Institutes of Health, June 26, 2008.

Gestational trophoblastic tumor, a rare cancer in women, is a disease in which cancer (malignant) cells grow in the tissues that are formed following conception (the joining of sperm and egg).

Gestational trophoblastic tumors start inside the uterus, the hollow, muscular, pear-shaped organ where a baby grows. This type of cancer occurs in women during the years when they are able to have children. There are two types of gestational trophoblastic tumors: hydatidiform mole and choriocarcinoma.

If a patient has a hydatidiform mole (also called a molar pregnancy), the sperm and egg cells have joined without the development of a baby in the uterus. Instead, the tissue that is formed resembles grape-like cysts. Hydatidiform mole does not spread outside of the uterus to other parts of the body.

If a patient has a choriocarcinoma, the tumor may have started from a hydatidiform mole or from tissue that remains in the uterus following an abortion or delivery of a baby. Choriocarcinoma can spread from the uterus to other parts of the body. A very rare type of gestational trophoblastic tumor starts in the uterus where the placenta was attached. This type of cancer is called placental-site trophoblastic disease.

Gestational trophoblastic tumor is not always easy to find. In its early stages, it may look like a normal pregnancy. A doctor should be seen if the there is vaginal bleeding (not menstrual bleeding) and if a woman is pregnant and the baby hasn't moved at the expected time.

If there are symptoms, a doctor may use several tests to see if the patient has a gestational trophoblastic tumor. An internal (pelvic) examination is usually the first of these tests. The doctor will feel for any lumps or strange feeling in the shape or size of the uterus. The doctor may then do an ultrasound, a test that uses sound waves to find tumors. A blood test will also be done to look for high levels of a hormone called beta-hCG (beta human chorionic gonadotropin) which is present during normal pregnancy. If a woman is not pregnant and HCG is in the blood, it can be a sign of gestational trophoblastic tumor.

The chance of recovery (prognosis) and choice of treatment depend on the type of gestational trophoblastic tumor, whether it has spread to other places, and the patient's general state of health.

Chapter 33

For Women with Diabetes: Your Guide to Pregnancy

You have type 1 or type 2 diabetes and you are pregnant or hoping to get pregnant soon. You can learn what to do to have a healthy baby. You can also learn how to take care of yourself and your diabetes before, during, and after your pregnancy.

Pregnancy and new motherhood are times of great excitement, worry, and change for any woman. If you have diabetes and are pregnant, your pregnancy is automatically considered a high-risk pregnancy. Women carrying twins—or more—or who are beyond a certain age are also considered to have high-risk pregnancies. High risk doesn't mean you'll have problems. Instead, high risk means you need to pay special attention to your health and you may need to see specialized doctors. Millions of high-risk pregnancies produce perfectly healthy babies without the mom's health being affected. Special care and attention are the keys.

Taking Care of Your Baby and Yourself

Keeping your blood glucose as close to normal as possible before you get pregnant and during your pregnancy is the most important thing you can do to stay healthy and have a healthy baby. Your health care team can help you learn how to use meal planning, physical activity,

Excerpted from "For Women with Diabetes: Your Guide to Pregnancy," by the National Institute on Diabetes and Digestive and Kidney Diseases (NIDDK, www.niddk.nih.gov), February 2008.

and medications to reach your blood glucose goals. Together, you'll create a plan for taking care of yourself and your diabetes.

Pregnancy causes a number of changes in your body, so you might need to make changes in the ways you manage your diabetes. Even if you've had diabetes for years, you may need changes in your meal plan, physical activity routine, and medications. In addition, your needs might change as you get closer to your delivery date.

High blood glucose levels before and during pregnancy can:

- worsen your long-term diabetes complications, such as vision problems, heart disease, and kidney disease;

- increase the chance of problems for your baby, such as being born too early, weighing too much or too little, and having low blood glucose or other health problems at birth;

- increase the risk of your baby having birth defects;

- increase the risk of losing your baby through miscarriage or stillbirth.

However, research has shown that when women with diabetes keep blood glucose levels under control before and during pregnancy, the risk of birth defects is about the same as in babies born to women who don't have diabetes.

Glucose in a pregnant woman's blood passes through to the baby. If your blood glucose level is too high during pregnancy, so is your baby's glucose level before birth.

Your Diabetes: Before and during Your Pregnancy

As you know, in diabetes, blood glucose levels are above normal. Whether you have type 1 or type 2 diabetes, you can manage your blood glucose levels and lower the risk of health problems.

A baby's brain, heart, kidneys, and lungs form during the first 8 weeks of pregnancy. High blood glucose levels are especially harmful during this early part of pregnancy. Yet many women don't realize they're pregnant until 5 or 6 weeks after conception. Ideally, you will work with your health care provider to get your blood glucose under control before you get pregnant.

If you're already pregnant, see your health care provider as soon as possible to make a plan for taking care of yourself and your baby. Even if you learn you're pregnant later in your pregnancy, you can still do a lot for your baby's health and your own.

Planning Ahead

Before you get pregnant, talk with your health care team about your wish to have a baby. Your team can work with you to make sure your blood glucose levels are on target. If you have questions or worries, bring them up. If you're already pregnant, see your doctor right away.

Daily Blood Glucose Levels

You'll check your blood glucose levels using a blood glucose meter several times a day. Most health care providers recommend testing at least four times a day. Ask your health care provider when you should check your blood glucose levels. Generally, you should check blood glucose levels at the following times:

- fasting—when you wake up, before you eat or drink anything;

- before each meal;

- 1 hour after the start of a meal;

- 2 hours after the start of a meal;

- before bedtime;

- in the middle of the night—for example, at 2 or 3 a.m.

The daily goals recommended by the American Diabetes Association for most pregnant women are shown in Table 33.1. Write down the goals you and your health care team have chosen.

The A1C Test

Another way to see whether you're meeting your goals is to have an A1C blood test. Results of the A1C test show your average blood glucose levels during the past 2 to 3 months.

Low Blood Glucose

When you're pregnant, you're at increased risk of having low blood glucose, also called hypoglycemia. When blood glucose levels are too low, your body can't get the energy it needs. Usually hypoglycemia is mild and can easily be treated by eating or drinking something with carbohydrate. But left untreated, hypoglycemia can make you pass out.

Although hypoglycemia can happen suddenly, it can usually be treated quickly, bringing your blood glucose level back to normal. Low blood glucose can be caused by:

- meals or snacks that are too small, delayed, or skipped;
- doses of insulin that are too high;
- increased activity or exercise.

Low blood glucose also can be caused by drinking too much alcohol. However, women who are trying to get pregnant or who are already pregnant should avoid all alcoholic beverages.

Table 33.1. Blood Glucose Goals for Pregnant Women Recommended by the American Diabetes Association

When	Plasma Blood Glucose (mg/dL)
Before meals and when you wake up	80 to 110
2 hours after the start of a meal	Below 155

Source: American Diabetes Association. Preconception care of women with diabetes. *Diabetes Care.* 2004;27(Supplement 1):S76–78.

Table 33.2. Blood Glucose Goals Recommended by the American College of Obstetricians and Gynecologists

When	Plasma Blood Glucose (mg/dL)
Fasting	105 or less
Before meals	110 or less
1 hour after the start of a meal	155 or less
2 hours after the start of a meal	135 or less
During the night	Not less than 65

Source: American College of Obstetricians and Gynecologists (ACOG) Committee on Practice Bulletins. ACOG Practice Bulletin Number 60: Pregestational diabetes mellitus. *Obstetrics and Gynecology.* 2005;105(3):675–685.

Using Glucagon for Severe Low Blood Glucose

If you have severe low blood glucose and pass out, you'll need help to bring your blood glucose level back to normal. Your health care team can teach your family members and friends how to give you an injection of glucagon, a hormone that raises blood glucose levels right away.

High Blood Glucose

High blood glucose, also called hyperglycemia, can happen when you don't have enough insulin or when your body isn't able to use insulin correctly. High blood glucose can result from:

- a mismatch between food and medication;
- eating more food than usual;
- being less active than usual;
- illness;
- stress.

In addition, if your blood glucose level is already high, physical activity can make it go even higher. Symptoms of high blood glucose include:

- frequent urination;
- thirst;
- weight loss.

Talk with your health care provider about what to do when your blood glucose is too high—whether it happens once in a while or at the same time every day for several days in a row. Your provider might suggest a change in your insulin, meal plan, or physical activity routine.

Ketone Levels

When your blood glucose is too high or if you're not eating enough, your body might make chemicals called ketones. Ketones are produced when your body doesn't have enough insulin and glucose can't be used for energy. Then the body uses fat instead of glucose for energy. Burning fat instead of glucose can be harmful to your health and your baby's health. Harmful ketones can pass from you to your baby. Your health care provider can teach you how and when to test your urine or blood for ketones.

If ketones build up in your body, you can develop a condition called ketosis. Ketosis can quickly turn into diabetic ketoacidosis, which can be very dangerous. Symptoms of ketoacidosis are:

- stomach pain;
- frequent urination or frequent thirst, for a day or more;
- fatigue;
- nausea and vomiting;
- muscle stiffness or aching;
- feeling dazed or in shock;
- rapid deep breathing;
- breath that smells fruity.

Checking Your Urine or Blood Ketone Levels

Your health care provider might recommend you test your urine or blood daily for ketones and also when your blood glucose is high, such as higher than 200 mg/dL.

You can prevent serious health problems by checking for ketones as recommended. Ask your health care team about when to check for ketones and what to do if you have them.

If you use an insulin infusion pump, your health care provider might also recommend that you test for ketones when your blood glucose level is unexpectedly high.

Your health care provider might teach you how to make changes in the amount of insulin you take or when you take it. Or your provider may prefer that you call for advice when you have ketones.

Checkups

Pregnancy can make some diabetes-related health problems worse. Your health care provider can talk with you about how pregnancy might affect any problems you had since before pregnancy. If you plan your pregnancy enough in advance, you may want to work with your health care provider to arrange for treatments, such as laser treatment for eye problems, before you get pregnant. Your diabetes-related health conditions can also affect your pregnancy.

Have a complete checkup before you get pregnant or at the start of your pregnancy. Your doctor should check for:

- high blood pressure, also called hypertension;
- eye disease, also called diabetic retinopathy;
- heart and blood vessel disease, also called cardiovascular disease;
- nerve damage, also called diabetic neuropathy;
- kidney disease, also called diabetic nephropathy;
- thyroid disease.

You'll also get regular checkups throughout your pregnancy to check your blood pressure and average blood glucose levels and to monitor the protein in your urine.

Medications for Diabetes

During pregnancy, the safest diabetes medication is insulin. Your health care team will work with you to make a personalized plan for your insulin routine. If you've been taking diabetes pills to control your blood glucose levels, you'll need to stop taking them. Researchers have not yet determined whether diabetes pills are safe for use throughout pregnancy. Instead, your health care team will show you how to take insulin.

If you're already taking insulin, you might need a change in the kind, the amount, and how or when you take it. The amount of insulin you take is likely to increase as you go through pregnancy because your body becomes less able to respond to the action of insulin, a condition called insulin resistance. Your insulin needs may double or even triple as you get closer to your delivery date. Insulin can be taken in several ways. Your health care team can help you decide which way is best for you.

301

Chapter 34

Epilepsy and Pregnancy

What Is Epilepsy?

Epilepsy is a brain disorder in which clusters of nerve cells, or neurons, in the brain sometimes signal abnormally. Neurons normally generate electrochemical impulses that act on other neurons, glands, and muscles to produce human thoughts, feelings, and actions. In epilepsy, the normal pattern of neuronal activity becomes disturbed, causing strange sensations, emotions, and behavior, or sometimes convulsions, muscle spasms, and loss of consciousness. During a seizure, neurons may fire as many as 500 times a second, much faster than normal. In some people, this happens only occasionally; for others, it may happen up to hundreds of times a day.

More than 2 million people in the United States—about 1 in 100— have experienced an unprovoked seizure or been diagnosed with epilepsy. For about 80 percent of those diagnosed with epilepsy, seizures can be controlled with modern medicines and surgical techniques. However, about 25 to 30 percent of people with epilepsy will continue to experience seizures even with the best available treatment. Doctors call this situation intractable epilepsy. Having a seizure does not necessarily mean that a person has epilepsy. Only when a person has had two or more seizures is he or she considered to have epilepsy.

From "Seizures and Epilepsy: Hope Through Research," by the National Institute of Neurological Disorders and Stroke (NINDS, www.ninds.nih.gov), part of the National Institutes of Health, March 23, 2009.

Epilepsy is not contagious and is not caused by mental illness or mental retardation. Some people with mental retardation may experience seizures, but seizures do not necessarily mean the person has or will develop mental impairment. Many people with epilepsy have normal or above-average intelligence.

Seizures sometimes do cause brain damage, particularly if they are severe. However, most seizures do not seem to have a detrimental effect on the brain. Any changes that do occur are usually subtle, and it is often unclear whether these changes are caused by the seizures themselves or by the underlying problem that caused the seizures.

While epilepsy cannot currently be cured, for some people it does eventually go away. One study found that children with idiopathic epilepsy, or epilepsy with an unknown cause, had a 68 to 92 percent chance of becoming seizure-free by 20 years after their diagnosis. The odds of becoming seizure-free are not as good for adults or for children with severe epilepsy syndromes, but it is nonetheless possible that seizures may decrease or even stop over time. This is more likely if the epilepsy has been well-controlled by medication or if the person has had epilepsy surgery.

Eclampsia

Eclampsia is a life-threatening condition that can develop in pregnant women. Its symptoms include sudden elevations of blood pressure and seizures. Pregnant women who develop unexpected seizures should be rushed to a hospital immediately. Eclampsia can be treated in a hospital setting and usually does not result in additional seizures or epilepsy once the pregnancy is over.

Pregnancy and Motherhood

Women with epilepsy are often concerned about whether they can become pregnant and have a healthy child. This is usually possible. While some seizure medications and some types of epilepsy may reduce a person's interest in sexual activity, most people with epilepsy can become pregnant. Moreover, women with epilepsy have a 90 percent or better chance of having a normal, healthy baby, and the risk of birth defects is only about 4 to 6 percent. The risk that children of parents with epilepsy will develop epilepsy themselves is only about 5 percent unless the parent has a clearly hereditary form of the disorder.

Parents who are worried that their epilepsy may be hereditary may wish to consult a genetic counselor to determine what the risk might be. Amniocentesis and high-level ultrasound can be performed during pregnancy to ensure that the baby is developing normally, and a procedure called a maternal serum alpha-fetoprotein test can be used for prenatal diagnosis of many conditions if a problem is suspected.

There are several precautions women can take before and during pregnancy to reduce the risks associated with pregnancy and delivery. Women who are thinking about becoming pregnant should talk with their doctors to learn any special risks associated with their epilepsy and the medications they may be taking.

Some seizure medications, particularly valproate, trimethadione, and phenytoin, are known to increase the risk of having a child with birth defects such as cleft palate, heart problems, or finger and toe defects. For this reason, a woman's doctor may advise switching to other medications during pregnancy.

Whenever possible, a woman should allow her doctor enough time to properly change medications, including phasing in the new medications and checking to determine when blood levels are stabilized, before she tries to become pregnant. Women should also begin prenatal vitamin supplements—especially with folic acid, which may reduce the risk of some birth defects—well before pregnancy.

Women who discover that they are pregnant but have not already spoken with their doctor about ways to reduce the risks should do so as soon as possible. However, they should continue taking seizure medication as prescribed until that time to avoid preventable seizures. Seizures during pregnancy can harm the developing baby or lead to miscarriage, particularly if the seizures are severe. Nevertheless, many women who have seizures during pregnancy have normal, healthy babies.

Women with epilepsy sometimes experience a change in their seizure frequency during pregnancy, even if they do not change medications. About 25 to 40 percent of women have an increase in their seizure frequency while they are pregnant, while other women may have fewer seizures during pregnancy. The frequency of seizures during pregnancy may be influenced by a variety of factors, including the woman's increased blood volume during pregnancy, which can dilute the effect of medication. Women should have their blood levels of seizure medications monitored closely during and after pregnancy, and the medication dosage should be adjusted accordingly.

Pregnant women with epilepsy should take prenatal vitamins and get plenty of sleep to avoid seizures caused by sleep deprivation. They also should take vitamin K supplements after 34 weeks of pregnancy to reduce the risk of a blood-clotting disorder in infants called neonatal coagulopathy that can result from fetal exposure to epilepsy medications. Finally, they should get good prenatal care, avoid tobacco, caffeine, alcohol, and illegal drugs, and try to avoid stress.

Labor and delivery usually proceed normally for women with epilepsy, although there is a slightly increased risk of hemorrhage, eclampsia, premature labor, and cesarean section. Doctors can administer antiepileptic drugs intravenously and monitor blood levels of anticonvulsant medication during labor to reduce the risk that the labor will trigger a seizure. Babies sometimes have symptoms of withdrawal from the mother's seizure medication after they are born, but these problems wear off in a few weeks or months and usually do not cause serious or long-term effects. A mother's blood levels of anticonvulsant medication should be checked frequently after delivery as medication often needs to be decreased.

Epilepsy medications need not influence a woman's decision about breast-feeding her baby. Only minor amounts of epilepsy medications are secreted in breast milk, usually not enough to harm the baby and much less than the baby was exposed to in the womb. On rare occasions, the baby may become excessively drowsy or feed poorly, and these problems should be closely monitored. However, experts believe the benefits of breast-feeding outweigh the risks except in rare circumstances.

Women with epilepsy should be aware that some epilepsy medications can interfere with the effectiveness of oral contraceptives. Women who wish to use oral contraceptives to prevent pregnancy should discuss this with their doctors, who may be able to prescribe a different kind of antiepileptic medication or suggest other ways of avoiding an unplanned pregnancy.

Chapter 35

Lupus and Pregnancy

Twenty years ago, medical textbooks said that women with lupus should not get pregnant because of the risks to both the mother and unborn child. Today, most women with lupus can safely become pregnant. With proper medical care, you can decrease the risks associated with pregnancy and deliver a normal, healthy baby.

To increase the chances of a happy outcome, however, you must carefully plan your pregnancy. Your disease should be under control or in remission before conception takes place. Getting pregnant when your disease is active could result in a miscarriage, a stillbirth, or serious complications for you. It is extremely important that your pregnancy be monitored by an obstetrician who is experienced in managing high-risk pregnancies and who can work closely with your primary doctor. Delivery should be planned at a hospital that can manage a high-risk patient and provide the specialized care you and your baby will need. Be aware that a vaginal birth may not be possible. Very premature babies, babies showing signs of stress, and babies of mothers who are very ill will probably be delivered by cesarean section.

One problem that can affect a pregnant woman is the development of a lupus flare. In general, flares are not caused by pregnancy. Flares that do develop often occur during the first or second trimester or

Excerpted from *Lupus: A Patient Care Guide for Nurses and Other Health Professionals, 3rd Edition*, National Institute of Arthritis and Musculoskeletal and Skin Diseases. NIH Publication No. 06-4262, September 2006.

during the first few months following delivery. Most flares are mild and easily treated with small doses of corticosteroids.

Another complication is pregnancy-induced hypertension. If you develop this serious condition, you will experience a sudden increase in blood pressure, protein in the urine, or both. Pregnancy-induced hypertension is a serious condition that requires immediate treatment, usually including delivery of the infant.

The most important question asked by pregnant women with lupus is, "Will my baby be okay?" In most cases, the answer is yes. Babies born to women with lupus have no greater chance of birth defects or mental retardation than do babies born to women without lupus. As your pregnancy progresses, the doctor will regularly check the baby's heartbeat and growth with sonograms. About 10 percent of lupus pregnancies end in unexpected miscarriages or stillbirths. Another 30 percent may result in premature birth of the infant. Although prematurity presents a danger to the baby, most problems can be successfully treated in a hospital that specializes in caring for premature newborns.

About 3 percent of babies born to mothers with lupus will have neonatal lupus. This lupus consists of a temporary rash and abnormal blood counts. Neonatal lupus usually disappears by the time the infant is 3 to 6 months old and does not recur. About one-half of babies with neonatal lupus are born with a heart condition called heart block. This condition is permanent, but it can be treated with a pacemaker.

Caring for Yourself

- Keep all of your appointments with your primary doctor and your obstetrician.

- Get enough rest. Plan for a good night's sleep and rest periods throughout the day.

- Eat a sensible, well-balanced diet. Avoid excessive weight gain. Have your obstetrician refer you to a registered dietitian if necessary.

- Take your medications as prescribed. Your doctor may have you stop some medications and start or continue others.

- Don't smoke, and don't drink alcoholic beverages.

- Be sure your doctor or nurse reviews with you the normal body changes that occur during pregnancy. Some of these changes may be similar to those that occur with a lupus flare. Although it is up to the doctor to determine whether the changes are normal or represent the development of a flare, you must be familiar with them so that you can report them as soon as they occur.

- If you are not sure about a problem or begin to notice a change in the way you feel, talk to your doctor right away.

- Ask your doctor or nurse about participating in childbirth preparation and parenting classes. Although you have lupus, you have the same needs as any other new mother-to-be.

Planning Your Pregnancy

You and your spouse or partner should talk to your doctor about the possibility of pregnancy. You and the doctor should be satisfied that your lupus condition is under good control or in remission. Your doctor should also review potential problems or complications that could arise during the pregnancy, their treatment, and outcomes for both you and the unborn child.

You should select an obstetrician who has experience in managing high-risk pregnancies. Additional experience in managing women with lupus is also good. The obstetrician should be associated with a hospital that specializes in high-risk deliveries and has the facilities to care for newborns with special needs. It is a good idea to meet with the obstetrician before you become pregnant so that he or she has an opportunity to evaluate your overall condition before conception. This meeting also will give you the opportunity to decide if this obstetrician is right for you.

Check your health insurance plan. Make sure that it covers your health care needs and those of the baby and any problems that may arise.

Review your work and activities schedule. Be prepared to make changes if you are not feeling well or need more rest.

Consider your financial status. If you work outside the home, your pregnancy and motherhood could affect your ability to work.

Develop a plan for help at home during the pregnancy and after the baby is born. Motherhood can be overwhelming and tiring, and even more so for a woman with lupus. Although most women with lupus do well, some may become ill and find it difficult to care for their child.

Chapter 36

Sickle Cell Disease and Pregnancy

Impact of Hydroxyurea on Pregnancy

Women and men who are taking hydroxyurea should use contraceptive methods and discontinue the drug if they plan to conceive a child, since hydroxyurea has been shown to be teratogenic in animal models. However, it remains unclear whether the drug causes birth defects in humans. Approximately 55 cases of hydroxyurea use during pregnancy have been reported. Based on these cases, the risk of birth defects appears to be much lower than animal studies have suggested. A 2007 expert panel concluded that hydroxyurea probably does not cause short-term negative effects on offspring, but that there is not enough data to completely exclude risk.

Management of Pregnancy

Prenatal Care

The prenatal assessment visit serves to provide counseling and outline continued care for the duration of the pregnancy. The primary focus is to identify maternal risks for low birth weight, preterm delivery, and genetic risks for fetal abnormalities. At this time, the physician

Excerpted from "The Management of Sickle Cell Disease," a publication by the Centers for Disease Control and Prevent (CDC, www.cdc.gov), and the National Heart, Lung and Blood Institute (NHLBI, www.nhlbi.nih.gov), June 2002. Revised by David A. Cooke, MD, FACP, April 29, 2009.

reviews and discusses the behavior and social patterns that place the patient at risk for sexually transmitted diseases, illicit drug use, alcohol and tobacco use, and physical abuse.

A history of previous cesarean section and uterine curettage should be obtained at prenatal evaluation because of the correlation of the occurrence of placenta previa in patients with previous uterine surgery. Adequate nutritional assessment and the avoidance of precipitating factors that cause painful events should be outlined with this initial visit as well as all subsequent visits. The patient's prepregnant weight, height, and optimal weight gain in pregnancy will be recorded. Physical exam should also include determination of splenic size.

Initial comprehensive laboratory studies include complete blood count with a reticulocyte index, hemoglobin electrophoresis, serum iron, total iron binding capacity (TIBC), ferritin levels, liver function tests, urine examination and culture, electrolytes, blood urea nitrogen (BUN), creatinine, blood type and group, red cell antibody screen, and measurement of antibodies to hepatitis A, B, and C, as well as to HIV [human immunodeficiency virus]. Rubella antibody titre, tuberculin skin test, Pap smear, cervical smear, and gonococcus culture and screening for other sexually transmitted diseases, and bacterial vaginosis also should be performed.

Hepatitis vaccine should be administered when appropriate for patients who are negative for hepatitis B. If asymptomatic bacteriuria is found, the patient should receive antibiotics in order to prevent urinary tract infection and pyelonephritis.

Return visits are recommended 2 weeks after the initial visit. Low-risk patients are scheduled for monthly visits until the second trimester, when they should be seen every two weeks; in the third trimester, they should be seen every week.

Recognition of Pregnancy-Induced Hypertension and Diabetes

For women with SCD, preeclampsia and severe anemia have been identified as risk factors for delivering infants that are small for their gestational age. The incidence of preeclampsia (defined as blood pressure >140/90 mmHg, proteinuria of >300 mg/2 hours, and pathologic edema), and eclampsia (seizures in addition to features of preeclampsia) in pregnant women with SCD was 15 percent. The mechanisms for the high incidence of hypertension in this patient population remain unclear; multiple factors such as placental ischemia and endothelial injury have been implicated. Other known risk factors for

312

preeclampsia, even in women without SCD, are nulliparity, a history of renal disease or hypertension, multiple gestation, and diabetes.

Pregnant women with SCD should be observed closely if blood pressure rises above 125/75 mmHg, if the systolic blood pressure increases by 30 mmHg, or diastolic blood pressure increases by 15 mmHg, in association with edema and proteinuria in the second trimester. Preeclampsia, which requires frequent monitoring, can be treated with bed rest at home or in the hospital, if needed.

If preeclampsia is worsening, delivery of the fetus may be required if the gestational age is greater than 32 weeks. Expedited delivery is recommended for uncontrolled hypertension.

Labor, Delivery, Postpartum Care, and Counseling

Cardiac function can be compromised because of chronic hypoxemia and anemia. During labor, fetal monitoring is useful to detect fetal distress, which can trigger prompt delivery by cesarean section. If surgery appears imminent, simple transfusion or rapid exchange transfusion can be of benefit depending on the baseline hemoglobin levels. The postpartum patient may require transfusion if she has undergone extensive blood loss during parturition.

Venous thromboembolism can also complicate the postpartum course. To prevent this, early ambulation is initiated.

Counseling is also an important component of postpartum care. Results of the screen for SCD in the infant should be made available to the mother and father, as well as to the pediatrician.

Contraception and plans for future pregnancies also should be discussed. If a woman is considering no future pregnancies, she can receive preliminary counseling about tubal ligation for permanent birth control.

Chapter 37

Thyroid Disease and Pregnancy

What is thyroid disease?

The thyroid gland's production of thyroid hormones (T3 and T4) is triggered by thyroid-stimulating hormone (TSH), which is made by the pituitary gland. Thyroid disease is a disorder that results when the thyroid gland produces more or less thyroid hormone than the body needs. Too much thyroid hormone is called hyperthyroidism and can cause many of the body's functions to speed up. Too little thyroid hormone is called hypothyroidism, in which many of the body's functions slow down.

How does pregnancy normally affect thyroid function?

Two pregnancy-related hormones—human chorionic gonadotropin (hCG) and estrogen—cause increased thyroid hormone levels in the blood. Made by the placenta, hCG is similar to TSH and mildly stimulates the thyroid to produce more thyroid hormone. Increased estrogen produces higher levels of thyroid-binding globulin, a protein that transports thyroid hormone in the blood. These normal hormonal changes can sometimes make thyroid function tests during pregnancy difficult to interpret.

Excerpted from "Pregnancy and Thyroid Disease," by the National Institute of Diabetes and Digestive and Kidney Diseases (NIDDK, www.niddk.nih.gov), part of the National Institutes of Health, June 2008.

Thyroid hormone is critical to normal development of the baby's brain and nervous system. During the first trimester, the fetus depends on the mother's supply of thyroid hormone, which it gets through the placenta. At 10 to 12 weeks, the baby's thyroid begins to function on its own. The baby gets its supply of iodine, which the thyroid gland uses to make thyroid hormone, through the mother's diet.

Women need more iodine when they are pregnant—about 250 micrograms (µg) a day. In the United States, about 7 percent of pregnant women may not get enough iodine in their diet or through prenatal vitamins. Choosing iodized salt—salt supplemented with iodine—over plain salt is one way to ensure adequate intake.

The thyroid gland enlarges slightly in healthy women during pregnancy, but not enough to be detected by a physical exam. A noticeably enlarged gland can be a sign of thyroid disease and should be evaluated. Higher levels of thyroid hormone in the blood, increased thyroid size, and other symptoms common to both pregnancy and thyroid disorders—such as fatigue—can make thyroid problems hard to diagnose in pregnancy.

What causes hyperthyroidism in pregnancy?

Hyperthyroidism in pregnancy is usually caused by Graves disease and occurs in about one of every 500 pregnancies. Graves disease is an autoimmune disorder, which means the body's immune system makes antibodies that act against its own healthy cells and tissues.

In Graves disease, the immune system makes an antibody called thyroid stimulating immunoglobulin, sometimes called TSH receptor antibody, which mimics TSH and causes the thyroid to make too much thyroid hormone. Although Graves disease may first appear during pregnancy, a woman with preexisting Graves disease could actually see an improvement in her symptoms in her second and third trimesters. Remission of Graves disease in later pregnancy may result from the general suppression of the immune system that occurs during pregnancy. The disease usually worsens again in the first few months after delivery.

Rarely, hyperthyroidism in pregnancy is caused by hyperemesis gravidarum—severe nausea and vomiting that can lead to weight loss and dehydration. This extreme nausea and vomiting is believed to be triggered by high levels of hCG, which can also lead to temporary hyperthyroidism that usually resolves by the second half of pregnancy.

316

How does hyperthyroidism affect the mother and baby?

Uncontrolled hyperthyroidism during pregnancy can lead to:

- congestive heart failure;
- preeclampsia—a dangerous rise in blood pressure in late pregnancy;
- thyroid storm—a sudden, severe worsening of symptoms;
- miscarriage;
- premature birth; and
- low birthweight.

If a woman has Graves disease or was treated for Graves disease in the past, the thyroid-stimulating antibodies she produces may travel across the placenta to the baby's bloodstream and stimulate the fetal thyroid. If the mother is being treated with antithyroid drugs, hyperthyroidism in the baby is less likely because these drugs also cross the placenta. But if she was treated for Graves disease with surgery or radioactive iodine, both of which destroy all or part of the thyroid, she can still have antibodies in her blood even though her thyroid levels are normal. Women who received either of these treatments for Graves disease should inform their doctor so the baby can be monitored for thyroid-related problems later in the pregnancy.

Hyperthyroidism in a newborn can result in rapid heart rate that can lead to heart failure, poor weight gain, irritability, and sometimes an enlarged thyroid that can press against the windpipe and interfere with breathing. Women with Graves disease and their newborns should be closely monitored by their health care team.

What causes hypothyroidism in pregnancy?

Hypothyroidism in pregnancy is usually caused by Hashimoto disease and occurs in one to three of every 1,000 pregnancies. Like Graves disease, Hashimoto disease is an autoimmune disorder. In Hashimoto disease, the immune system makes antibodies that attack cells in the thyroid and interfere with their ability to produce thyroid hormones. White blood cells also invade the thyroid and decrease thyroid hormone production.

Hypothyroidism in pregnancy can also result from existing hypothyroidism that is inadequately treated or from prior destruction or removal of the thyroid as a treatment for hyperthyroidism.

317

How does hypothyroidism affect the mother and baby?

Some of the same problems caused by hyperthyroidism can occur in hypothyroidism. Uncontrolled hypothyroidism during pregnancy can lead to:

- congestive heart failure;
- preeclampsia;
- anemia—a disorder in which the blood does not carry enough oxygen to the body's tissues;
- miscarriage;
- low birthweight; and
- stillbirth.

Because thyroid hormones are crucial to fetal brain and nervous system development, uncontrolled hypothyroidism—especially during the first trimester—can lead to cognitive and developmental disabilities in the baby.

Chapter 38

Eating Disorders during Pregnancy

Chapter Contents

Section 38.1

How Do Eating Disorders Impact Pregnancy?

"Eating Disorders during Pregnancy," © 2008 American Pregnancy
Association (www.americanpregnancy.org). Reprinted with permission.

Eating disorders affect approximately seven million American women each year and tend to peak during child-bearing years. Pregnancy is a time when body image concerns are more prevalent, and for those who are struggling with an eating disorder, the nine months of pregnancy can cause disorders to worsen.

Two of the most common types of eating disorders are anorexia and bulimia. Anorexia involves obsessive dieting or starvation to control weight gain. Bulimia involves binge eating and vomiting or using laxatives to rid the body of excess calories. Both types of eating disorders may negatively affect the reproductive process and pregnancy.

How Do Eating Disorders Affect Fertility?

Eating disorders, particularly anorexia, affect fertility by reducing your chances of conceiving. Most women with anorexia do not have menstrual cycles, and approximately 50% of women struggling with bulimia do not have normal menstrual cycles. The absence of menstruation is caused by reduced calorie intake, excessive exercise, and/or psychological stress. If a woman is not having regular periods, getting pregnant can be difficult.

How Do Eating Disorders Affect Pregnancy?

Eating disorders affect pregnancy negatively in a number of ways. The following complications are associated with eating disorders during pregnancy:

- premature labor;
- low birth weight;

- stillbirth or fetal death;
- likelihood of cesarean birth;
- delayed fetal growth;
- respiratory problems;
- gestational diabetes;
- complications during labor;
- depression;
- miscarriage;
- preeclampsia.

Women who are struggling with bulimia will often gain excess weight, which places them at risk for hypertension. Women with eating disorders have higher rates of postpartum depression and are more likely to have problems with breastfeeding.

The laxatives, diuretics, and other medications taken may be harmful to the developing baby. These substances take away nutrients and fluids before they are able to feed and nourish the baby. It is possible they may lead to fetal abnormalities as well, particularly if they are used on a regular basis.

Reproductive Recommendations for Women with Eating Disorders

If you are struggling with an eating disorder, you have an increased risk of complications, and it is recommended that you try to resolve weight and behavior problems. The good news is that the majority of women with eating disorders can have healthy babies. Also, if you gain normal weight throughout your pregnancy, there should be no greater risk of complications.

Here are some suggested guidelines for women with eating disorders who are trying to conceive or have discovered that they are pregnant.

Prior to Pregnancy

- Achieve and maintain a healthy weight.
- Avoid purging.
- Consult your health care provider for a pre-conception appointment.

- Meet with a nutritionist and start a healthy pregnancy diet, which may include prenatal vitamins.

- Seek counseling to address your eating disorder and any underlying concerns; seek both individual and group therapy.

During Pregnancy

- Schedule a prenatal visit early in your pregnancy and inform your health care provider that you have been struggling with an eating disorder.

- Strive for healthy weight gain.

- Eat well-balanced meals with all the appropriate nutrients.

- Find a nutritionist who can help you with healthy and appropriate eating.

- Avoid purging.

- Seek counseling to address your eating disorder and any underlying concerns; seek both individual and group therapy.

After Pregnancy

- Continue counseling to improve physical and mental health.

- Inform your safe network (health care provider, spouse, and friends) of your eating disorder and the increased risk of postpartum depression; ask them to be available after the birth.

- Contact a lactation consultant to help with early breastfeeding.

- Find a nutritionist who can help work with you to stay healthy, manage your weight, and invest in your baby.

Section 38.2

Pica

Definition

Pica is a pattern of eating non-food materials (such as dirt or paper).

Causes

Pica is seen more in young children than adults. Between 10 and 32% of children ages 1–6 have these behaviors.

Pica can occur during pregnancy. In some cases, a lack of certain nutrients, such as iron deficiency anemia and zinc deficiency, may trigger the unusual cravings. Pica may also occur in adults who crave a certain texture in their mouth.

Symptoms

Children and adults with pica may eat:

- animal feces;
- clay;
- dirt;
- hairballs;
- ice;
- paint;
- sand.

This pattern of eating should last at least 1 month to fit the diagnosis of pica.

Exams and Tests

There is no single test that confirms pica. However, because pica can occur in people who have lower-than-normal nutrient levels and poor nutrition (malnutrition), the health care provider should test blood levels of iron and zinc.

Hemoglobin can also be checked to test for anemia. Lead levels should always be checked in children who may have eaten paint or objects covered in lead-paint dust. The health care provider should test for infection if the person has been eating contaminated soil or animal waste.

Treatment

Treatment should first address any missing nutrients and other medical problems, such as lead exposure.

Treatment involves behavior and development, environmental, and family education approaches. Other successful treatments include associating the pica behavior with bad consequences or punishment (mild aversion therapy) followed by positive reinforcement for eating the right foods.

Medications may help reduce the abnormal eating behavior, if pica occurs as part of a developmental disorder such as mental retardation.

Outlook (Prognosis)

Treatment success varies. In many cases, the disorder lasts several months, then disappears on its own. In some cases, it may continue into the teen years or adulthood, especially when it occurs with developmental disorders.

Possible Complications

- bezoar
- infection
- intestinal obstruction
- lead poisoning
- malnutrition

When to Contact a Medical Professional

Call your health care provider if you notice that a child (or adult) often eats non-food materials.

Prevention

There is no specific prevention. Getting enough nutrition may help.

Chapter 39

Overweight, Obesity, and Pregnancy

Chapter Contents

Section 39.1

Pregnancy and the Overweight Woman

If a woman is overweight or obese before pregnancy, she faces special health risks. But she can take steps to protect her own health and the health of her baby. To find out if you are overweight or obese, you'll need to know your height and weight. You then can calculate your body mass index (BMI). BMI helps to determine if your weight is appropriate for your height.

Health Risks during Pregnancy for Overweight and Obese Women

Women who have a high BMI are more likely to have high blood pressure and diabetes during pregnancy. They are also more likely to have problems in childbirth. Their babies may also have serious health problems.

Gestational hypertension (high blood pressure): Gestational hypertension happens when a pregnant woman has a sudden rise in blood pressure during the second half of her pregnancy. Health care providers can find this condition during regular blood pressure checks.

If a pregnant woman has high blood pressure, she may need medicine and more frequent checkups in the weeks before delivery. Gestational hypertension usually goes away after the baby is born. High blood pressure during pregnancy can be a sign of preeclampsia.

Preeclampsia and eclampsia: Preeclampsia is a potentially serious illness marked by high blood pressure and protein in the urine. If untreated, it can become a rare, life-threatening condition called eclampsia. Eclampsia can cause seizures and, in some cases, coma. Fortunately, eclampsia is rare in women who receive regular prenatal care.

After delivery, a woman with preeclampsia may need to stay in the hospital longer than usual. This is done for the safety of both her and her baby.

Pregnant women should be on the lookout for these warning signs:

- Headaches
- Vision trouble
- Quick weight gain
- Swelling of the hands and face
- Pain in the right upper belly

Gestational diabetes: Gestational diabetes occurs when a pregnant woman's system has trouble controlling the level of glucose (sugar) in her body. Glucose is the body's main source of fuel. If your glucose levels are too high, serious health problems can arise for you and your baby.

Out of every 100 pregnant women, 3 to 5 develop gestational diabetes. While gestational diabetes usually goes away once the baby is born, over half of the women develop diabetes later in life.

Childbirth

An overweight woman is at increased risk of having problems during and after childbirth. The higher her BMI, the more likely she may need a cesarean delivery, which is major surgery. Compared to other pregnant women, very overweight women may have more trouble recovering from a c-section. Also, they may need to stay in the hospital longer.

Babies Born to Overweight and Obese Mothers

Babies born to overweight and obese mothers may face their own challenges. These newborns are at increased risk of:

- Being born prematurely;
- Having certain birth defects;
- Needing special care in a neonatal intensive care unit (NICU);
- Being obese in childhood.

What You Can Do

Before pregnancy: To help avoid these health problems, have regular medical checkups before getting pregnant. If you're overweight or obese, your health care provider or a registered dietitian can help you lose pounds so that you reach a healthier weight before trying to get pregnant. They will talk with you about exercise and eating healthy.

Check out MyPyramid, an online tool from the U.S. Department of Agriculture. It can help you plan a healthy diet based on your age, weight, height and physical activity.

During pregnancy: If you are overweight at the start of pregnancy, do not start dieting. Fad diets can reduce the nutrients your baby needs for his growth and health. Generally, overweight women should gain between 15–25 pounds during pregnancy.

Remember: Every woman's body is unique. Always talk to your health care provider about the healthiest steps for you and your baby.

Section 39.2

Obesity before Pregnancy Linked to Childhood Weight Problems

Excerpted from "Obesity Before Pregnancy Linked to Childhood Weight Problems," by the National Institutes of Health, December 5, 2005.

A study shows that a child's weight may be influenced by the mother even before the child is actually born. The study, conducted by researchers from Ohio State University (OSU) College of Nursing and School of Public Health, appears in the December 5, 2005 issue of the journal *Pediatrics* and was supported by the National Institute of Nursing Research (NINR), one of the National Institutes of Health (NIH).

The study showed that a child is more likely to be overweight at a very young age—at 2 or 3 years old—if the mother was overweight or obese before she became pregnant. The data also indicate that other prenatal characteristics, particularly race, ethnicity, and maternal smoking during pregnancy, place a child at greater risk of becoming overweight. Specifically, a child is at greater risk of becoming overweight if born to a black or Hispanic mother, or to a mother who smoked during her pregnancy, according to the study.

Pamela Salsberry, PhD, the study's lead author and an associate professor at OSU, noted that "there's a good chance that an overweight child will stay overweight for the rest of his or her life." "A child who is overweight by her second birthday is more likely to be overweight at a later age," said Dr. Salsberry. "Prevention of childhood obesity needs to begin before a woman becomes pregnant," she added.

"Dr. Salsberry's work underscores the importance of prenatal care and how the health habits of the mother prior to and during pregnancy may impact the health of her child through the early years of childhood and possibly through adulthood," said NINR Director Dr. Patricia A. Grady. "Understanding how these factors may contribute to obesity very early in life will better equip us to fight the increasing problem of obesity in America and help to prevent diseases associated with obesity, such as type 2 diabetes, heart disease, and some forms of cancer," Dr. Grady added.

The researchers analyzed the data for 3,022 children included in the National Longitudinal Survey of Youth's (NLSY) Child-Mother file. In this study, children were weighed at three age intervals—3, 5 and 7 years. The survey also gathered information on each child's race and ethnicity as well as the mother's prepregnancy weight. Each mother was also asked if she had smoked while pregnant and if she had breast-fed her child.

Children were considered overweight if their body mass index (BMI) was greater than or equal to the 95th percentile for their age and gender. BMI is a calculation that takes into account both height and weight. A child in the 95th percentile for his or her weight is heavier than 95 percent of children at that age.

The study showed a significant relationship between a mother's weight prior to pregnancy and her child's weight. A mother's weight within 1 to 2 months before she became pregnant had the greatest impact on a child's weight at all three age intervals.

If a woman was overweight before she became pregnant, her child was nearly three times more likely to be overweight by age 7 compared to a child whose mother was not overweight or obese, according to the study. The risk that a child would be overweight at a young age increased with the degree of the mother's obesity.

The investigators reported that at each age interval, about 4 to 6 percent more black and Hispanic children were overweight than white children. However, the percentage of all children who were overweight, regardless of race or ethnicity, decreased with age. "Some children lose extra body weight and become leaner as they grow," Salsberry said.

Children of mothers who smoked during pregnancy were more likely to be heavy at all three age intervals. "Obviously smoking during pregnancy causes a host of serious problems, but this finding adds to the growing body of evidence that suggests that smoking during pregnancy may be a key risk factor that increases a child's chances of being overweight," Salsberry said.

Breast-feeding had a slight effect on weight at each measurement: As much as 5 percent fewer children who were breast-fed were also overweight, compared to bottle-fed babies.

The researchers also looked at other factors that may affect a child's weight, such as the age of the mother when she gave birth, the child's gender, and whether or not the mother was married. None of these factors had the same degree of effect on childhood weight as a mother's weight prior to pregnancy, race, ethnicity, or smoking.

Two out of three children who were overweight at their final weighing were also overweight during at least one prior weighing. Three out of four children who were at a normal weight at the final weighing had always been at a normal weight.

"A child's weight at 3 years is a good prediction of what his weight will be at age 5, and so on," Salsberry said. "Weight states tend to persist over time. "Obesity continues to rise in adults," she said. "And that risk has increased in children, too. Interventions should begin immediately for children who are already overweight at these young ages."

Section 39.3

Pregnancy after Weight-Loss Surgery

"Pregnancy after Weight-Loss Surgery," by John G. Kral, MD, PhD, FACS, Obesity Action Coalition, April 2007. © 2007 Obesity Action Coalition. Reprinted with permission.

According to some U.S. statistics 40–50 percent of pregnancies are unplanned, so it is difficult to warn obese young women to delay pregnancy until after weight loss.

Taking into consideration that obesity causes earlier menarche and is more common among the poor and uneducated, and among African American and Hispanic women, it is obvious that huge educational, cultural, and societal resources are required to limit the growing obesity epidemic.

Women's health education in schools and homes should emphasize the importance of planning pregnancies and should encourage medical consultation while planning a pregnancy. This is especially important in the obese.

How Does Surgical Treatment of Obesity Fit into the Picture? Or Does It?

Not knowing the dangers of obese pregnancies is only part of the problem. The other part is lacking access to effective means of achieving weight loss, or even maintaining a stable weight among those prone to weight gain. Regardless of reason(s) for undergoing weight-loss surgery, the fact is that rapidly increasing numbers of younger and younger women are having weight-loss operations. The majority of them are expected to become pregnant. In fact, obesity is a common cause of infertility, and weight loss by surgery or other means often cures such infertility.

What should obese women considering surgery, or having undergone weight-loss surgery, know about its effects on pregnancy outcomes?

First, it is important to understand the differences between the two major types of operations. Most operations nowadays are (or should be) performed using a laparoscope and three or four instruments inserted through half-inch cuts in the belly wall, instead of one large cut eight to 12 inches long.

One type of operation is purely "gastric restrictive," creating a small stomach pouch by placing an adjustable band around the top of the stomach. The inflated band makes a very small opening for the food to pass into the large stomach below the band. This causes small amounts of solid food to stretch the stomach pouch wall creating a sense of fullness as well as slowing the emptying of solid food from the small pouch. Liquids and melting foods (chocolate, cookies, chips) go straight through unless solid food is blocking the opening.

The other type of operation combines restriction (a small pouch) with bypass of more than 95 percent of the stomach and the first portions of the small bowel. The restrictive sense of fullness disappears over the first 10–18 months because the pouch and the opening between the pouch and the small bowel stretch.

The bypass operations work better because the undigested solid food and liquids cause fullness even after the pouch and opening have stretched. Clearly the restrictive action of the operations can cause vomiting, especially if the patient eats quickly and chews poorly. Pills or capsules can similarly cause vomiting if they are sufficiently large.

331

Weight-loss operations are designed to cause rapid weight loss which obviously is what the "customer" desires. I've already answered the question: "Will weight-loss surgery influence my ability to become pregnant?" But, what about the effects on the pregnancy, the fetus, the delivery, and the developing infant on its way into childhood, adolescence, and adulthood?

Effects on Pregnancy Outcomes

It is always recommended that young women, who have undergone weight-loss surgery and have the capacity to conceive, should take precautions to prevent pregnancy during the phase of rapid weight loss, and at least for 18 months to two years after their surgery.

Pregnancy outcomes after all types of weight-loss surgery—even the problematic old intestinal bypass operations and the complex modern aggressive operations with the ability to cause deficiencies and other nutritional problems—are universally safer and better than outcomes of obese pregnancies. Even if mothers are still obese after their surgery, the outcomes are better than if they haven't had surgery.

Having said this, it is important to recognize that there are risks caused by weight-loss operations if the mother fails to follow recommendations about responding to vomiting, diarrhea, or feelings of weakness. Patients must take recommended supplements, and blood levels of critical nutrients must be monitored as part of responsible prenatal care. As is the case for all patients who have had obesity surgery, the rules of eating and vomiting must be followed.

The most recent information about outcomes after obesity surgery suggests that guidelines for "healthy weight gain" should be revised. Commonly, normal-weight women with a body mass index (BMI) of 19.8–26 are recommended to gain 25–35 pounds, while those in the "high range" (BMI of 26.1–29) should have a "recommended target weight gain of at least 15 pounds" according to the Institute of Medicine of the National Academy of Sciences.

The dramatically increasing numbers of obese women have provided more statistics on pregnancy weight change in severely obese women (BMI greater than 35) allowing the development of new guidelines. Severely obese women often lose weight during pregnancy and the outcomes after weight-loss surgery, even during the non-recommended early rapid weight-loss phase, are healthy despite the absence of any weight gain.

Thus, it is important to "spread the word" that severely obese women (those with a BMI greater than 35) and those who have undergone weight-loss surgery can actually lose weight with a healthy outcome for the offspring. However, never forget that essential vitamins, minerals, and other nutrients must be monitored and supplemented as needed to optimize pregnancy outcomes in the obese, before and after surgery.

Effects on the Child

Obese mothers give birth to small for age or underweight infants more often than lean mothers. After having weight-loss surgery, mothers do not have any increase in the numbers of small offspring compared to when they were obese. Only recently it has been recognized that small children are "healthy." In fact, it is dangerous for small (or even premature) infants to gain weight quickly. Rapid weight often leads to childhood obesity. It is important to realize that obese pregnancies and early rearing practices can cause many problems. No more, are the old expressions as acceptable: "cute baby fat," "she'll grow out of it." Round pudgy cheeks are not the signs of a "healthy baby."

Obese women do not breast-feed as commonly as non-obese women. When they do breast-feed, obese women do so for a much shorter period of time. Shorter breast-feeding practices are associated with greater postnatal body weight in the mother and increased obesity in the child. Everything must be done to encourage breast-feeding. It is a very healthy and rewarding practice, and it has a role in preventing obesity in the mother and child.

Conclusions

- Obese pregnancies are dangerous pregnancies.
- Pregnancies following weight-loss surgery are safer than obese pregnancies for mother and child.
- Pregnancies after weight-loss surgery, regardless of weight: a.) should be prevented during the first 18 months after surgery; b.) should be monitored for nutrient deficiencies to guide taking supplements.

Recommendations for Pregnant Women Who Have Undergone Gastric Restrictive Weight-Loss Operations

Eating Behavior

To reduce the risk of vomiting:

- Eat slowly with minimal stress and distraction.

- Progress your diet from liquids to semisolid food to solid food.
- Eat small portions.
- Chew well before swallowing.
- If you feel your pouch, stop eating.
- Do not drink with your food—wait at least one hour after eating.

Response to Vomiting

If you vomit or regurgitate:

- Try to identify the reasons.
- Do not drink for four hours.
- Progress your diet slowly, starting with liquids.
- If nausea or vomiting during progression occurs, consume nothing by mouth for 12 hours.
- If you continue to vomit, despite above measures, contact your surgeon.

About the Author

John G. Kral, MD, PhD, FACS, received his MA degree in Psychology in 1961 from the University of Göteborg, Sweden, where he then attended medical school, completed specialty training in surgery and subsequently defended a PhD thesis entitled, Surgical Reduction of Adipose Tissue in 1976. In 1980, Dr. Kral was recruited to St. Luke's Hospital Center, Columbia University College of Physicians and Surgeons, to develop a program of surgical metabolism and anti-obesity surgery where he investigated eating behavior and continued studies on severe obesity and effects of long-term maintenance of significant weight-loss on body composition after malabsorptive and gastric restrictive operations.

Part Five

Pregnancy Complications

Chapter 40

What Are Pregnancy Complications?

Chapter Contents

Section 40.1

Overview of Pregnancy Complications

Excerpted from "Pregnancy Complications," by the Office of Women's
Health (www.womenshealth.gov), part of the U.S. Department of Health
and Human Services, March 2009.

Complications of pregnancy are health problems that occur during pregnancy. They can involve the mother's health, the baby's health, or both. Some women have health problems before they become pregnant that could lead to complications. Other problems arise during the pregnancy. Keep in mind that whether a complication is common or rare, there are ways to manage problems that come up during pregnancy.

Health Problems before Pregnancy

If you have an ongoing health problem, make sure to talk to your doctor before pregnancy. Your doctor might want to change the way your health problem is managed. Some medicines used to treat health problems could be harmful if taken during pregnancy. At the same time, stopping medicines that you need could be more harmful than the risks posed should you become pregnant. Be assured that you are likely to have a normal, healthy baby when health problems are under control and you get good prenatal care for health problems such as:

- **Asthma:** Poorly controlled asthma may increase risk of preeclampsia, poor weight gain in the fetus, preterm birth, cesarean birth, and other complications.

- **Depression:** Depression that persists during pregnancy can make it hard for a woman to care for herself and her unborn baby. Having depression before pregnancy also is a risk factor for postpartum depression.

- **Diabetes:** High blood glucose (sugar) levels during pregnancy can harm the fetus and worsen a woman's long-term diabetes complications. Doctors advise getting diabetes under control at least 3 to 6 months before trying to conceive.

- **Eating disorders:** Body image changes during pregnancy can cause eating disorders to worsen. Eating disorders are linked to many pregnancy complications, including birth defects and premature birth. Women with eating disorders also have higher rates of postpartum depression.

- **Epilepsy and other seizure disorders:** Seizures during pregnancy can harm the fetus, and increase the risk of miscarriage or stillbirth. But using medicine to control seizures might cause birth defects. For most pregnant women with epilepsy, using medicine poses less risk to their own health and the health of their babies than stopping medicine.

- **High blood pressure:** Having chronic high blood pressure puts a pregnant woman and her baby at risk for problems. Women with high blood pressure have a higher risk of preeclampsia and placental abruption (when the placenta separates from the wall of the uterus). The likelihood of preterm birth and low birth weight also is higher.

- **Human immunodeficiency virus (HIV):** HIV can be passed from a woman to her baby during pregnancy or delivery. Some HIV medicines can lower the chances of HIV being passed to the baby. But the effects of some medicines on the fetus are not clear or not known. Good prenatal care will help protect a woman's baby from HIV and keep her healthy.

- **Migraine:** Migraine symptoms tend to improve during pregnancy. Some women have no migraine attacks during pregnancy. Certain medicines commonly used to treat headaches should not be used during pregnancy. A woman who has severe headaches should speak to her doctor about ways to relieve symptoms safely.

- **Overweight and obesity:** Recent studies suggest that the heavier a woman is before she becomes pregnant, the greater her risk of a range of pregnancy complications, including preeclampsia and preterm delivery. Overweight and obese women who lose weight before pregnancy are likely to have healthier pregnancies.

- **Sexually transmitted infections (STIs):** Some STIs can cause early labor, a woman's water to break too early, and infection in the uterus after birth. Some STIs also can be passed from a woman to her baby during pregnancy or delivery. Some ways STIs can harm the baby include: low birth weight, dangerous infections, brain damage, blindness, deafness, liver problems, or stillbirth.

- **Thyroid disease:** Uncontrolled hyperthyroidism (overactive thyroid) can be dangerous to the mother and cause health problems such as heart failure and poor weight gain in the fetus. Uncontrolled hypothyroidism (underactive thyroid) also threatens the mother's health and can lead to intellectual disabilities in the baby.

- **Uterine fibroids:** Uterine fibroids are not uncommon, but few cause symptoms that require treatment. Uterine fibroids rarely cause miscarriage. Sometimes, fibroids can cause preterm or breech birth. Cesarean delivery may be needed if a fibroid blocks the birth canal.

Pregnancy-Related Problems

Sometimes pregnancy problems arise—even in healthy women. Some prenatal tests done during pregnancy can help prevent these problems or spot them early. Use Table 40.1 to learn about some common pregnancy complications. Call your doctor if you have any of the symptoms on this chart. If a problem is found, make sure to follow your doctor's advice about treatment. Doing so will boost your chances of having a safe delivery and a strong, healthy baby.

When to Call the Doctor

When you are pregnant don't wait to call your doctor or midwife if something is bothering or worrying you. Sometimes physical changes can be signs of a problem. Call your doctor or midwife as soon as you can if you:

- are bleeding or leaking fluid from the vagina;
- have sudden or severe swelling in the face, hands, or fingers;
- get severe or long-lasting headaches;
- have discomfort, pain, or cramping in the lower abdomen;
- have a fever or chills;
- are vomiting or have persistent nausea;

340

- feel discomfort, pain, or burning with urination;

- have problems seeing or blurred vision;

- feel dizzy;

- suspect your baby is moving less than normal after 28 weeks of pregnancy (if you count less than 10 movements within 2 hours);

- have thoughts of harming yourself or your baby.

Table 40.1. Common Pregnancy Complications (continued on next page)

Anemia—Lower than normal number of healthy red blood cells

Symptoms: Feel tired or weak; look pale; feel faint; shortness of breath

Treatment: Treating the underlying cause of the anemia will help restore the number of healthy red blood cells. Women with pregnancy related anemia are helped by taking iron and folic acid supplements. Your doctor will check your iron levels throughout pregnancy to be sure anemia does not happen again.

Depression—Extreme sadness during pregnancy or after birth (postpartum)

Symptoms: Intense sadness; helplessness and irritability; appetite changes; thoughts of harming self or baby

Treatment: Women who are pregnant might be helped with one or a combination of treatment options, including therapy, support groups, and medicines. A mother's depression can affect her baby's development, so getting treatment is important for both mother and baby.

Ectopic pregnancy—When a fertilized egg implants outside of the uterus, usually in the fallopian tube

Symptoms: Abdominal pain; shoulder pain; vaginal bleeding; feeling dizzy or faint

Treatment: With ectopic pregnancy, the egg cannot develop. Drugs or surgery is used to remove the ectopic tissue so your organs are not damaged.

Fetal problems—Unborn baby has a health issue, such as poor growth or heart problems

Symptoms: Baby moving less; baby is smaller than normal for gestational age; fewer than 10 kicks per day after 26 weeks; some problems have no symptoms, but are found with prenatal tests

Treatment: Treatment depends on results of tests to monitor baby's health. If a test suggests a problem, this does not always mean the baby is in trouble. It may only mean that the mother needs special care until the baby is delivered. This can include a wide variety of things, such as bed rest, depending on the mother's condition. Sometimes, the baby has to be delivered early.

341

Table 40.1. Common Pregnancy Complications (continued from previous page)

Gestational diabetes—Too high blood sugar levels during pregnancy

Symptoms: Usually, there are no symptoms. Sometimes, extreme thirst, hunger, or fatigue; screening test shows high blood sugar levels

Treatment: Most women with pregnancy related diabetes can control their blood sugar levels by a following a healthy meal plan from their doctor. Some women also need insulin to keep blood sugar levels under control. Doing so is important because poorly controlled diabetes increases the risk of preeclampsia; early delivery; cesarean birth; having a big baby, which can complicate delivery; baby born with low blood sugar, breathing problems, and jaundice.

High blood pressure (pregnancy related)—High blood pressure that starts after 20 weeks of pregnancy and goes away after birth

Symptoms: High blood pressure without other signs and symptoms of pre-eclampsia

Treatment: The health of the mother and baby are closely watched to make sure high blood pressure is not preeclampsia.

Hyperemesis gravidarum (HG)—Severe, persistent nausea and vomiting during pregnancy

Symptoms: More extreme than morning sickness; nausea that does not go away; vomiting several times every day; weight loss; reduced appetite; dehydration; feeling faint or fainting

Treatment: Dry, bland foods and fluids is the first line of treatment. Sometimes, medicines are prescribed to help nausea. Many women with HG have to be hospitalized so they can be fed fluids and nutrients through a tube in their veins. Usually, women with HG begin to feel better by the 20th week of pregnancy. But some women vomit and feel nauseated throughout all three trimesters.

Miscarriage—Pregnancy loss from natural causes before 20 weeks. As many as 20 percent of pregnancies end in miscarriage. Often, miscarriage occurs before a woman even knows she is pregnant

Symptoms: Signs of a miscarriage can include vaginal spotting or bleeding; cramping or abdominal pain; fluid or tissue passing from the vagina

Treatment: In most cases, miscarriage cannot be prevented. Sometimes, a woman must undergo treatment to remove pregnancy tissue in the uterus. Counseling can help with emotional healing.

Table 40.1. Common Pregnancy Complications (continued from previous page)

Placenta previa—Placenta covers part or entire opening of cervix inside of the uterus

Symptoms: Painless vaginal bleeding during second or third trimester; for some, no symptoms

Treatment: If diagnosed after the 20th week of pregnancy, but with no bleeding, a woman will need to cut back on her activity level and increase bed rest. If bleeding is heavy, hospitalization may be needed until mother and baby are stable. If the bleeding stops or is light, continued bed rest is resumed until baby is ready for delivery. If bleeding doesn't stop or if preterm labor starts, baby will be delivered by cesarean.

Placental abruption—Placenta separates from uterine wall before delivery, which can mean the fetus doesn't get enough oxygen

Symptoms: Vaginal bleeding; cramping, abdominal pain, and uterine tenderness

Treatment: When the separation is minor, bed rest for a few days usually stops the bleeding. Moderate cases may require complete bed rest. Severe cases (when more than half of the placenta separates) can require immediate medical attention and early delivery of the baby.

Preeclampsia—A condition starting after 20 weeks of pregnancy that causes high blood pressure and problems with the kidneys and other organs. Also called toxemia.

Symptoms: High blood pressure; swelling of hands and face; too much protein in urine; stomach pain; blurred vision; dizziness; headaches

Treatment: The only cure is delivery, which may not be best for the baby. Labor will probably be induced if condition is mild and the woman is near term (37 to 40 weeks of pregnancy). If it is too early to deliver, the doctor will watch the health of the mother and her baby very closely. She may need medicines and bed rest at home or in the hospital to lower her blood pressure. Medicines also might be used to prevent the mother from having seizures.

Preterm labor—Going into labor before 37 weeks of pregnancy

Symptoms: Increased vaginal discharge; pelvic pressure and cramping; back pain radiating to the abdomen; contractions

Treatment: Medicines can stop labor from progressing. Bed rest is often advised. Sometimes, a woman must deliver early. Giving birth before 37 weeks is called preterm birth.

Section 40.2

Bed Rest May Reduce Risk of Pregnancy Complications

Until this point in your pregnancy, you've probably been going about your normal activities of work, chores at home, spending time with family and friends, and exercise. But one day, suddenly or perhaps planned in advance, your doctor tells you that for your health and the health of your baby, you'll be restricted to bed rest.

Even though your friends and family may envy you for what they see as a mini-vacation, don't be fooled—bed rest during pregnancy is no walk in the park. Fortunately, though, there are plenty of ways to make your time in bed more enjoyable and productive, so keep reading and find out how to make the best of bed rest.

Doctor's Orders

There are several situations that might cause your doctor to recommend bed rest for some portion of your pregnancy. If your medical history, including previous pregnancies, contains information that might point to a medical complication, your doctor might recommend bed rest. Or, you might experience symptoms, such as bleeding or contractions, that require you to go on bed rest.

Even if your medical history is clear and you experience no symptoms, your doctor may require bed rest if the results of a test or procedure indicate a medical complication or if your baby's growth is determined to be poor.

So what are some common pregnancy complications that often result in bed rest? A few include: high blood pressure (including pregnancy-induced hypertension, preeclampsia, and eclampsia), vaginal bleeding (including placenta previa), premature labor, and cervical changes (such as incompetent cervix and cervical effacement).

If you're having multiples, your pregnancy may be termed high risk and will require close monitoring by your doctor. If you develop any problems, your doctor might place you on bed rest. Bed rest might also be recommended if you've had previous pregnancies that ended in miscarriage, stillbirth, or a premature birth.

Just as every pregnancy is different, every woman's experience with bed rest is different. Some women may know early on that because of their medical histories, they will have to go on bed rest at some point in their pregnancies. Other women may be surprised to hear their doctors announce, after a routine appointment, that they'll be on bed rest for a few weeks.

Some women are on bed rest early in their pregnancies and then released, whereas others spend their entire pregnancies confined to their beds. Your doctor can give you specific information about the duration of your bed rest.

How Does Bed Rest Help?

Women with pregnancy conditions related to high blood pressure may be placed on bed rest to decrease stress, both physical and emotional, with the hope of lowering their blood pressure. Vaginal bleeding can be aggravated by activity, lifting, or exercise, so bed rest may also be used to reduce bleeding. Women experiencing premature labor and contractions may also be restricted, because activity and stress can also aggravate these conditions.

Depending on your condition, your doctor may ask you to lie on your side to facilitate blood flow to the placenta or to rest with your feet up and your back elevated.

What Can—and Can't—You Do on Bed Rest?

Sometimes, doctors recommend modified bed rest or "house arrest," which generally allows women to stay on the couch, bed, or in a sitting position, but restricts them from sexual intercourse, exercise, or lifting. Other women may be told to remain in bed, only sitting up for meals or standing to take quick showers. Some women have to remain in bed in the hospital because their pregnancies require closer monitoring by a trained hospital staff.

Whatever kind of bed rest your doctor recommends, if it's long-term, you'll need to remember to exercise your legs to keep the blood circulating and prevent clots. Because every woman who experiences bed rest is different, be sure to get answers to the following questions from your doctor:

- Can I get up to use the bathroom?
- Can I get up to prepare quick meals or to do light chores?
- Can I take a bath or shower?
- What position should I be in while I'm resting?
- Can I go to work or work from home?
- Is driving OK?
- How much walking is safe?
- How much and what kind of sexual activity is OK?
- What activities can I do to increase blood circulation safely?

Tips for Surviving Bed Rest

Fortunately, there are plenty of ways to make your bed rest enjoyable without becoming addicted to daytime TV. Try these tips:

- **Stick to a schedule.** Even if you have to stay in bed all day, you'll feel better if you take care of yourself. After you wake up, change into comfortable clothes and plan what to do for the day. Having a plan will make you feel as if you're accomplishing something and will give you something to look forward to.

- **Catch up while you can.** Let's face it, after the baby arrives, you'll be too busy to think about catching up on correspondence or reading your favorite author's latest novel. Try these time passers:

  - Choose a doctor for your child, find quality child care, or write up a birth plan (if you haven't already done these things).

  - Start a journal chronicling your pregnancy—and your bed rest.

  - Start a family tree that you can share with your child someday.

  - Firm up your baby-name choices—use books and websites for ideas.

  - Organize photo albums.

346

- Read anything—newspapers, magazines, classic novels, the latest bestsellers, compilations of fiction or poetry—you could even revisit some of your favorite childhood stories or try out some books from the library for your little one.

- Watch rented videos/DVDs or taped TV shows.

- Answer letters or correspondence.

- Write thank-you cards if you've already had a baby shower—if not, start addressing the envelopes to people (friends and family) whom you know will probably give gifts.

- Build an e-mail and phone list of people to call when the baby comes, if you haven't already done so.

- Start a calendar of important dates to remember (birthdays, anniversaries, etc.).

- Contact your job about your maternity-leave benefits.

- Fill out health insurance paperwork for your baby in advance.

- Designate a guardian for your child and have your lawyer draft a new will.

- **Stock up.** Just because you're on your back doesn't mean you have to be unprepared. You can fully stock your baby's nursery and layette by phone or the Internet. Order all the items you think you'll need for the first 3 months—including diapers! In addition to baby stores and centers, online drugstores often carry a wide variety of baby care items that they'll deliver right to your door.

- **Don't be afraid to ask visitors for assistance.** Your friends and family would probably love to help you with household chores, errands, or meal preparation. Create a task list so that when someone offers help, you can assign him or her a task. Visits from your friends and family can boost your spirits—just make sure you ask them to come at a time that's convenient and comfortable for you.

- **Become a parenting expert.** Plenty of parenting books and websites can help to answer many of your parenting and children's health questions. If you feel uncomfortable reading about high-risk pregnancy issues, learn about breastfeeding or how to encourage your child's development instead. You could also get subscriptions to local and national parenting magazines and start clipping out useful articles and tips. File your clippings in folders (i.e., new baby care, feeding, crying, sleeping, safety, development, etc.) for future reference when the baby comes. Also file away any articles you print out from the Internet.

- **Seek out a support system.** The Internet is a great place to find support from other moms on bed rest. Check out bed rest message boards and chat rooms, where you can share tips and get advice.

- **Support your support person.** You're probably relying heavily on your spouse or partner to tend to household chores, child care, and errands during your bed rest. Make sure you take the time to show your appreciation—you can always order a nice gift by phone or online!

Chapter 41

Amniotic Fluid Abnormalities

Chapter Contents

Section 41.1

Polyhydramnios (Excessive Amniotic Fluid)

"Polyhydramnios," © 2009 A.D.A.M., Inc. Reprinted with permission.

Definition

Polyhydramnios is the presence of excessive amniotic fluid surrounding the unborn infant.

Considerations

Amniotic fluid surrounds and cushions the infant throughout development. There may be too little or too much amniotic fluid due to problems in the fetus.

Polyhydramnios can occur if the fetus does not swallow and absorb amniotic fluid in normal amounts. This can happen due to gastrointestinal disorders, brain and nervous system (neurological) problems, or a variety of other causes. Polyhydramnios may also be related to increased fluid production, as is the case with certain fetal lung disorders.

Sometimes, no specific cause for polyhydramnios is found.

Causes

- Achondroplasia
- Anencephaly
- Beckwith-Wiedemann syndrome
- Diaphragmatic hernia
- Duodenal atresia
- Esophageal atresia
- Gastroschisis
- Gestational diabetes
- Hydrops fetalis
- Multiple gestation (for example, twins or triplets)

What to Expect at Your Office Visit

This condition is discovered during pregnancy, and evaluated before delivery. If the health care provider finds a fetal abnormality, the baby will be delivered in a hospital with specialists who can provide immediate evaluation and treatment.

Documenting polyhydramnios may include:

- history of this pregnancy;
- history of previous pregnancies and health of the children delivered;
- other family history;
- ultrasound scans of the fetus.

Section 41.2

Potter Syndrome and Oligohydramnios (Inadequate Amniotic Fluid)

Alternative Names

Potter phenotype

Definition

Potter syndrome and Potter phenotype refers to a group of findings associated with a lack of amniotic fluid and kidney failure in an unborn infant.

Causes

In Potter syndrome, the primary problem is kidney failure. The kidneys fail to develop properly as the baby is growing in the womb. The kidneys normally produce the amniotic fluid (as urine).

Potter phenotype refers to a typical facial appearance that occurs in a newborn when there is no amniotic fluid. The lack of amniotic fluid is called oligohydramnios. Without amniotic fluid, the infant is not cushioned from the walls of the uterus. The pressure of the uterine wall leads to an unusual facial appearance, including widely separated eyes.

Potter phenotype may also lead to abnormal limbs, or limbs that are held in abnormal positions or contractures.

Oligohydramnios also stops development of the lungs, so the lungs do not work properly at birth.

Symptoms

- Widely separated eyes with epicanthal folds, broad nasal bridge, low set ears, and receding chin
- Absence of urine output
- Difficulty breathing

Exams and Tests

A pregnancy ultrasound may show lack of amniotic fluid, absence of fetal kidneys, or severely abnormal kidneys in the unborn baby.

The following tests may be used to help diagnose the condition in a newborn:

- X-ray of the abdomen
- X-ray of the lungs

Treatment

Resuscitation at delivery may be attempted pending the diagnosis. Treatment will be provided for any urinary outlet obstruction.

Outlook (Prognosis)

This is a very serious condition, usually deadly. The short term outcome depends on the severity of lung involvement. Long-term outcome depends on the severity of kidney involvement.

Prevention

There is no known prevention.

References

Behrman RE. *Nelson Textbook of Pediatrics*. 17th ed. Philadelphia, Pa: WB Saunders; 2004.

Chapter 42

Birth Defects

Chapter Contents

Section 42.1

Birth Defects That May Be Diagnosed during Pregnancy

"Overview of Birth Defects," © 2008 Children's Hospital of Pittsburgh (www.chp.edu). Reprinted with permission.

What is a birth defect?

A birth defect is a health problem or physical change, which is present in a baby at the time he/she is born. Birth defects may be very mild, where the baby looks and acts like any other baby, or birth defects may be very severe, where you can immediately tell there is a health problem present. Some of the severe birth defects can be life threatening, where a baby may only live a few months, or may die at a young age (in their teens, for example).

Birth defects are also called congenital anomalies or congenital abnormalities. The word congenital means present at birth. The words anomalies and abnormalities mean that there is a problem present in a baby.

What causes birth defects to occur?

There are many reasons why birth defects happen. Most occur due to environmental and genetic factors, but often the cause is unknown.

Who is affected by birth defects?

Birth defects have been present in babies from all over the world, in families of all nationalities and backgrounds. Anytime a couple becomes pregnant, there is a chance that their baby will have a birth defect. Most babies are born healthy. In fact, 97 out of 100 babies are born healthy. Anytime a couple becomes pregnant, there is a 3 to 4 percent chance that their baby will have a birth defect. The 3 to 4 percent number is sometimes called the background rate for birth defects, or the population risk for birth defects. In a family where birth defects are already present in family members or the parents themselves, the chance for a couple to have a child with a birth defect may be higher than the background rate of 3 to 4 percent.

What are the genetic and environmental causes of birth defects?

When a baby is born with a birth defect, the first question usually asked by the parents is "how did this happen?" Sometimes, this question cannot be answered. This can be very upsetting for parents because it is normal to seek an answer as to why your baby has a health problem. For some birth defects, however, there is a known cause, which may have to do with either genetic or environmental factors, or a combination of the two. Here is some general information and terms related to the different causes of birth defects:

- **Inheritance:** Inheritance is a word used to describe a trait given to you or passed on to you from one of your parents. Examples of inherited traits would be your eye color or blood type.

- **Chromosome abnormalities:** Chromosomes are stick-like structures in the center of each cell (called the nucleus) that contain your genes.

- **Single gene defects:** Genes are what determine your traits. Sometimes, a child can inherit not only those genes responsible for their normal traits such as the color of their eyes, but also disease causing genes that result in a birth defect.

- **Multifactorial inheritance:** Multifactorial inheritance means that "many factors" (multifactorial) are involved in causing a birth defect. The factors are usually both genetic and environmental.

- **Teratogens:** A teratogen is an agent, which can cause a birth defect. It is usually something in the environment that the mother may be exposed to during her pregnancy. It could be a prescribed medication, a street drug, alcohol use, or a disease that the mother has, which could increase the chance for the baby to be born with a birth defect.

Why are birth defects a concern?

Although some birth defects have a single abnormality, others have abnormalities in multiple body systems or organs. Birth defects may cause life-long disability and illness, and with some, survival is not possible.

Some birth defects, such as mental retardation, are non-treatable disabilities. However, many physical defects can be treated with surgery. Repair is possible with many defects including cleft lip or palate and certain heart defects.

How are birth defects diagnosed?

Many birth defects can be diagnosed before birth with special tests (prenatal diagnosis). Chromosomal abnormalities such as Down syndrome can be diagnosed before birth by analyzing cells in the amniotic fluid or from the placenta.

Fetal ultrasound during pregnancy can also give information about the possibility of certain birth defects, but ultrasound is not 100 percent accurate, since some babies with birth defects may look the same on ultrasound as those without problems. A chromosome analysis, whether performed on a blood sample or cells from the amniotic fluid or placenta, is over 99.9 percent accurate.

Tests that help screen for birth defects include the following:

- **Alpha-fetoprotein:** This blood test measures the levels of alpha-fetoprotein (AFP), a protein released by the fetal liver and found in the mother's blood. AFP is sometimes called MSAFP (maternal serum AFP). AFP screening may be included as one part of a two, three, or four-part screening, often called a multiple marker screen. The other parts may include the following.

  - **hCG:** Human chorionic gonadotropin (hCG) is a hormone secreted by the early placental cells. High hCG levels may indicate a fetus with Down syndrome (a chromosomal abnormality that includes mental retardation and distinct physical features).

  - **Estriol:** A hormone produced by the placenta and by the fetal liver and adrenal glands. Low levels may indicate a fetus with Down syndrome.

  - **Inhibin:** A hormone produced by the placenta.

- **Chorionic villus sampling (CVS):** a prenatal test that involves taking a sample of some of the placental tissue. This tissue contains the same genetic material as the fetus and can be tested for chromosomal abnormalities and some other genetic problems. Testing is available for other genetic defects and disorders depending on the family history and availability of laboratory testing at the time of the procedure. In comparison to amniocentesis (another type of prenatal test), CVS does not provide information on neural tube defects such as spina bifida. For this reason, women who undergo CVS also need a follow-up blood test between 16 to 18 weeks of their pregnancy, to screen for neural tube defects.

- **Amniocentesis:** a procedure used to obtain a small sample of the amniotic fluid that surrounds the fetus to diagnose chromosomal disorders and open neural tube defects (ONTDs) such as spina bifida. Testing is available for other genetic defects and disorders depending on the family history and availability of laboratory testing at the time of the procedure. The American College of Obstetricians and Gynecologists (ACOG) recommends amniocentesis around 15 weeks to 20 weeks of pregnancy for those women who are at increased risk for chromosome abnormalities, such as women who are over age 35 years of age at delivery, or those who have had an abnormal maternal serum screening test, indicating an increased risk for a chromosomal abnormality or neural tube defect. However, in some situations, amniocentesis may be performed as early as 14 weeks.

- **Ultrasound:** a diagnostic technique that uses high-frequency sound waves to create an image of the internal organs. Many birth defects can be detected with ultrasound. Sometimes, birth defects are not diagnosed until physical examination of the baby after birth. To confirm the physical findings, a small blood sample can be taken and the chromosomes can be analyzed. This information is important in determining the risk for that birth defect in future pregnancies.

Prevention of Birth Defects

Research is ongoing to find and treat the causes of many birth defects. Immunizations of the mother against certain infections, such as rubella, can prevent infection. Much has been learned about the dangerous effects of alcohol on the developing baby and women are now advised to not drink during pregnancy.

In recent years, a strong link has been discovered between the lack of the B-vitamin folic acid and the development of neural tube defects such as spina bifida. Taking a vitamin containing sufficient folic acid before conception and in early pregnancy can often help prevent many serious defects.

Section 42.2

Birth Defects and Developmental Disabilities

Excerpted from "Birth Defects and Developmental Disabilities," by the National Institute of Child Health and Human Development (NICHD, www.nichd.nih.gov), part of the U.S. Department of Health and Human Services, September 18, 2006.

The March of Dimes Birth Defects Foundation defines "birth defects" as: an abnormality of structure, function, or metabolism (body chemistry) present at birth that results in physical or mental disability, or is fatal. To date, researchers have identified thousands of different birth defects. Currently, birth defects rank as the leading cause of death for infants during the first year of life. Birth defects can be caused by different factors, such as the following:

• Genetic problems that result from the failure of one or more genes to work properly

• Problems with the number or structure of chromosomes, such as extra or missing groups of genes

• Things that happen to a woman during pregnancy, such as getting rubella or German measles while pregnant, having untreated or uncontrolled diabetes while pregnant, being around or in contact with dangerous chemicals in the environment while pregnant, or using drugs or alcohol during pregnancy

These factors can change normal infant growth or development resulting in different types of birth defects, such as the following:

• Physical problems with body parts or structures: Some physical problems include cleft (has a gap or split) lip or cleft palate, heart defects, and abnormal limbs, such as a club foot

• Functional problems with how a body part or body system works: These problems are often called developmental disabilities and can include things like these:

358

- Nervous system or brain problems, such as learning disabilities, behavioral disorders, speech or language difficulties, muscle spasms or convulsions, and movement trouble

- Sensory problems, such as cataracts of the eyes, blindness, hearing loss, or deafness

- Metabolic disorders involve a body process or chemical pathway or reaction, such as conditions that limit the body's ability to get rid of waste materials or harmful chemicals.

- Degenerative disorders are conditions that might not be obvious at birth, but steadily make worse one or more aspects of health.

In some cases, birth defects can result from a combination of these factors, or they can affect many parts or processes in the body, which may lead to both physical and functional problems, to different degrees.

Some of these types of birth defects and developmental disabilities are described below.

Physical Birth Defects

Researchers and health care providers use the term neural tube defects to describe one important category of birth defects. These problems are related to the growth and development of the brain and spinal cord. Neural tube defects can include conditions like anencephaly, a fatal condition in which much of the brain does not develop; and spina bifida, in which the membranes around the spinal cord don't close properly, or the cord itself is not completely normal. People with spina bifida may have difficulty walking or be unable to walk without help, or they may have abnormal limbs. The condition is also associated with other structural problems with the body. In half of all babies born with spina bifida, the resulting problems are severe enough to result in death.

Research in this area has shown that getting the right amount of folic acid before and during pregnancy can prevent most neural tube defects. The U.S. Public Health Service recommends that women of childbearing age get at least 400 micrograms of folic acid each day, through food sources and/or supplements. Health care providers recommend that women supplement their diets with folic acid for 3 months before conception, and then for at least the 3 three months of pregnancy. Findings from research supported by the National Institute of Child Health and Human Development (NICHD) and other agencies indicate that the right amount of folic acid can help prevent certain birth defects and other problems during pregnancy.

In some cases, spina bifida can be detected in the womb. This early detection may allow surgeons to correct the spinal cord problems before birth, but researchers have yet to confirm this idea. If this research proves effective, it could alleviate many of the lasting effects of these problems. To learn more about this type of surgery, the NICHD is supporting the MOMS (Management of Meningomyelocele Study) trial, a clinical trial that will compare the safety and effectiveness of surgery before birth, with surgery performed right after birth in correcting spinal cord problems. The research is part of the Maternal-Fetal Medicine Unit (MFMU) Network, an NICHD-supported program that uses 14 sites around the country to conduct clinical trials related to the mechanisms of pregnancy and birth.

Functional Birth Defects/Developmental Disabilities

This complex group of birth defects involves a problem with the operation of a part of the body, a system in the body, or a process or pathway in the body. Although this information groups these developmental disabilities into general categories, many functional birth defects affect multiple body parts or systems. For example, a metabolic disorder may lead to nervous system or brain problems. This website groups the information to make it easier to remember.

Nervous System/Brain Problems

As mentioned above, some birth defects affect the functioning of the brain, which can impact intelligence and learning. This section describes some of the more commonly known functional birth defects.

Mental retardation: The term "mental retardation" describes a certain range of scores on an IQ (intelligence quotient) test. Mental retardation can result from a number of different birth defects, including:

- In the past, a specific type of bacterial infection, called Hib, was a leading cause of mental retardation in the United States. But, as a result of NICHD-supported research on this infection, researchers funded by the NICHD were able to develop a vaccine to prevent the infection from occurring. Since the discovery of the vaccine, Hib has been nearly eliminated in the United States, and in other areas where the vaccine is available. As a result,

Hib is also no longer a cause of mental retardation in the United States and other areas.

- Down syndrome describes a set of mental and physical characteristics related to having an extra copy of a specific chromosome, Chromosome 21. This set of symptoms includes mental retardation. Interventions and treatments for the symptoms of Down syndrome can allow many individuals with this condition to live healthy, productive lives. NICHD-supported work in Down syndrome includes efforts to understand some of the other problems associated with the condition, such as heart defects and early mental decline.

- Fragile X syndrome is the most common inherited form of mental retardation. Parents with few or no symptoms can pass the condition on to their children through genes. A defect in a specific part of a specific gene, called the Fragile X Mental Retardation 1 gene, or FMR1, causes the body to produce low amounts or none of a certain protein. This protein is vital to normal brain development; without enough of it, the brain doesn't grow properly, leading to the symptoms of Fragile X. In 1991, NICHD-supported researchers were the first to identify that a change in the FMR1 gene caused Fragile X. This and other NICHD-supported research has continued in hopes of finding out what the protein that is lacking or missing does in the brain. In response to the Children's Health Act of 2000, the NICHD created three centers for Fragile X research, to ensure that this work can continue. In addition, the NICHD is working with other agencies and organizations dedicated to understanding Fragile X to further knowledge about this condition. The Institute's Families and Fragile X Syndrome publication describes what is currently known about and what research is being done to learn more about Fragile X.

Autism spectrum disorders: Other developmental disabilities include problems like autism spectrum disorders, a range of problems that can affect a person's ability to communicate, social skills, and intelligence. Because autism is diagnosed on a spectrum, people with this condition can be severely affected, or have only mild symptoms; but they all have a type of autism.

Sensory-Related Developmental Disabilities

Sensory-related problems are often an important part of complex birth defect patterns. For instance, children with congenital rubella, a collection of problems that a child whose mother had rubella or German measles while pregnant may have, are likely to be deaf, and to develop cataracts of the eyes. Children with Williams syndrome have trouble seeing spatial relationships between objects around them. Those with Fragile X syndrome are often very sensitive to loud noises; they may overreact or have outbursts in reaction to such sounds.

Metabolic Disorders

This group of functional birth defects affects a person's metabolism, which is the way the body builds up, breaks down, and otherwise processes the materials it needs to function. For example, digestion, how your body breaks down food into its smaller parts, is a metabolic process. Two commonly known metabolic disorders include:

• Phenylketonuria, also called PKU, is a condition in which a problem with a specific enzyme, a protein that speeds up certain chemical reactions, causes mental retardation. NICHD-supported researchers developed a dietary therapy that helps to balance the amount of this enzyme in the body, which has almost eliminated mental retardation in people with PKU. Conclusions from the NIH Consensus Development Conference on PKU: Screening and Management recommend that this dietary therapy continue throughout life. Women known to have PKU should follow the diet while they are pregnant to prevent mental retardation in their children. The NICHD hopes to use its successes with PKU research as a model for efforts on other diseases.

• Hypothyroidism is a hormonal condition that, if left untreated in a pregnant woman, can cause mental retardation in her baby. The thyroid is a gland in the body that makes a chemical signal called a hormone. Hormones help to regulate certain functions in the body, including puberty and pregnancy. Without enough thyroid hormone in the mother's body, the fetus' brain won't develop correctly, resulting in mental retardation. NICHD-supported researchers found that, by identifying women who have this condition early in or before pregnancy, treatments to get the level of thyroid hormone back to normal can prevent mental retardation in some cases. In addition, NICHD research found that children who are born with hypothyroidism could also be treated with thyroid hormone to prevent many of the long-term effects of this condition.

Degenerative Disorders

Some infants born with degenerative disorders appear normal at birth, but then lose abilities or functions due to the condition. In these cases, the defect is usually not detected until an older age, when the child or person starts to show signs of a problem. Degenerative disorder can cause physical, mental, and sensory problems, depending on the specific defect.

In one type of degenerative disorder, early onset X-linked adrenoleukodystrophy, also called X-ALD, boys develop normally until between ages 4 and 8. After this point, they begin to lose brain and nervous system function. Eventually, boys with X-ALD lose so much of their brain and neural abilities that they appear to be in a "frozen" state, unable to move and communicate. X-ALD was the focus of the movie Lorenzo's Oil, which described one family's efforts to spur scientific progress.

Another type of degenerative birth defect is Rett syndrome. This disorder, which usually affects girls, is caused by a specific genetic abnormality. The NICHD's efforts to understand these types of birth defects focus on screening techniques that allow early detection of these problems, and strategies to treat or relieve some of the symptoms of these conditions. Other work is underway to find the cellular mechanisms or genetic markers for these conditions.

Additional Research and Other Resources on Birth Defects

Research on birth defects often begins by focusing on the specific effects of the problem on an infant. Sometimes, the effects of birth defects can be severe, such as not being able to walk, having organ systems that aren't complete, or even death. Once scientists know the outcomes of a certain problem, they can backtrack, following the problem back to early stages of development to isolate when it might have happened. Knowing when the problem first occurred can offer insight into how it occurred.

Through this general scheme, NICHD-supported researchers and their colleagues have made great progress in understanding the characteristics of certain birth defects, the patterns that these problems take, and possible points in growth and development where the problems might occur. And, armed with this understanding, researchers have developed interventions to prevent some birth defects, methods of identifying birth defects early in development, and possible treatments for birth defects.

The NICHD's research on birth defects has not only improved the chances of survival for those affected, but has also improved the quality of life for many people impacted by birth defects and their families.

The NICHD and other Institute are currently conducting a number of clinical trials related to birth defects.

Chapter 43

Bleeding and Blood Clots in Pregnancy

Chapter Contents

Section 43.1

Bleeding during Early Pregnancy

Many women have some bleeding from the vagina in pregnancy. Sometimes the pregnancy continues with no ill effects. But bleeding could be an early sign of miscarriage. If you are pregnant and have bleeding, call your doctor or midwife.

Symptoms to Watch For

- If you have any bleeding, apply a pad and call your doctor or midwife. Write down the time and the amount of bleeding. Call the doctor or midwife again if you have to change your pad more often than once an hour. Rest with your feet up until the bleeding slows down.

- If you have cramping with the bleeding, you can take acetaminophen (such as Tylenol).

- If you pass anything that looks like tissue onto the pad or into the toilet, call your doctor. He or she probably will have you come to the emergency department. You will be asked to bring a sample of the tissue with you.

- If you have a fever of 101 degrees Fahrenheit or higher, call your doctor.

If you call your doctor or midwife with any of these symptoms, he or she probably will want to examine you. You also may need to have blood tests.

If you have any questions or concerns about these symptoms, talk to your doctor or midwife.

Section 43.2

Blood Clots

Excerpted from "Deep Vein Thrombosis," by the National
Heart, Lung and Blood Institute (NHLBI, www.nhlbi.nih.gov),
part of the National Institutes of Health, November 2007.

What Is Deep Vein Thrombosis?

Deep vein thrombosis, or DVT, is a blood clot that forms in a vein deep in the body. Blood clots occur when blood thickens and clumps together.

Most deep vein blood clots occur in the lower leg or thigh. They also can occur in other parts of the body.

A blood clot in a deep vein can break off and travel through the bloodstream. The loose clot is called an embolus. When the clot travels to the lungs and blocks blood flow, the condition is called pulmonary embolism, or PE.

PE is a very serious condition. It can damage the lungs and other organs in the body and cause death.

Blood clots in the thigh are more likely to break off and cause PE than blood clots in the lower leg or other parts of the body.

Blood clots also can form in the veins closer to the skin's surface. However, these clots won't break off and cause PE.

Other Names for Deep Vein Thrombosis

- Blood clot in the legs
- Venous thrombosis
- Venous thromboembolism (VTE). This term is used for both deep vein thrombosis and pulmonary embolism.

What Causes Deep Vein Thrombosis?

Blood clots can form in your body's deep veins when:

- damage occurs to a vein's inner lining. This damage may result from injuries caused by physical, chemical, and biological factors.

367

Such factors include surgery, serious injury, inflammation, or an immune response.

- blood flow is sluggish or slow. Lack of motion can cause sluggish or slowed blood flow. This may occur after surgery, if you're ill and in bed for a long time, or if you're traveling for a long time.

- your blood is thicker or more likely to clot than usual.

Certain inherited conditions (such as factor V Leiden) increase blood's tendency to clot. This also is true of treatment with hormone replacement therapy or birth control pills.

Who Is at Risk for Deep Vein Thrombosis?

Many factors increase your risk for deep vein thrombosis (DVT). They include:

- a history of DVT.

- disorders or factors that make your blood thicker or more likely to clot than normal. Certain inherited blood disorders (such as factor V Leiden) will do this. This also is true of treatment with hormone replacement therapy or using birth control pills.

- injury to a deep vein from surgery, a broken bone, or other trauma.

- slow blood flow in a deep vein from lack of movement. This may occur after surgery, if you're ill and in bed for a long time, or if you're traveling for a long time.

- pregnancy and the first 6 weeks after giving birth.

- recent or ongoing treatment for cancer.

- a central venous catheter. This is a tube placed in vein to allow easy access to the bloodstream for medical treatment.

- being older than 60 (although DVT can occur in any age group).

- being overweight or obese.

- your risk for DVT increases if you have more than one of the risk factors listed above.

What Are the Signs and Symptoms of Deep Vein Thrombosis?

The signs and symptoms of deep vein thrombosis (DVT) may be related to DVT itself or to pulmonary embolism (PE). See your doctor right away if you have symptoms of either. Both DVT and PE can cause serious, possibly life-threatening complications if not treated.

Deep Vein Thrombosis

Only about half of the people with DVT have symptoms. These symptoms occur in the leg affected by the deep vein clot. They include:

- swelling of the leg or along a vein in the leg;
- pain or tenderness in the leg, which you may feel only when standing or walking;
- increased warmth in the area of the leg that's swollen or in pain; and
- red or discolored skin on the leg.

Pulmonary Embolism

Some people don't know they have DVT until they have signs or symptoms of PE. Symptoms of PE include:

- unexplained shortness of breath;
- pain with deep breathing; and
- coughing up blood.

Rapid breathing and a fast heart rate also may be signs of PE.

Chapter 44

Cholestasis of Pregnancy

Some women experience a very severe itching in late pregnancy. The most common cause of this is cholestasis, a common liver disease that only happens in pregnancy. Cholestasis of pregnancy is a condition in which the normal flow of bile in the gallbladder is affected by the high amounts of pregnancy hormones. Cholestasis is more common in the last trimester of pregnancy when hormones are at their peak, but it usually goes away within a few days after delivery. According to Cincinnati Children's Hospital Medical Center, cholestasis occurs in about 1 out of 1,000 pregnancies but is more common in Swedish and Chilean ethnic groups. Cholestasis is sometimes referred to as extrahepatic cholestasis which occurs outside the liver, intrahepatic cholestasis which occurs inside the liver, or obstetric cholestasis.

What causes cholestasis of pregnancy?

Pregnancy hormones affect gallbladder function, resulting in slowing or stopping the flow of bile. The gallbladder holds bile that is produced in the liver, which is necessary in the breakdown of fats in digestion. When the bile flow is stopped or slowed down, this causes a build up of bile acids in the liver which can spill into the bloodstream.

What are the symptoms of cholestasis of pregnancy?

- Itching, particularly on the hands and feet (often is the only symptom noticed)
- Dark urine color
- Light coloring of bowel movements
- Fatigue or exhaustion
- Loss of appetite
- Depression

Less common symptoms include:

- Jaundice (yellow coloring of skin, eyes, and mucous membranes);
- Upper-right quadrant pain;
- Nausea.

Who is at risk for cholestasis of pregnancy?

One to 2 pregnancies in 1000 are affected by cholestasis. The following women have a higher risk of getting cholestasis during pregnancy:

- Women carrying multiples
- Women who have previous liver damage
- Women whose mother or sisters had cholestasis

How is cholestasis of pregnancy diagnosed?

A diagnosis of cholestasis can be made by doing a complete medical history, physical examination, and blood tests that evaluate liver function, bile acids, and bilirubin.

How will the baby be affected if the mother is diagnosed with cholestasis?

Cholestasis may increase the risks for fetal distress, preterm birth, or stillbirth. A developing baby relies on the mother's liver to remove bile acids from the blood; therefore, the elevated levels of maternal bile cause stress on the baby's liver. Women with cholestasis should be monitored closely and serious consideration should be given to inducing labor once the baby's lungs have reached maturity.

What is the treatment for cholestasis of pregnancy?

The treatment goals for cholestasis of pregnancy are to relieve itching. Some treatment options include:

- Topical anti-itch medications or medication with corticosteroids;

- Medication to decrease the concentration of bile acids such as ursodeoxycholic acid;

- Cold baths and ice water slow down the flow of blood in the body by decreasing its temperature;

- Dexamethasone is a steroid that increases the maturity of the baby's lungs;

- Vitamin K supplements administered to the mother before delivery and again once the baby is born to prevent intracranial hemorrhaging;

- Dandelion root and milk thistle are natural substances that are beneficial to the liver;

- Bi-weekly non-stress tests which involve fetal heart monitoring and contraction recordings;

- Regular blood tests monitoring both bile serum levels and liver function.

Treatment for cholestasis of pregnancy needs to be determined by your physician who will take the following criteria into consideration:

- Your pregnancy, overall health, and medical history

- The extent of the disease

- Your tolerance of specific medications, procedures, or therapies

- Expectations for the course of the disease

- Your opinion or preference

Treatments that should not be used for cholestasis include:

- Antihistamines

- Aveeno and oatmeal bath

There are conflicting views on using the medication cholestyramine for treatment of cholestasis. In the past, this medication was readily used to treat this condition, but some studies have shown that chole-styramine may not be as effective as other treatments and potentially has some adverse side effects such as blocking essential vitamins like Vitamin K (a vitamin that is already deficient in women with chole-stasis).

What are the chances of the mother getting cholestasis in another pregnancy?

Whether or not a woman will get cholestasis in future pregnan-cies is debatable. However, some sources claim that women who have had cholestasis of pregnancy have up to a 90% chance of having this repeat in future pregnancies.

Chapter 45

Gestational Diabetes

What is gestational diabetes?

Gestational diabetes is diabetes that is found for the first time when a woman is pregnant. Out of every 100 pregnant women in the United States, three to eight get gestational diabetes. Diabetes means that your blood glucose (also called blood sugar) is too high. Your body uses glucose for energy. But too much glucose in your blood can be harmful. When you are pregnant, too much glucose is not good for your baby.

What causes gestational diabetes?

Changing hormones and weight gain are part of a healthy pregnancy. But both changes make it hard for your body to keep up with its need for a hormone called insulin. When that happens, your body doesn't get the energy it needs from the food you eat.

What is my risk of gestational diabetes?

To learn your risk for gestational diabetes, check each item that applies to you. Talk with your doctor about your risk at your first prenatal visit.

- I have a parent, brother, or sister with diabetes.

"What I Need to Know about Gestational Diabetes," by the National Institute of Diabetes and Digestive and Kidney Diseases (NIDDK, www.niddk.nih .gov), part of the National Institutes of Health, April 2006.

- I am African American, American Indian, Asian American, Hispanic/Latino, or Pacific Islander.

- I am 25 years old or older.

- I am overweight.

- I have had gestational diabetes before, or I have given birth to at least one baby weighing more than 9 pounds.

- I have been told that I have "pre-diabetes," a condition in which blood glucose levels are higher than normal, but not yet high enough for a diagnosis of diabetes. Other names for it are "impaired glucose tolerance" and "impaired fasting glucose."

If you checked any of these risk factors, ask your health care team about testing for gestational diabetes.

- You are at high risk if you are very overweight, have had gestational diabetes before, have a strong family history of diabetes, or have glucose in your urine.

- You are at average risk if you checked one or more of the risk factors.

- You are at low risk if you did not check any of the risk factors.

When will I be checked for gestational diabetes?

Your doctor will decide when you need to be checked for diabetes depending on your risk factors.

- If you are at high risk, your blood glucose level may be checked at your first prenatal visit. If your test results are normal, you will be checked again sometime between weeks 24 and 28 of your pregnancy.

- If you have an average risk for gestational diabetes, you will be tested sometime between weeks 24 and 28 of pregnancy.

- If you are at low risk, your doctor may decide that you do not need to be checked.

How is gestational diabetes diagnosed?

Your health care team will check your blood glucose level. Depending on your risk and your test results, you may have one or more of the following tests.

Fasting blood glucose or random blood glucose test: Your doctor may check your blood glucose level using a test called a fasting blood glucose test. Before this test, your doctor will ask you to fast, which means having nothing to eat or drink except water for at least 8 hours. Or your doctor may check your blood glucose at any time during the day. This is called a random blood glucose test.

These tests can find gestational diabetes in some women, but other tests are needed to be sure diabetes is not missed. Your health care provider will check your blood glucose level to see if you have gestational diabetes.

Screening glucose challenge test: For this test, you will drink a sugary beverage and have your blood glucose level checked an hour later. This test can be done at any time of the day. If the results are above normal, you may need further tests.

Oral glucose tolerance test: If you have this test, your health care provider will give you special instructions to follow. For at least 3 days before the test, you should eat normally. Then you will fast for at least 8 hours before the test.

The health care team will check your blood glucose level before the test. Then you will drink a sugary beverage. The staff will check your blood glucose levels 1 hour, 2 hours, and 3 hours later. If your levels are above normal at least twice during the test, you have gestational diabetes.

How will gestational diabetes affect my baby?

Untreated or uncontrolled gestational diabetes can mean problems for your baby, such as:

- being born very large and with extra fat—this can make delivery difficult and more dangerous for your baby;
- low blood glucose right after birth; and

Table 45.1. Above-Normal Results for the Oral Glucose Tolerance Test

Fasting	95 or higher
At 1 hour	180 or higher
At 2 hours	155 or higher
At 3 hours	140 or higher

Note: Some labs use other numbers for this test. These numbers are for a test using a drink with 100 grams of glucose.

- breathing problems.

If you have gestational diabetes, your health care team may recommend some extra tests to check on your baby, such as:

- an ultrasound exam, to see how your baby is growing; and
- "kick counts" to check your baby's activity (the time between the baby's movements) or special "stress" tests.

Working closely with your health care team will help you give birth to a healthy baby.

Both you and your baby are at increased risk for type 2 diabetes for the rest of your lives.

How will gestational diabetes affect me?

Often, women with gestational diabetes have no symptoms. However, gestational diabetes may:

- increase your risk of high blood pressure during pregnancy; and
- increase your risk of a large baby and the need for cesarean section at delivery.

The good news is your gestational diabetes will probably go away after your baby is born. However, you will be more likely to get type 2 diabetes later in your life. You may also get gestational diabetes again if you get pregnant again.

Some women wonder whether breastfeeding is OK after they have had gestational diabetes. Breastfeeding is recommended for most babies, including those whose mothers had gestational diabetes.

Gestational diabetes is serious, even if you have no symptoms. Taking care of yourself helps keep your baby healthy.

How is gestational diabetes treated?

Treating gestational diabetes means taking steps to keep your blood glucose levels in a target range. You will learn how to control your blood glucose using:

- a meal plan;
- physical activity; and
- insulin (if needed).

Meal plan: You will talk with a dietitian or a diabetes educator who will design a meal plan to help you choose foods that are healthy for you and your baby. Using a meal plan will help keep your blood glucose in your target range. The plan will provide guidelines on which foods to eat, how much to eat, and when to eat. Choices, amounts, and timing are all important in keeping your blood glucose levels in your target range.

You may be advised to:

- limit sweets;

- eat three small meals and one to three snacks every day;

- be careful about when and how much carbohydrate-rich food you eat—your meal plan will tell you when to eat carbohydrates and how much to eat at each meal and snack; and

- include fiber in your meals in the form of fruits, vegetables, and whole-grain crackers, cereals, and bread.

Physical activity: Physical activity, such as walking and swimming, can help you reach your blood glucose targets. Talk with your health care team about the type of activity that is best for you. If you are already active, tell your health care team what you do.

Insulin: Some women with gestational diabetes need insulin, in addition to a meal plan and physical activity, to reach their blood glucose targets. If necessary, your health care team will show you how to give yourself insulin. Insulin is not harmful for your baby. It cannot move from your bloodstream to the baby's.

How will I know whether my blood glucose levels are on target?

Your health care team may ask you to use a small device called a blood glucose meter to check your levels on your own. You will learn:

- how to use the meter;

- how to prick your finger to obtain a drop of blood;

- what your target range is; and

- when to check your blood glucose.

You may be asked to check your blood glucose:

- when you wake up;

379

- just before meals;
- 1 or 2 hours after breakfast;
- 1 or 2 hours after lunch; and
- 1 or 2 hours after dinner.

Table 45.2 shows blood glucose targets for most women with gestational diabetes. Talk with your health care team about whether these targets are right for you.

Table 45.2. Blood Glucose Targets for Most Women with Gestational Diabetes

On awakening	not above 95
1 hour after a meal	not above 140
2 hours after a meal	not above 120

Each time you check your blood glucose, write down the results in a record book. Take the book with you when you visit your health care team. If your results are often out of range, your health care team will suggest ways you can reach your targets.

Will I need to do other tests on my own?

Your health care team may teach you how to test for ketones in your morning urine or in your blood. High levels of ketones are a sign that your body is using your body fat for energy instead of the food you eat. Using fat for energy is not recommended during pregnancy. Ketones may be harmful for your baby.

If your ketone levels are high, your health care providers may suggest that you change the type or amount of food you eat. Or you may need to change your meal times or snack times.

After I have my baby, how can I find out whether my diabetes is gone?

You will probably have a blood glucose test 6 to 12 weeks after your baby is born to see whether you still have diabetes. For most women, gestational diabetes goes away after pregnancy. You are, however, at risk of having gestational diabetes during future pregnancies or getting type 2 diabetes later.

Chapter 46

Gestational Hypertension

What is high blood pressure?

Blood pressure is the amount of force exerted by the blood against the walls of the arteries. A person's blood pressure is considered high when the readings are greater than 140 mm Hg systolic (the top number in the blood pressure reading) or 90 mm Hg diastolic (the bottom number). In general, high blood pressure, or hypertension, contributes to the development of coronary heart disease, stroke, heart failure, and kidney disease.

What are the effects of high blood pressure in pregnancy?

Although many pregnant women with high blood pressure have healthy babies without serious problems, high blood pressure can be dangerous for both the mother and the fetus. Women with pre-existing, or chronic, high blood pressure are more likely to have certain complications during pregnancy than those with normal blood pressure. However, some women develop high blood pressure while they are pregnant (often called gestational hypertension).

The effects of high blood pressure range from mild to severe. High blood pressure can harm the mother's kidneys and other organs, and

---

From "High Blood Pressure in Pregnancy," by the National Heart, Lung and Blood Institute (NHLBI, www.nhlbi.nih.gov), part of the National Institutes of Health. The date of this document is unknown. Reviewed by David A. Cooke, MD, FACP, April 12, 2009 it can cause low birth weight and early delivery. In the most serious cases, the mother develops preeclampsia—or "toxemia of pregnancy"—which can threaten the lives of both the mother and the fetus.

What is preeclampsia?

Preeclampsia is a condition that typically starts after the 20th week of pregnancy and is related to increased blood pressure and protein in the mother's urine (as a result of kidney problems). Preeclampsia affects the placenta, and it can affect the mother's kidney, liver, and brain. When preeclampsia causes seizures, the condition is known as eclampsia—the second leading cause of maternal death in the United States. Preeclampsia is also a leading cause of fetal complications, which include low birth weight, premature birth, and stillbirth.

There is no proven way to prevent preeclampsia. Most women who develop signs of preeclampsia, however, are closely monitored to lessen or avoid related problems. The only way to "cure" preeclampsia is to deliver the baby.

How common are high blood pressure and preeclampsia in pregnancy?

High blood pressure problems occur in 6 percent to 8 percent of all pregnancies in the United States, about 70 percent of which are first-time pregnancies. In 1998, more than 146,320 cases of preeclampsia alone were diagnosed.

Although the proportion of pregnancies with gestational hypertension and eclampsia has remained about the same in the United States over the past decade, the rate of preeclampsia has increased by nearly one-third. This increase is due in part to a rise in the numbers of older mothers and of multiple births, where preeclampsia occurs more frequently. For example, in 1998 birth rates among women ages 30 to 44 and the number of births to women ages 45 and older were at the highest levels in three decades, according to the National Center for Health Statistics. Furthermore, between 1980 and 1998, rates of twin births increased about 50 percent overall and 1,000 percent among women ages 45 to 49; rates of triplet and other higher-order multiple births jumped more than 400 percent overall, and 1,000 percent among women in their 40s.

Who is more likely to develop preeclampsia?

- Women with chronic hypertension (high blood pressure before becoming pregnant)

- Women who developed high blood pressure or preeclampsia during a previous pregnancy, especially if these conditions occurred early in the pregnancy

- Women who are obese prior to pregnancy

- Pregnant women under the age of 20 or over the age of 40

- Women who are pregnant with more than one baby

- Women with diabetes, kidney disease, rheumatoid arthritis, lupus, or scleroderma

How is preeclampsia detected?

Unfortunately, there is no single test to predict or diagnose preeclampsia. Key signs are increased blood pressure and protein in the urine (proteinuria). Other symptoms that seem to occur with preeclampsia include persistent headaches, blurred vision or sensitivity to light, and abdominal pain.

All of these sensations can be caused by other disorders; they can also occur in healthy pregnancies. Regular visits with your doctor help him or her to track your blood pressure and level of protein in your urine, to order and analyze blood tests that detect signs of preeclampsia, and to monitor fetal development more closely.

How can women with high blood pressure prevent problems during pregnancy?

If you are thinking about having a baby and you have high blood pressure, talk first to your doctor or nurse. Taking steps to control your blood pressure before and during pregnancy—and getting regular prenatal care—go a long way toward ensuring your well-being and your baby's health.

Before becoming pregnant:

- Be sure your blood pressure is under control. Lifestyle changes such as limiting your salt intake, participating in regular physical activity, and losing weight if you are overweight can be helpful.

- Discuss with your doctor how hypertension might affect you and your baby during pregnancy, and what you can do to prevent or lessen problems.

- If you take medicines for your blood pressure, ask your doctor whether you should change the amount you take or stop taking them during pregnancy. Experts currently recommend avoiding angiotensin-converting enzyme (ACE) inhibitors and angiotensin II (AII) receptor antagonists during pregnancy; other blood pressure medications may be OK for you to use. Do not, however, stop or change your medicines unless your doctor tells you to do so.

While you are pregnant:

• Obtain regular prenatal medical care.

• Avoid alcohol and tobacco.

• Talk to your doctor about any over-the-counter medications you are taking or are thinking about taking.

Does hypertension or preeclampsia during pregnancy cause long-term heart and blood vessel problems?

The effects of high blood pressure during pregnancy vary depending on the disorder and other factors. According to the National High Blood Pressure Education Program (NHBPEP), preeclampsia does not in general increase a woman's risk for developing chronic hypertension or other heart-related problems. The NHBPEP also reports that in women with normal blood pressure who develop preeclampsia after the 20th week of their first pregnancy, short-term complications— including increased blood pressure—usually go away within about 6 weeks after delivery.

Some women, however, may be more likely to develop high blood pressure or other heart disease later in life. More research is needed to determine the long-term health effects of hypertensive disorders in pregnancy and to develop better methods for identifying, diagnosing, and treating women at risk for these conditions.

Even though high blood pressure and related disorders during pregnancy can be serious, most women with high blood pressure and those who develop preeclampsia have successful pregnancies. Obtaining early and regular prenatal care is the most important thing you can do for you and your baby.

Chapter 47

Hyperemesis Gravidarum (Severe Nausea and Vomiting)

Overview

Hyperemesis gravidarum (HG) is a severe form of nausea and vomiting in pregnancy. It is generally described as unrelenting, excessive pregnancy-related nausea and/or vomiting that prevents adequate intake of food and fluids. If severe and/or inadequately treated, it is typically associated with:

- loss of greater than 5% of pre-pregnancy body weight (usually over 10%);
- dehydration and production of ketones;
- nutritional deficiencies;
- metabolic imbalances;
- difficulty with daily activities.

HG usually extends beyond the first trimester and may resolve by 21 weeks; however, it can last the entire pregnancy in less than half of these women. Complications of vomiting (e.g. gastric ulcers, esophageal bleeding, malnutrition, etc.) may also contribute to and worsen ongoing nausea.

"Understanding Hyperemesis," © 2006 Hyperemesis Education & Research Foundation. All Rights Reserved. For additional information, visit the HER Foundation website at www.helpher.org.

There are numerous theories regarding the etiology of hyperemesis gravidarum. Unfortunately, HG is not fully understood and conclusive research on its potential cause is rare. New theories and findings emerge every year, substantiating that it is a complex physiological disease likely caused by multiple factors.

Diagnosis is usually made by measuring weight loss, checking for ketones, and assessing the overall condition of the mother. If she meets the standard criteria and is having difficulty performing her daily activities, medications and/or other treatments are typically offered.

Treating HG is very challenging and early intervention is critical. HG is a multifaceted disease that should be approached with a broad view of possible etiologies and complications. When treating mothers with HG, preventing and correcting nutritional deficiencies is a high priority to promote a healthy outcome for mother and child.

Most studies examining the risks and outcomes for a pregnant woman with nausea and vomiting in pregnancy find no detrimental effects long-term for milder cases. Those with more severe symptoms that lead to complications, severe weight loss, and/or prolonged nausea and vomiting are at greatest risk of adverse outcomes for both mother and child. The risk increases if medical intervention is inadequate or delayed.

The list of potential complications due to repeated vomiting or severe nausea is extensive, all of which may worsen symptoms. Common complications from nausea and vomiting include debilitating fatigue, gastric irritation, ketosis, and malnutrition. Aggressive care early in pregnancy is very important to prevent these and more life-threatening complications such as central pontine myelinolysis or Wernicke's encephalopathy. After pregnancy and in preparation of future ones, it is important to address any resulting physical and psychological complications.

Hyperemesis gravidarum impacts societies, families, and individuals. Recent, conservative estimations suggest HG costs nearly $200 million annually just for inpatient hospitalization. Considering many women are treated outside the hospital to save costs, the actual cost is likely many times greater. Beyond financial impact, many family relationships dissolve and future family plans are almost always limited. Women often lose their employment because of HG, and women are frequently undertreated and left feeling stigmatized by a disease erroneously presumed to be psychological.

Treatment

Hyperemesis is no doubt a physiological disease. Treating it as anything else is not therapeutic and can be detrimental to the mother and her unborn child. Early, aggressive therapy can often result in fewer complications and reduce overall medical costs. Medications, bed rest, IV (intravenous) fluids, and nutritional therapy are typically the most effective therapies for HG. HG may last throughout pregnancy in varying severity. As each woman is different, it is most critical that therapies target a mother's symptoms and response to treatment.

Women left untreated may terminate a wanted pregnancy to end the misery. Often secondary psychosocial challenges such as depression and anxiety result and complicate management. Depression is a natural consequence of being confined to home or bed, and unable to perform even simple daily activities, much less care for one's family. Further, the accompanying anxiety often results from the thought of vomiting and retching relentlessly for hours, as well as feeling severely nauseous in between. Many women fear dying and feel guilty that they may cause the death of their unborn child if they don't force feed themselves, despite the inevitable vomiting that will follow. Treating the complex physiological changes that cause such severe symptoms can be very challenging.

Further, each woman will respond differently to treatments since the cause is multifactorial, so a single medication cannot be prescribed. It is becoming clear that proactive intervention with a treatment plan, can decrease both severity and duration, not to mention prevent many complications for many women. The challenge is finding the treatment that works for each woman.

The general good care of women with severe hyperemesis extends beyond the use of steroid therapy. Thiamine replacement, possibly with other water-soluble vitamins is required if vomiting has been prolonged in order to avoid Wernicke's encephalopathy. Deficiency can arise after lack of food intake for several weeks. Thiamine is an essential cofactor for critical enzymes of carbohydrate metabolism and it is important that it is replaced before carbohydrate is given. However, once thiamine has been replaced, provision of calories as IV 10% Dextrose (which provides 400 kcal/L) hastens recovery. Significant heartburn is frequently caused by the regurgitated gastric acid and this requires treatment with ranitidine. Finally, mobilization must be gradual as physical movement exacerbates the underlying nausea. Discharge is not wise as soon as IV fluids are no longer necessary, as this may be associated with loss of control precipitated by the journey home. Full and sympathetic explanation of the condition and likely prognosis is also part of routine management. [Al-Ozairi MBChB MRCP, E., Waugh MBBS MRCOG, J. J. S. , & Taylor MD FRCP, R. (2009). Termination is not the treatment of choice for severe hyperemesis gravidarum: Successful management using prednisolone. *Obstetric Medicine.* 2, 34–37.]

The HER Foundation Survey found bed rest and IV hydration to be two of the most beneficial treatments for HG. This does not mean these alone are adequate, rather these are nearly universally beneficial in women with HG. IV fluids can be given at home in some countries at very low cost and minimal risk. Fluids can also include much-needed vitamins. Insurance coverage often includes home IV care which allows the mother to have continuous fluids instead of cycling from hydration to vomiting and dehydration. This cycle worsens HG and delays recovery. Many women state they feel so much better after their trip to the emergency room for IV fluids, only to begin vomiting and have to return a few days later for more fluids. Home IV fluids can prevent this. A regular IV can be left in for up to a week, provided it does not infiltrate or become infected. Many doctors are not aware of the concept of stopping the dehydration cycle to avoid exacerbation of HG. Any mother producing ketones or exhibiting signs of dehydration should receive IV fluids, preferably with IV vitamins. Vitamins are critical in mothers vomiting more than a few weeks to prevent life-altering complications.

- **Medications:** Antiemetic (anti-vomiting) medications are the most common and typically most effective treatments for HG. The risks are often outweighed by the benefits.

- **Allergy treatments:** Sometimes HG symptoms can be managed with allergy management procedures.

- **Complementary and alternative medicine (CAM):** CAM is sometimes effective in easing nausea and vomiting in milder cases of HG, however, it most often is used in conjunction with allopathic medicine (traditional medical care).

- **Nutritional therapies:** Research shows that nausea and vomiting for more than a few weeks causes significant deficiency of important nutrients, which can worsen nausea and vomiting. If not replaced, a woman is at risk for more complications and a prolonged recovery. These can be replaced via an intravenous (IV) line or directly into the gastrointestinal (stomach/intestines) system.

- **Behavioral therapy:** This therapy uses stimulus control and imaging procedures and is sometimes used in mild cases with positive effects.

- **Bed rest:** Prolonged bed rest can produce negative effects like atrophy and a delayed recovery time after delivery. The best strategy is to do all you can to get effective care and stay as mobile as possible. Physical therapy may be beneficial.

- **Sensory deprivation therapy (SDT):** This is essentially placing a woman in a room without any interaction or stimulation of any kind. She is denied any visitors such as her family for days or weeks. This is cruel and ineffective for true cases of HG. Isolation and secondary depression only worsen HG and increase the stress on a woman. It should not be used. However, since odors, noise, and light may worsen her symptoms, it is helpful to minimize as much as she requests.

- **Psychotherapy:** This treatment may be effective for secondary complications such as depression and anxiety, if used in conjunction with antiemetic medications and hydration. It should never be used as a primary modality for cases of HG. It is helpful to some women to manage feelings related to HG, or with normal adjustments related to pregnancy and motherhood. Further, it is often very helpful postpartum to manage PPD [postpartum depression] and PTSD [posttraumatic stress disorder]. Since HG is not a psychological disorder, this therapy must follow symptom management.

- **Therapeutic abortion:** Abortion in most cases of HG is avoidable with aggressive use of the available treatment options. Women who choose abortion do so most often because of ineffective or inadequate treatment. Women left untreated sometimes become so metabolically imbalanced, abortion is chosen to save the life of the mother. However, it should be considered only a last resort. The long term consequences cannot be overlooked or underestimated.

- **Other treatments:** Women with HG have numerous other symptoms that often cause significant distress. One is ptyalism (also called hypersalivation, sialorrhea, or hyperptyalism). Ptyalism is essentially an overproduction of saliva thought to be caused by increased hormone levels. It happens in non-HG pregnancies as well and worsens nausea. There are few treatments and most women just tolerate it by spitting into a cup or tissue. In severe cases, a suction machine may be prescribed to avoid skin irritation on the lips and chin from constant exposure to saliva. Other issues are pain from prolonged periods of inactivity, which are typically managed with over the counter pain relievers like Tylenol.

Complications

Although numerous depending on one's individual biochemistry, severity of symptoms, and the medical interventions given, many potential complications may result from HG. With an aggressive and proactive approach to treatment, many sequelae can be avoided. If care is inadequate, ineffective, or delayed, cases of morning sickness or mild HG may progress to moderate or severe HG. Women suffer greatly with HG, and effective intervention early in pregnancy can greatly ease the misery and stress associated with this disease.

Long term complications (often with vague, chronic symptomology) will likely occur without proper intervention in the early stages. Fortunately, there are usually few immediate, adverse effects of HG on the baby unless weight gain continues to be poor during the second half of pregnancy, or symptoms are severe and prolonged. Acute or chronic complications reported by women to the HER Foundation include gall bladder disease, temporomandibular joint disorders, depression, anxiety, difficulty with weight management, diabetes, motion sickness, and dental caries. Some just say they never have felt the same as before they were pregnant. Women with prolonged HG are also at greater risk for preterm labor, and pre-eclampsia.

Emerging research is showing the possibility of potential future health risks to the infant if the mother is malnourished during pregnancy. This should strongly be considered when caring for women with HG, as the care provided affects not only the mother, but also the child for decades to come.

Signs of Severe HG

- Debilitating, chronic nausea
- Frequent vomiting of bile or blood
- Chronic ketosis and dehydration
- Muscle weakness and extreme fatigue
- Medication does not stop vomiting/nausea
- Inability to care for self (shower, prepare food)
- Loss of over 5–10% of your pre-pregnancy weight
- Weight loss (or little gain) after the first trimester
- Inability to eat/drink sufficiently by about 14 weeks

Chapter 48

Placental Complications

The placenta is an unborn baby's life support system. It forms from the same cells as the embryo and attaches to the wall of the uterus. The placenta forms connections with the mother's blood supply, from which it supplies oxygen and nutrients to the fetus. The placenta also connects with the fetus's blood supply, from which it removes wastes and returns them to the mother's blood. The mother's kidneys dispose of the waste. The placenta has other important functions in pregnancy. It produces hormones that play a role in triggering labor and delivery. The placenta also helps protect the fetus from infections and potentially harmful substances. After the baby is delivered, the placenta's job is done, and it is delivered as the afterbirth.

The mature placenta is flat and circular and weighs about 1 pound. But sometimes the placenta:

- is structured abnormally;

- is poorly positioned in the uterus;

- does not function properly.

Placental problems are among the most common complications of the second half of pregnancy. Here are some of the most frequent placental problems and how they can affect mother and baby.

"Placental Complications," © 2007 March of Dimes Birth Defects Foundation. All rights reserved. For additional information, contact the March of Dimes at their website www.marchofdimes.com.

What is placental abruption?

Placental abruption (sometimes called abruptio placentae) is a condition in which the placenta peels away from the uterine wall, partially or almost completely, before delivery. Mild cases may cause few problems, but severe cases can deprive the fetus of oxygen and nutrients. Severe cases also can cause bleeding in the mother that can endanger both her and the baby.

Placental abruption increases the risk of premature birth (birth before 37 completed weeks gestation). Studies suggest that abruption contributes to about 10 percent of premature births.[1] Premature babies are at increased risk for health problems during the newborn period, lasting disabilities, and even death. Abruption also increases the risk for poor fetal growth and stillbirth.[1]

How common is placental abruption?

Abruption occurs in about 1 in 100 pregnancies.[2] It occurs most often in the third trimester, but it can happen any time after about 20 weeks of pregnancy.

What are the symptoms of abruption?

The main sign of placental abruption is vaginal bleeding. A pregnant woman should contact her health care provider if she has vaginal bleeding.

The pregnant woman also may experience uterine discomfort and tenderness or sudden, continuous abdominal pain. In a few cases, these symptoms may occur without vaginal bleeding because the blood is trapped behind the placenta.

How is placental abruption diagnosed?

If the health care provider suspects an abruption, she probably will recommend that the woman go to the hospital for a complete evaluation. The provider will do a physical examination and, most likely, an ultrasound examination. An ultrasound can detect many, but not all, cases of abruption.

How is placental abruption treated?

How a woman is treated depends on the severity of the abruption and her stage of pregnancy.

A mild abruption usually is not dangerous unless it progresses. If a woman has a mild abruption at term, her health care provider may recommend prompt delivery (either by inducing labor or by c- [Cesarean] section) to avoid any risks associated with a worsening abruption.

If a woman has a mild abruption and her fetus would be very premature if delivered immediately, her provider will probably admit her to the hospital for careful monitoring. If tests show that neither mother nor baby is having difficulties, the provider may try to prolong the pregnancy to avoid prematurity-related complications for the baby.

If the provider suspects that the abruption is likely to result in premature delivery between 24 and 34 weeks of pregnancy, she will probably recommend treatment with drugs called corticosteroids. These drugs speed maturation of the fetal lungs and significantly reduce the risk of prematurity-related complications and infant deaths.

Some women with mild abruptions may be able to go home after the bleeding stops, while others may need to stay in the hospital until delivery.[1]

If an abruption progresses, a woman is bleeding heavily, or the baby is having difficulties, a prompt delivery, usually by c-section, probably will be necessary.

What causes placental abruption?

The cause of abruption is unknown. However, the following factors can increase a woman's risk for abruption.[1,3]

- High blood pressure
- Cocaine use
- Cigarette smoking
- Abdominal trauma (such as may occur with an automobile accident or abuse)
- Certain abnormalities of the uterus or umbilical cord
- Being more than 35 years of age
- Pregnant with twins, triplets, or more
- Premature rupture of the membranes (bag of waters)
- Having too little amniotic fluid
- Having certain inherited disorders of blood clotting
- Having an infection involving the uterus

What is the risk of an abruption happening again in another pregnancy?

A woman who has had an abruption has about a 10 percent chance of it happening again in a later pregnancy.[1]

What can a woman do to reduce her risk for abruption?

In most cases, abruption cannot be prevented. However, these steps may help a woman reduce her risk:

- Keep high blood pressure under control. Women who have high blood pressure should see their health care provider regularly and take medication, if recommended. Women who are not yet pregnant should see their provider for a preconception checkup to get their blood pressure under control right from the start.

- Avoid cigarettes and cocaine. These contribute to abruption and other pregnancy complications.

- Wear a seat belt. This can help prevent trauma resulting from auto accidents.

- Discuss possible treatments for blood clotting disorders with a health care provider. Some women with inherited blood clotting disorders may benefit from treatment, for example with blood-thinning drugs, during pregnancy.[1] Some providers recommend treatment to affected women who have had an abruption or other pregnancy complication that may be linked with a blood-clotting disorder.

What is placenta previa?

Placenta previa is a low-lying placenta that covers part or all of the opening of the cervix. This positioning of the placenta can block the baby's exit from the uterus. As the cervix begins to thin and dilate in preparation for labor, blood vessels that connect the abnormally placed placenta to the uterus may tear, resulting in bleeding. During labor and delivery, bleeding can be severe, endangering mother and baby.

As with placental abruption, placenta previa can result in the birth of a premature baby.

How common is placenta previa?

Placenta previa occurs in about 1 in 200 pregnancies.[4]

What are the symptoms of placenta previa?

The most common symptom of placenta previa is painless uterine bleeding during the second half of pregnancy. Women who experience vaginal bleeding in pregnancy should contact their health care provider.

How is placenta previa diagnosed?

An ultrasound examination can diagnose placenta previa and pinpoint the placenta's location. The provider usually avoids doing a vaginal examination when placenta previa is suspected because the examination may trigger heavy bleeding.

Some women who have not experienced vaginal bleeding learn during a routine ultrasound examination that they have a low-lying placenta. A pregnant woman should not be too worried if this happens to her, especially if she is in the first half of pregnancy. More than 90 percent of the time, placenta previa diagnosed in the second trimester corrects itself by term.[3,4]

How is placenta previa treated?

How a woman with placenta previa is treated depends on her stage of pregnancy, the severity of the bleeding, and the condition of mother and baby. The goal, whenever possible, is to prolong pregnancy until the baby is at or near full term. Cesarean delivery is recommended for nearly all women with placenta previa because c-sections usually can prevent severe bleeding.

When a woman develops significant bleeding due to placenta previa after about 34 weeks of pregnancy, her provider may recommend a prompt c-section. Babies born after this time usually do well, though some have mild prematurity-related health problems during the newborn period.

Women who develop bleeding as a result of placenta previa before about 34 weeks are generally admitted to the hospital, where they can be monitored closely. If tests show that mother and baby are doing well, the provider will probably attempt to prolong the pregnancy. In some cases, when there has been a significant amount of bleeding, the mother may be treated with blood transfusions. She also will be treated with corticosteroid drugs if she is likely to deliver before 34 weeks.

Some women are able to go home after bleeding stops, but others must remain in the hospital until delivery. At 36 to 37 weeks, if she hasn't delivered, the provider may suggest a test of the amniotic fluid (obtained by amniocentesis) to see if the baby's lungs are mature. If they are, the provider will likely recommend a c-section at that time to prevent risks associated with any future bleeding episodes.

At any stage of pregnancy, a prompt c-section may be necessary if the mother develops dangerously heavy bleeding, or if mother or baby is having difficulties.

What causes placenta previa?

The cause of placenta previa is unknown. However, certain factors can increase a woman's risk.[3,4]

- Cigarette smoking

- Cocaine use

- Being more than 35 years of age

- Second or later pregnancy

- Previous uterine surgery, including a c-section; a D&C (dilation and curettage, in which the lining of the uterus is scraped), which is often done following a miscarriage or during an abortion

- Pregnant with twins, triplets, or more

What is the risk of placenta previa happening again in another pregnancy?

A woman who has had a placenta previa in a previous pregnancy has a two to three percent chance of a recurrence.[3]

Can a woman reduce her risk for placenta previa?

There is no way to prevent placenta previa. However, a woman may be able to reduce her risk by avoiding using cigarettes and cocaine. She also may be able to reduce her risk in future pregnancies by avoiding having an elective c-section (i.e., a c-section scheduled for convenience), unless there is a medical reason.

What is placenta accreta?

Placenta accreta refers to a placenta that implants too deeply and too firmly into the uterine wall. Similarly, placenta increta and percreta refer to a placenta that imbeds itself even more deeply into

uterine muscle or through the entire thickness of the uterus, sometimes extending into nearby structures, such as the bladder.

How common are placenta accreta and related disorders?

These disorders occur in about 1 in 2,500 deliveries.[4] They sometimes lead to the birth of a premature baby.

What are the symptoms of placenta accreta and related disorders?

Like placenta previa, these disorders often cause vaginal bleeding
in the third trimester.

Who is at risk for placenta accreta and related disorders?

These disorders occur most frequently in women who have placenta
previa in the current pregnancy and also have a history of one or more
c-sections or other uterine surgery.[4]

How are placenta accreta and related disorders diagnosed?

These disorders can be diagnosed with an ultrasound examination.
In some cases, another imaging technique called magnetic resonance
imaging (MRI) may be recommended.[4]

How are placenta accreta and related disorders treated?

In these disorders, the placenta does not completely separate from
the uterus as it should following the delivery of the baby. This can lead
to dangerous hemorrhage following vaginal delivery. The placenta
usually must be surgically removed to stop the bleeding, and often a
hysterectomy (removal of the uterus) is necessary.

When placenta accreta is diagnosed before birth, a c-section immediately followed by a hysterectomy may be planned in order to reduce blood loss and complications in the mother. In some cases, other
surgical procedures can be used to save the uterus.

What are some other placental problems?

In some cases the placenta may not develop correctly or function
as well as it should. It may be too thin, too thick or have an extra lobe,

or the membranes may be improperly attached. Or problems can occur during pregnancy that damage the placenta, including infections, blood clots, and areas of tissue destruction (infarcts). These placental abnormalities can contribute to a number of complications, such as miscarriage, poor fetal growth, prematurity, maternal hemorrhage at delivery and, possibly, birth defects. A doctor often will examine the placenta following delivery or send it to the laboratory, especially if the newborn has certain complications, such as poor growth, to help diagnose the cause of the problem.

Does the March of Dimes support research on placental conditions?

March of Dimes grantees are studying how certain infections, such as cytomegalovirus (CMV), may damage the placenta, possibly contributing to miscarriage, poor fetal growth, and birth defects, such as cerebral palsy.

Others are exploring how certain genes regulate the development and function of the placenta in order to develop ways to prevent miscarriages, growth problems, and premature births, which may result from placental abnormalities.

References

1. Oyelese, Y. and Ananth, C.V. Placental Abruption. *Obstetrics and Gynecology*, volume 108, number 4, October 2006, pages 1005–1016.

2. Ananth, C.V., et al. Placental Abruption in Term and Preterm Gestations. *Obstetrics and Gynecology,* volume 107, number 4, April 2006, pages 785–792.

3. Kay, H.H. Placenta Previa and Abruption, in Scott, J.R., et al. (eds.): *Danforth's Obstetrics and Gynecology,* Ninth Edition, Philadelphia, Lippincott Williams & Wilkins, 2003, pages 365–379.

4. Oyelese, Y. and Smulian, J.C. Placenta Previa, Placenta Accreta, and Vasa Previa. *Obstetrics and Gynecology,* volume 107, number 4, April 2006, pages 927–941.

Chapter 49

Rh Incompatibility

If you just found out you're pregnant, one of the first—and most important—tests you should expect is a blood-type test. This basic test determines your blood type and Rh factor. Your Rh factor may play a role in your baby's health, so it's important to know this information early in your pregnancy.

About the Rh Factor

People with different blood types have proteins specific to that blood type on the surfaces of their red blood cells (RBCs). There are four blood types—A, B, AB, and O.

Each of the four blood types is additionally classified according to the presence of another protein on the surface of RBCs that indicates the Rh factor. If you carry this protein, you are Rh positive. If you don't carry the protein, you are Rh negative.

Most people—about 85%—are Rh positive. But if a woman who is Rh negative and a man who is Rh positive conceive a baby, there is the potential for a baby to have a health problem. The baby growing inside the Rh-negative mother may have Rh-positive blood, inherited from the father. Approximately half of the children born to an Rh-negative mother and Rh-positive father will be Rh positive.

Rh incompatibility usually isn't a problem if it's the mother's first pregnancy because, unless there's some sort of abnormality, the fetus's blood does not normally enter the mother's circulatory system during the course of the pregnancy.

However, during delivery, the mother's and baby's blood can intermingle. If this happens, the mother's body recognizes the Rh protein as a foreign substance and can begin producing antibodies (protein molecules in the immune system that recognize, and later work to destroy, foreign substances) against the Rh proteins introduced into her blood.

Other ways Rh-negative pregnant women can be exposed to the Rh protein that might cause antibody production include blood transfusions with Rh-positive blood, miscarriage, and ectopic pregnancy.

Rh antibodies are harmless until the mother's second or later pregnancies. If she is ever carrying another Rh-positive child, her Rh antibodies will recognize the Rh proteins on the surface of the baby's blood cells as foreign, and pass into the baby's bloodstream and attack those cells. This can lead to swelling and rupture of the baby's RBCs. A baby's blood count can get dangerously low when this condition, known as hemolytic or Rh disease of the newborn, occurs.

Preventing and Treating Rh Disease of the Newborn

In generations past, Rh incompatibility was a very serious problem. Fortunately, significant medical advances have been made to help prevent complications from Rh incompatibility and to treat any newborn affected by Rh disease.

Today, when a woman with the potential to develop Rh incompatibility is pregnant, doctors administer a series of two Rh immune-globulin shots during her first pregnancy. The first shot is given around the 28th week of pregnancy and the second within 72 hours after giving birth. Rh immune-globulin acts like a vaccine, preventing the mother's body from producing any potentially dangerous Rh antibodies that can cause serious complications in the newborn or complicate any future pregnancies.

A dose of Rh immune-globulin may also be given if a woman has a miscarriage, an amniocentesis, or any bleeding during pregnancy.

If a doctor determines that a woman has already developed Rh antibodies, then the pregnancy will be closely monitored to make sure that those levels are not too high. In rare cases, if the incompatibility is severe and the baby is in danger, a series of special blood transfusions (called exchange transfusions) can be performed either while the baby is still in the uterus or after delivery.

Exchange transfusions replace the baby's blood with RBCs that are Rh-negative. This procedure stabilizes the baby's level of red blood cells and minimizes further damage caused by circulating Rh antibodies already present in the baby's bloodstream.

Because of the success rate of the Rh immune-globulin shots, exchange transfusions are needed in fewer than 1% of Rh-incompatible pregnancies in the United States today.

If Rh Disease Is Not Prevented

Rh incompatibility rarely causes complications in a first pregnancy and does not affect the health of the mother. But Rh antibodies that develop during subsequent pregnancies can be potentially dangerous to mother and child. Rh disease can result in severe anemia, jaundice, brain damage, and heart failure in a newborn. In extreme cases, it can cause the death of the fetus because too many RBCs have been destroyed.

If you're not sure what your Rh factor is and think you're pregnant, it's important to start regular prenatal care as soon as possible— including blood-type testing. With early detection and treatment of Rh incompatibility, you can focus on more important things—like welcoming a new, healthy baby into your household.

Chapter 50

Umbilical Cord Abnormalities

The umbilical cord is a narrow tube-like structure that connects the fetus (developing baby) to the placenta (afterbirth). The cord is sometimes called the baby's "supply line" because it carries the baby's blood back and forth, between the baby and the placenta. It delivers nutrients and oxygen to the baby and removes the baby's waste products.

The umbilical cord begins to form at five weeks after conception. It becomes progressively longer until 28 weeks of pregnancy, reaching an average length of 22 to 24 inches.[1] As the cord gets longer, it generally coils around itself. The cord contains three blood vessels: two arteries and one vein.

- The vein carries oxygen and nutrients from the placenta (which connects to the mother's blood supply) to the baby.

- The two arteries transport waste from the baby to the placenta (where waste is transferred to the mother's blood and disposed of by her kidneys).

A gelatin-like tissue called Wharton's jelly cushions and protects these blood vessels.

A number of abnormalities can affect the umbilical cord. The cord may be too long or too short. It may connect improperly to the placenta or become knotted or compressed. Cord abnormalities can lead to problems during pregnancy or during labor and delivery.

In some cases, cord abnormalities are discovered before delivery during an ultrasound. However, they usually are not discovered until after delivery when the cord is examined directly. The following are the most frequent cord abnormalities and their possible effects on mother and baby.

What is single umbilical artery?

About 1 percent of singleton and about 5 percent of multiple pregnancies (twins, triplets, or more) have an umbilical cord that contains only two blood vessels, instead of the normal three. In these cases, one artery is missing.[2] The cause of this abnormality, called single umbilical artery, is unknown.

Studies suggest that babies with single umbilical artery have an increased risk for birth defects, including heart, central nervous system and urinary-tract defects, and chromosomal abnormalities.[2,3] A woman whose baby is diagnosed with single umbilical artery during a routine ultrasound may be offered certain prenatal tests to diagnose or rule out birth defects. These tests may include a detailed ultrasound, amniocentesis (to check for chromosomal abnormalities) and in some cases, echocardiography (a special type of ultrasound to evaluate the fetal heart). The provider also may recommend that the baby have an ultrasound after birth.

What is umbilical cord prolapse?

Umbilical cord prolapse occurs when the cord slips into the vagina after the membranes (bag of waters) have ruptured, before the baby descends into the birth canal. This complication affects about 1 in 300 births.[1] The baby can put pressure on the cord as he passes through the cervix and vagina during labor and delivery. Pressure on the cord reduces or cuts off blood flow from the placenta to the baby, decreasing the baby's oxygen supply. Umbilical cord prolapse can result in stillbirth unless the baby is delivered promptly, usually by cesarean section.

If the woman's membranes rupture and she feels something in her vagina, she should go to the hospital immediately or, in the United States, call 911. A health care provider may suspect umbilical cord prolapse if the fetus develops heart rate abnormalities after the membranes have ruptured. The provider can confirm a cord prolapse by doing a pelvic examination. Cord prolapse is an emergency. Pressure on the cord must be relieved immediately by lifting the presenting fetal part away from the cord while preparing the woman for prompt cesarean delivery.

The risk of umbilical cord prolapse increases if:

- the baby is in a breech (foot-first) position;

- the woman is in preterm labor;

- the umbilical cord is too long;

- there is too much amniotic fluid;

- the provider ruptures the membranes to start or speed up labor;

- the woman is delivering twins vaginally. The second twin is more commonly affected.

What is vasa previa?

Vasa previa occurs when one or more blood vessels from the umbilical cord or placenta cross the cervix underneath the baby. The blood vessels, unprotected by the Wharton's jelly in the umbilical cord or the tissue in the placenta, sometimes tear when the cervix dilates or the membranes rupture. This can result in life-threatening bleeding in the baby. Even if the blood vessels do not tear, the baby may suffer from lack of oxygen due to pressure on the blood vessels. Vasa previa occurs in 1 in 2,500 births.[4]

When vasa previa is diagnosed unexpectedly at delivery, more than half of affected babies are stillborn.[4] However, when vasa previa is diagnosed by ultrasound earlier in pregnancy, fetal deaths generally can be prevented by delivering the baby by cesarean section at about 35 weeks of gestation.[4]

Pregnant women with vasa previa sometimes have painless vaginal bleeding in the second or third trimester. A pregnant woman who experiences vaginal bleeding should always report it to her health care provider so that the cause can be determined and any necessary steps taken to protect the baby.

A pregnant woman may be at increased risk for vasa previa if she:

- has a velamentous insertion of the cord (the umbilical cord inserts abnormally into the fetal membranes, instead of the center of the placenta);

- has placenta previa (a low-lying placenta that covers part or all of the cervix) or certain other placental abnormalities;

- is expecting more than one baby.

What is a nuchal cord?

About 25 percent of babies are born with a nuchal cord (the umbilical cord wrapped around the baby's neck).[1] A nuchal cord, also called nuchal loops, rarely causes any problems. Babies with a nuchal cord are generally healthy.

Sometimes fetal monitoring shows heart rate abnormalities during labor and delivery in babies with a nuchal cord. This may reflect pressure on the cord. However, the pressure is rarely serious enough to cause death or any lasting problems, although occasionally a cesarean delivery may be needed.

Less frequently, the umbilical cord becomes wrapped around other parts of the baby's body, such as a foot or hand. Generally, this doesn't harm the baby.

What are umbilical cord knots?

About 1 percent of babies are born with one or more knots in the umbilical cord.[1] Some knots form during delivery when a baby with a nuchal cord is pulled through the loop. Others form during pregnancy when the baby moves around. Knots occur most often when the umbilical cord is too long and in identical-twin pregnancies. Identical twins share a single amniotic sac, and the babies' cords can become entangled.

As long as the knot remains loose, it generally does not harm the baby. However, sometimes the knot or knots can be pulled tight, cutting off the baby's oxygen supply. Cord knots result in miscarriage or stillbirth in 5 percent of cases.[1] During labor and delivery, a tightening knot can cause the baby to have heart rate abnormalities that are detected by fetal monitoring. In some cases, a cesarean delivery may be necessary.

What is an umbilical cord cyst?

Umbilical cord cysts are outpockets in the cord. They are found in about 3 percent of pregnancies.[2]

There are true and false cysts:

- True cysts are lined with cells and generally contain remnants of early embryonic structures.

- False cysts are fluid-filled sacs that can be related to a swelling of the Wharton's jelly.

Studies suggest that both types of cysts are sometimes associated with birth defects, including chromosomal abnormalities and kidney and abdominal defects.[2] When a cord cyst is found during an ultrasound, the provider may recommend additional tests, such as amniocentesis and a detailed ultrasound, to diagnose or rule out birth defects.

Does the March of Dimes support research on umbilical cord abnormalities?

The March of Dimes continues to support research aimed at preventing umbilical cord abnormalities and the complications they cause. One grantee is studying the development of blood vessels in the umbilical cord for insight into the causes of single umbilical artery and other cord abnormalities. The goals of this study are to:

- develop a better understanding of the causes of birth defects;

- develop treatments to help prevent oxygen deprivation before and during delivery, which may contribute to cerebral palsy and other forms of brain damage.

References

1. Cruikshank, D.W. Breech, Other Malpresentations, and Umbilical Cord Complications, in: Scott, J.R., et al. (eds.), *Danforth's Obstetrics and Gynecology,* 9th Edition. Philadelphia, Lippincott Williams and Wilkins, 2003, pages 381–395.

2. Morgan, B.L.G. and Ross, M.G. Umbilical Cord Complications. emedicine.com, March 1, 2006.

3. Gossett, D.R., et al. Antenatal Diagnosis of Single Umbilical Artery: Is Fetal Echocardiography Warranted? *Obstetrics and Gynecology,* volume 100, number 5, November 2002, pages 903–908.

4. Oyelese, Y. and Smulian, J.C. Placenta Previa, Placenta Accreta, and Vasa Previa. *Obstetrics and Gynecology,* volume 107, number 4, April 2006, pages 927–941.

Chapter 51

Overview of Sexually Transmitted Diseases (STDs) during Pregnancy

Can pregnant women become infected with STDs?

Yes, women who are pregnant can become infected with the same sexually transmitted diseases (STDs) as women who are not pregnant. Pregnancy does not provide women or their babies any protection against STDs. The consequences of an STD can be significantly more serious, even life threatening, for a woman and her baby if the woman becomes infected with an STD while pregnant. It is important that women be aware of the harmful effects of STDs and know how to protect themselves and their children against infection.

How common are STDs in pregnant women in the United States?

Some STDs, such as genital herpes and bacterial vaginosis, are quite common in pregnant women in the United States. Other STDs, notably HIV [human immunodeficiency virus] and syphilis, are much less common in pregnant women. Table 51.1 shows the estimated number of pregnant women in the United States who are infected with specific STDs each year.

From "STDs & Pregnancy," by the Centers for Disease Control and Prevention (CDC, www.cdc.gov), January 4, 2008.

Table 51.1. Pregnant Women Infected with STDs Each Year

STDs	Estimated Number of Pregnant Women
Bacterial vaginosis	1,080,000
Herpes simplex virus 2	880,000
Chlamydia	100,000
Trichomoniasis	124,000
Gonorrhea	13,200
Hepatitis B	16,000
HIV	6,400
Syphilis	<1,000

How do STDs affect a pregnant woman and her baby?

STDs can have many of the same consequences for pregnant women as women who are not pregnant. STDs can cause cervical and other cancers, chronic hepatitis, pelvic inflammatory disease, infertility, and other complications. Many STDs in women are silent; that is, without signs or symptoms.

STDs can be passed from a pregnant woman to the baby before, during, or after the baby's birth. Some STDs (like syphilis) cross the placenta and infect the baby while it is in the uterus (womb). Other STDs (like gonorrhea, chlamydia, hepatitis B, and genital herpes) can be transmitted from the mother to the baby during delivery as the baby passes through the birth canal. HIV can cross the placenta during pregnancy, infect the baby during the birth process, and unlike most other STDs, can infect the baby through breastfeeding.

A pregnant woman with an STD may also have early onset of labor, premature rupture of the membranes surrounding the baby in the uterus, and uterine infection after delivery.

The harmful effects of STDs in babies may include stillbirth (a baby that is born dead), low birth weight (less than five pounds), conjunctivitis (eye infection), pneumonia, neonatal sepsis (infection in the baby's blood stream), neurologic damage, blindness, deafness, acute hepatitis, meningitis, chronic liver disease, and cirrhosis. Most of these problems can be prevented if the mother receives routine prenatal care, which includes screening tests for STDs starting early in pregnancy and repeated close to delivery, if necessary. Other problems can be treated if the infection is found at birth.

Should pregnant women be tested for STDs?

Yes, STDs affect women of every socioeconomic and educational level, age, race, ethnicity, and religion. The CDC 2006 Guidelines for Treatment of Sexually Transmitted Diseases recommend that pregnant women be screened on their first prenatal visit for STDs which may include the following:

- Chlamydia
- Gonorrhea
- Hepatitis B
- HIV
- Syphilis

In addition, some experts recommend that women who have had a premature delivery in the past be screened and treated for bacterial vaginosis at the first prenatal visit.

Pregnant women should ask their doctors about getting tested for these STDs, since some doctors do not routinely perform these tests. New and increasingly accurate tests continue to become available. Even if a woman has been tested in the past, she should be tested again when she becomes pregnant.

Can STDs be treated during pregnancy?

Chlamydia, gonorrhea, syphilis, trichomoniasis, and bacterial vaginosis (BV) can be treated and cured with antibiotics during pregnancy. There is no cure for viral STDs, such as genital herpes and HIV, but antiviral medication may be appropriate for pregnant women with herpes and definitely is for those with HIV. For women who have active genital herpes lesions at the time of delivery, a cesarean delivery (C-section) may be performed to protect the newborn against infection. C-section is also an option for some HIV-infected women. Women who test negative for hepatitis B, may receive the hepatitis B vaccine during pregnancy.

How can pregnant women protect themselves against infection?

The surest way to avoid transmission of sexually transmitted diseases is to abstain from sexual contact, or to be in a long-term

411

mutually monogamous relationship with a partner who has been tested and is known to be uninfected.

Latex condoms, when used consistently and correctly, are highly effective in preventing transmission of HIV, the virus that causes AIDS. Latex condoms, when used consistently and correctly, can reduce the risk of transmission of gonorrhea, chlamydia, and trichomoniasis. Correct and consistent use of latex condoms can reduce the risk of genital herpes, syphilis, and chancroid only when the infected area or site of potential exposure is protected by the condom. Correct and consistent use of latex condoms may reduce the risk for genital human papillomavirus (HPV) and associated diseases (e.g., warts and cervical cancer).

Chapter 52

Hepatitis B and Pregnancy

Chapter Contents

Section 52.1

What Is Hepatitis?

From "Viral Hepatitis," by the Centers for Disease
Control and Prevention (CDC, www.cdc.gov), July 22, 2008.

Hepatitis A

Hepatitis A is an acute liver disease caused by the hepatitis A virus (HAV), lasting from a few weeks to several months. It does not lead to chronic infection.

- **Transmission:** Ingestion of fecal matter, even in microscopic amounts, from close person-to-person contact or ingestion of contaminated food or drinks.

- **Vaccination:** Hepatitis A vaccination is recommended for all children starting at age 1 year, travelers to certain countries, and others at risk.

Hepatitis B

Hepatitis B is a liver disease caused by the hepatitis B virus (HBV). It ranges in severity from a mild illness, lasting a few weeks (acute), to a serious long-term (chronic) illness that can lead to liver disease or liver cancer.

- **Transmission:** Contact with infectious blood, semen, and other body fluids from having sex with an infected person, sharing contaminated needles to inject drugs, or from an infected mother to her newborn.

- **Vaccination:** Hepatitis B vaccination is recommended for all infants, older children and adolescents who were not vaccinated previously, and adults at risk for HBV infection.

Hepatitis C

Hepatitis C is a liver disease caused by the hepatitis C virus (HCV). HCV infection sometimes results in an acute illness, but most often becomes a chronic condition that can lead to cirrhosis of the liver and liver cancer.

- **Transmission:** Contact with the blood of an infected person, primarily through sharing contaminated needles to inject drugs.

- **Vaccination:** There is no vaccine for hepatitis C.

Hepatitis D

Hepatitis D is a serious liver disease caused by the hepatitis D virus (HDV) and relies on HBV to replicate. It is uncommon in the United States.

- **Transmission:** Contact with infectious blood, similar to how HBV is spread.

- **Vaccination:** There is no vaccine for hepatitis D.

Hepatitis E

Hepatitis E is a serious liver disease caused by the hepatitis E virus (HEV) that usually results in an acute infection. It does not lead to a chronic infection. While rare in the United States, hepatitis E is common in many parts of the world.

- **Transmission:** Ingestion of fecal matter, even in microscopic amounts; outbreaks are usually associated with contaminated water supply in countries with poor sanitation.

- **Vaccination:** There is currently no FDA [U.S. Food and Drug Administration]-approved vaccine for hepatitis E.

Section 52.2

Frequently Asked Questions about Pregnancy and Hepatitis B

Should I be tested for hepatitis B if I am pregnant?

Yes. All pregnant women should be tested for hepatitis B. Testing is especially important for women who fall into high-risk groups such as health care workers, women from ethnic communities where hepatitis B is common, spouses or partners living with an infected person, etc. If you are pregnant, be sure your doctor tests you for hepatitis B before your baby is born.

Why are these tests so important for pregnant women?

If you test positive for hepatitis B and are pregnant, the virus can be passed on to your newborn baby during delivery. If your doctor is aware that you have hepatitis B, he or she can make arrangements to have the proper medications in the delivery room to prevent your baby from being infected. If the proper procedures are not followed, your baby has a 95% chance of developing chronic hepatitis B.

Will a hepatitis B infection affect my pregnancy?

A hepatitis B infection should not cause any problems for you or your unborn baby during your pregnancy. It is important for your doctor to be aware of your hepatitis B infection so that he or she can monitor your health and so your baby can be protected from an infection after it is born.

If I am pregnant and have hepatitis B, how can I protect my baby?

If you test positive for hepatitis B, then your newborn must be given two shots immediately in the delivery room:

- First dose of the hepatitis B vaccine
- One dose of the hepatitis B immune globulin (HBIG)

If these two medications are given correctly within the first 12 hours of life, a newborn has more than a 90% chance of being protected against a lifelong hepatitis B infection. You must make sure your baby receives the second and third dose of the hepatitis B vaccine at one and six months of age to ensure complete protection.

There is no second chance to protect your newborn baby.

Can I breastfeed my baby if I have hepatitis B?

The Centers for Disease Control (CDC) recommend that all women with hepatitis B should be encouraged to breastfeed their newborns.

The benefits of breastfeeding outweigh the potential risk of infection, which is minimal. In addition, since it is recommended that all infants be vaccinated against hepatitis B at birth, any potential risk is further reduced.

Chapter 53

Human Immunodeficiency Virus (HIV) during Pregnancy, Labor and Delivery, and Birth

I am pregnant, and I may have human immunodeficiency virus (HIV). Will I be tested for HIV when I visit a doctor?

In most cases, health care providers cannot test you for HIV without your permission. However, the U.S. Public Health Service recommends that all pregnant women be tested. If you are thinking about being tested, it is important to understand the different ways perinatal HIV testing is done. There are two main approaches to HIV testing in pregnant women: opt-in and opt-out testing.

In opt-in testing, a woman cannot be given an HIV test unless she specifically requests to be tested. Often, she must put this request in writing.

In opt-out testing, health care providers must inform pregnant women that an HIV test will be included in the standard group of tests pregnant women receive. A woman will receive that HIV test unless she specifically refuses. The CDC (Centers for Disease Control and Prevention) currently recommends that health care providers adopt an opt-out approach to perinatal HIV testing.

What are the benefits of being tested?

By knowing your HIV status, you and your doctor can decide on the best treatment for you and your baby and can take steps to prevent

Excerpted from "HIV During Pregnancy, Labor and Delivery, and After Birth," by AIDSinfo (http://www.aidsinfo.nih.gov), a part of the U.S. Department of Health and Human Services, February 2008.

mother-to-child transmission of HIV. It is also important to know your HIV status so that you can take the appropriate steps to avoid infecting others.

Will my baby be tested for HIV?

Health care providers recommend that all babies born to HIV positive mothers be tested for HIV. However, states differ in the ways they approach HIV testing for babies.

I am HIV positive and pregnant. Should I take anti-HIV medications?

Yes. If you are HIV positive and pregnant, it is recommended that you take anti-HIV medications to prevent your baby from becoming infected with HIV, and in some cases, for your own health. Anti-HIV medications are recommended for all pregnant women regardless of CD4 count and viral load. HIV treatment is an important part of preventing your baby from becoming infected with HIV and maintaining your health.

When should I consider starting anti-HIV treatment?

When you start treatment will depend mostly on whether you need treatment only to prevent your baby from becoming infected with HIV or if you also need treatment for your own health. In general, it is recommended that pregnant women who are starting therapy for their own health be treated as soon as possible, including in the first trimester. For women who are beginning therapy only to prevent mother-to-child transmission, delaying anti-HIV medication until after the first trimester can be considered. You should discuss when to begin treatment with your doctor.

How do I find out which HIV treatment regimen is best for me?

Decisions about which HIV treatment regimen you will start should be based on many of the same factors that women who are not pregnant must consider. These factors include:

- risk that the HIV infection may become worse;
- risks and benefits of delaying treatment;
- potential drug toxicities and interactions with other drugs you are taking;

- the need to adhere to a treatment regimen closely;
- the results of drug resistance testing.

In addition to these factors, pregnant women must consider the following issues:

- benefit of lowering viral load and reducing the risk of mother-to-child transmission of HIV;
- unknown long-term effects on your baby if you take anti-HIV medications during your pregnancy;
- information available about the use of anti-HIV medications during pregnancy.

You should discuss your treatment options with your doctor so that together you can decide which treatment regimen is best for you and your baby.

What treatment regimen should I follow during my pregnancy if I have never taken anti-HIV medications?

Your best treatment options depend on when you were diagnosed with HIV, when you found out you were pregnant, at what point you sought medical treatment during your pregnancy, and whether you need treatment for your own health. Women who are in the first trimester of pregnancy and who do not have symptoms of HIV disease may consider delaying treatment until after 10 to 12 weeks into their pregnancies. After the first trimester, pregnant women with HIV should receive at least AZT (Retrovir or zidovudine); your doctor may recommend additional medications depending on your CD4 count, viral load, and drug resistance testing.

I am currently taking anti-HIV medications, and I just learned that I am pregnant. Should I stop taking my medications?

Do not stop taking any of your medications without consulting your doctor first. Stopping HIV treatment could lead to problems for you and your baby. If you are taking anti-HIV medications and your pregnancy is identified during the first trimester, talk with your doctor about the risks and benefits of continuing your current regimen. Your doctor may recommend that you change the medications you take. If your pregnancy is identified after the first trimester, it is recommended that you continue with your current treatment. No matter what HIV treatment regimen you were on before your pregnancy, it is generally recommended that AZT become part of your regimen.

Will I need treatment during labor and delivery?

Most mother-to-child transmission of HIV occurs around the time of labor and delivery. Therefore, HIV treatment during this time is very important for protecting your baby from HIV infection. Several treatments can be used together to reduce the risk of transmission to your baby.

1. Highly active antiretroviral therapy (HAART) is recommended even for HIV-infected pregnant women who do not need treatment for their own health. If possible, HAART should include AZT (Retrovir or zidovudine).

2. During labor and delivery, you should receive intravenous (IV) AZT.

3. Your baby should take AZT (in liquid form) every 6 hours for 6 weeks after birth.

If you have been taking any other anti-HIV medications during your pregnancy, your doctor will probably recommend that you continue to take them on schedule during labor.

Better understanding of HIV transmission has contributed to dramatically reduced rates of mother-to-child transmission of HIV. Discuss the benefits of HIV treatment during pregnancy with your doctor; these benefits should be weighed against the risks to you and to your baby.

I am HIV positive and pregnant. Are there any anti-HIV medications that may be dangerous to me or my baby during my pregnancy?

Yes. Although information on anti-HIV medications in pregnant women is limited, enough is known to make recommendations about medications for you and your baby. However, the long-term effects of babies' exposure to anti-HIV medications in utero are unknown. Talk to your doctor about which medications may be harmful during your pregnancy and what medication and dose changes are possible.

In general, protease inhibitors (PIs) are associated with increased levels of blood sugar (hyperglycemia), development of diabetes mellitus or worsening of diabetes mellitus symptoms, and diabetic ketoacidosis. Pregnancy is also a risk factor for hyperglycemia, but it is not known whether PI use increases the risk for pregnancy-associated hyperglycemia or gestational diabetes.

Two non-nucleoside reverse transcriptase inhibitors (NNRTIs), Rescriptor (delavirdine) and Sustiva (efavirenz), are not recommended for the treatment of HIV-infected pregnant women. Use of these medications during pregnancy may lead to birth defects. Another NNRTI, Viramune (nevirapine), may be part of your HIV treatment regimen. Long-term use of Viramune may cause negative side effects, such as exhaustion or weakness; nausea or lack of appetite; yellowing of eyes or skin; or signs of liver toxicity, such as severe skin rash, chills, fever, sore throat, or other flu-like symptoms, liver tenderness or enlargement or elevated liver enzyme levels. These negative side effects are not normally seen with short-term use (one or two doses) of Viramune during pregnancy. However, because pregnancy and early symptoms of liver toxicity can be similar, your doctor should monitor you closely while you are taking Viramune. Also, Viramune should be used with caution in women who have never received HIV treatment and who have CD4 counts greater than 250 cells/mm^3. Liver toxicity has occurred more frequently in these patients.

Nucleoside reverse transcriptase inhibitors (NRTIs) may cause mitochondrial toxicity, which may lead to a buildup of lactic acid in the blood. This buildup is known as hyperlactatemia or lactic acidosis. This toxicity may be of particular concern for pregnant women and babies exposed to NRTIs in utero.

There is very little known about the use of the entry inhibitors Fuzeon (enfuvirtide) and Selzentry (maraviroc) and the integrase inhibitor, Isentress (raltegravir), during pregnancy.

I am HIV positive and pregnant. What delivery options are available to me when I give birth?

Depending on your health and treatment status, you may plan to have either a cesarean (also called c-section) or a vaginal delivery. The decision of whether to have a cesarean or a vaginal delivery is something that you should discuss with your doctor during your pregnancy.

How do I decide which delivery option is best for my baby and me?

It is important that you discuss your delivery options with your doctor as early as possible in your pregnancy so that he or she can help you decide which delivery method is most appropriate for you.

Cesarean delivery is recommended for an HIV positive mother when:

- her viral load is unknown or is greater than 1,000 copies/mL at 36 weeks of pregnancy;

- she has not taken any anti-HIV medications or has only taken AZT (Retrovir or zidovudine) during her pregnancy;

- she has not received prenatal care until 36 weeks into her pregnancy or later.

To be most effective in preventing transmission, the cesarean should be scheduled at 38 weeks or should be done before the rupture of membranes (also called water breaking).

Vaginal delivery is recommended for an HIV positive mother when:

- she has been receiving prenatal care throughout her pregnancy;

- she has a viral load less than 1,000 copies/mL at 36 weeks.

Vaginal delivery may also be recommended if a mother has ruptured membranes and labor is progressing rapidly.

What are the risks involved with these delivery options?

All deliveries have risks. The risk of mother-to-child transmission of HIV may be higher for vaginal delivery than for a scheduled cesarean. For the mother, cesarean delivery has an increased risk of infection, anesthesia-related problems, and other risks associated with any type of surgery. For the infant, cesarean delivery has an increased risk of infant respiratory distress.

Is there anything else I should know about labor and delivery?

Intravenous (IV) AZT should be started 3 hours before a scheduled cesarean delivery and should be continued until delivery. IV AZT should be given throughout labor and delivery for a vaginal delivery. It is also important to minimize the baby's exposure to the mother's blood. This can be done by avoiding any invasive monitoring and forceps- or vacuum-assisted delivery. All babies born to HIV positive mothers should receive anti-HIV medication to prevent mother-to-child transmission of HIV. The usual treatment for infants is 6 weeks of AZT; sometimes, additional medications are also given.

Chapter 54

Group B Streptococcus (GBS)

If you are pregnant—or know anyone who is—you need to know about group B strep. Group B streptococcal bacteria (also called GBS, group B strep, or baby strep) is very common to all types of women and can be passed on to your baby during childbirth. Your baby can get very sick and even die if you are not tested and treated.

Group B strep (sometimes called GBS) is a type of bacteria that is often found in the vagina and rectum of healthy women. In the United States, about 1 in 4 women carry this type of bacteria. Women of any race or ethnicity can carry these bacteria.

Being a carrier for these bacteria does not mean you have an infection. It only means that you have group B strep bacteria in your body, usually living in the rectum or vagina. You would not feel the bacteria or have symptoms like a yeast infection. These bacteria are usually not harmful to you—only to your baby during labor.

Preventing Group B Strep

Ask your doctor for a GBS test when you are 35 to 37 weeks pregnant (in your 9th month). The test is an easy swab of the vagina and rectum that should not hurt.

Each time you are pregnant, you need to be tested for GBS. It doesn't matter if you did or did not have this type of bacteria before—each pregnancy is different.

From "Are You Pregnant? Protect your baby from group B strep!" by the Centers for Disease Control and Prevention (CDC, www.cdc.gov), April 2008.

Finding the GBS bacteria does not mean that you are not clean, and it does not mean that you have a sexually transmitted disease. The bacteria are not spread from food, sex, water, or anything that you might have come into contact with. They can come and go naturally in the body.

The medicine to stop GBS from spreading to your baby is an antibiotic given during labor. The antibiotic (usually penicillin) is given to you through an IV (intravenous—in the vein) during childbirth. If you are allergic to penicillin, there are still other choices to help treat you during labor.

It does not work to take antibiotics for GBS before labor. The bacteria can grow back so fast that taking the medicine before you begin labor does not prevent the bacteria from spreading to your baby during childbirth.

Other people in the house, including kids, are not at risk of getting sick from GBS.

If you think you might have a cesarean section or go into labor early (premature), talk with your doctor or nurse about your personal GBS plan.

What You Can Do before Labor

- Ask your doctor for a GBS test when you are 35 to 37 weeks pregnant (9th month).

- If you are allergic to penicillin or other antibiotics, make sure to tell your doctor or nurse about any reactions you have had.

- If your test shows that you carry the bacteria, talk with your doctor about a plan for labor.

- Continue your regular check-ups, and always call your doctor or nurse if you have any problems.

When Your Water Breaks or When You Go into Labor

If you have not had your GBS test when labor starts, remind the staff that you do not know your GBS status.

If you are a GBS carrier:

- Go to the hospital. The antibiotics work best if you get them at least 4 hours before you deliver.

- Tell the labor and delivery staff at the hospital that you are a group B strep carrier.

- Speak up if you are allergic to penicillin.
- Expect to get IV antibiotics (medicine through the vein) during labor.
- It is fine to breastfeed after your baby is born.

Chapter 55

Pregnancy Loss: Ectopic Pregnancy, Miscarriage, and Stillbirth

Chapter Contents

Section 55.1

Ectopic Pregnancy

Most pregnancies happen in the uterus (womb). An ectopic pregnancy is one that happens outside of the uterus. Often, an ectopic pregnancy happens in one of the fallopian tubes, which run from the ovaries to the uterus.

If you have a positive pregnancy test, and the pregnancy cannot be seen on ultrasound, you may have an ectopic pregnancy. You also may have a normal pregnancy, but it's too early to see the fetus by ultrasound.

You will have a blood test. The test will be repeated in 2 days. The results can help tell if you have an ectopic pregnancy.

An ectopic pregnancy is rare, but it is a serious condition. It can be life-threatening if you do not get medical care. An ectopic pregnancy can grow until it breaks through the fallopian tube. This is very painful. It can cause serious bleeding inside your lower belly (abdomen).

If this happens, you need to be treated in a hospital right away. An ectopic pregnancy is removed either by taking medicines or by having surgery.

Signs that you may have an ectopic pregnancy include:

- severe lower belly pain;

- lower belly pain that gets worse;

- shoulder pain;

- fainting or dizzy spells;

- nausea or vomiting;

- heavy vaginal bleeding.

If you have any of these problems, call your doctor or go to an emergency room right away.

Tests after Treatment

After you are treated for an ectopic pregnancy, your doctor may have you come back for an ultrasound or blood tests. These tests are very important.

Losing a Pregnancy

There is no right way to react to losing a pregnancy. Many women are overcome with grief. You and your partner may want to seek a counselor or pregnancy loss support group.

Follow-Up

If you have any concerns about your diagnosis, treatment, or effects of the treatment, or if you have questions about future pregnancies, talk to your doctor.

Section 55.2

Blighted Ovum

"Blighted Ovum," © 2006 American Pregnancy Association (www.americanpregnancy.org). Reprinted with permission.

Chances are you didn't even know you were pregnant or had just found out you were expecting when you received the shattering news that there is no visible developing embryo on the ultrasound. You are probably feeling sad and confused. As you take time to understand what this means, also take time to grieve as you would for any loss. And remember you are not alone.

What is a blighted ovum?

A blighted ovum (also known as "anembryonic pregnancy") happens when a fertilized egg attaches itself to the uterine wall, but the embryo does not develop. Cells develop to form the pregnancy sac, but not the embryo itself. A blighted ovum usually occurs within the first trimester before a woman knows she is pregnant. A high level of chromosome abnormalities usually causes a woman's body to naturally miscarry.

How do I know if I am having or have had a blighted ovum?

A blighted ovum can occur very early in pregnancy, before most women even know that they are pregnant. You may experience signs of pregnancy such as a missed or late menstrual period and even a positive pregnancy test. It is possible that you may have minor abdominal cramps, minor vaginal spotting, or bleeding. As with a normal period, your body may flush the uterine lining, but your period may be a little heavier than usual.

Many women assume their pregnancies are on track because their hCG [human chorionic gonadotropin] levels are increasing. The placenta can continue to grow and support itself without a baby for a short time, and pregnancy hormones can continue to rise, which would lead a woman to believe she is still pregnant. A diagnosis is usually not made until an ultrasound test shows either an empty womb or an empty birth sac.

What causes a blighted ovum?

A blighted ovum is the cause of about 50% of first trimester miscarriages and is usually the result of chromosomal problems. A woman's body recognizes abnormal chromosomes in a fetus and naturally does not try to continue the pregnancy because the fetus will not develop into a normal, healthy baby. This can be caused by abnormal cell division, or poor quality sperm or egg.

Should I have a D&C or wait for a natural miscarriage?

This is a decision only you can make for yourself. Most doctors do not recommend a D&C [dilation and curettage] for an early pregnancy loss. It is believed that a woman's body is capable of passing tissue on its own and there is no need for an invasive surgical procedure with a risk of complications. A D&C would, however, be beneficial if you were planning on having a pathologist examine the tissues to determine a reason for the miscarriage. Some women feel a D&C procedure helps with closure, mentally and physically.

How can a blighted ovum be prevented?

Unfortunately, in most cases a blighted ovum cannot be prevented. Some couples will seek out genetic testing if multiple early pregnancy loss occurs. A blighted ovum is often a one time occurrence, and rarely will a woman experience more than one. Most doctors recommend couples wait at least 1–3 regular menstrual cycles before trying to conceive again after any type of miscarriage.

Section 55.3

What Is a Miscarriage?

From "Miscarriage," by the National Institute of Child Health and Human Development (NICHD, www.nichd.nih.gov), part of the National Institutes of Health, May 24, 2007.

What is a miscarriage?

A miscarriage, sometimes called pregnancy loss, is the loss of pregnancy from natural causes before the 20th week of pregnancy. Most miscarriages occur very early in the pregnancy, often before a woman even knows she is pregnant.

What causes a miscarriage?

There are many different causes for a miscarriage, some known and others unknown. In most cases, there is nothing a woman can do to prevent a miscarriage.

There are some factors that may contribute to miscarriage.

- The most common cause of miscarriage in the first trimester is a chromosomal abnormality in the fetus. This is usually results from a problem with the sperm or egg that prevents the fetus from developing properly.

- During the second trimester, problems with the uterus or cervix can contribute to miscarriage.

- Women with a disorder called polycystic ovary syndrome are three times more likely to miscarry during the early months of pregnancy than women who don't have the syndrome.

Women who have miscarriages can and often do become pregnant again, with normal pregnancy outcomes.

What are the symptoms of and treatments for miscarriage?

Signs of a miscarriage can include:

* vaginal spotting or bleeding;
* cramping or abdominal pain; and
* fluid or tissue passing from the vagina.

Although vaginal bleeding is a common symptom when a woman has a miscarriage, many pregnant women have spotting early in their pregnancy but do not miscarry. But, pregnant women who have symptoms such as bleeding should contact their health care provider immediately.

Women who miscarry early in their pregnancy usually do not need any treatment. In some cases, a woman may need a procedure called a dilatation and curettage (D&C) to remove tissue remaining in the uterus. A D&C can be done in a health care provider's office, an outpatient clinic, or a hospital.

Section 55.4

Incompetent Cervix Can Lead to Miscarriage

"Incompetent Cervix: Weakened Cervix," © 2007 American Pregnancy Association (www.americanpregnancy.org). Reprinted with permission.

During pregnancy, as the baby grows and gets heavier, it presses on the cervix. This pressure may cause the cervix to start to open before the baby is ready to be born. This condition is called incompetent cervix or weakened cervix, and it may lead to a miscarriage or premature delivery. However, an incompetent cervix happens in only about 1 out of 100 pregnancies.

What causes an incompetent or weakened cervix?

A weakened cervix can be caused by one or more of the following conditions:

- previous surgery on the cervix;
- damage during a difficult birth;
- malformed cervix or uterus from a birth defect;
- previous trauma to the cervix, such as a D&C (dilation and curettage) from a termination or a miscarriage;
- DES (diethylstilbestrol) exposure.

How will I know if I have an incompetent cervix?

Incompetent cervix is not routinely checked for during pregnancy and therefore is not usually diagnosed until after a second or third trimester miscarriage has occurred.

Women can be evaluated before pregnancy, or in early pregnancy by ultrasound, if they have any of the factors that are potential causes of incompetent cervix.

Diagnosis can be made by your physician though a pelvic exam or by an ultrasound. The ultrasound would be used to measure the cervical opening or the length of the cervix.

How often does an incompetent cervix happen?

An incompetent or weakened cervix happens in about 1–2% of pregnancies. Almost 25% of babies miscarried in the second trimester are due to incompetent cervix.

What is the treatment for a weakened cervix?

The treatment for an incompetent or weakened cervix is a procedure that sews the cervix closed to reinforce the weak cervix. This procedure is called a cerclage and is usually performed between week 14–16 of pregnancy. These sutures will be removed between 36–38 weeks to prevent any problems when you go into labor.

Removal of the cerclage does not result in spontaneous delivery of the baby. A woman would not be eligible for a cerclage if:

- there is increased irritation of the cervix;
- the cervix has dilated 4 cm;
- membranes have ruptured.

Possible complications of cervical cerclage include uterine rupture, maternal hemorrhage, bladder rupture, cervical laceration, preterm labor, and premature rupture of the membranes. The likelihood of these risks is very minimal, and most health care providers feel that a cerclage is a life saving procedure that is worth the possible risks involved.

Section 55.5

Drug Offers Alternative to Surgical Treatment after Miscarriage

From "Drug Offers Alternative to Surgical Treatment After Miscarriage," by the National Institutes of Health (NIH, www.nih.gov), August 24, 2005.

A drug first used to reduce the risk of stomach ulcers in people taking certain types of painkillers offers an alternative to surgery after miscarriage, according to a study by researchers at the National Institute of Child Health and Human Development of the National Institutes of Health and other research institutions.

The study appeared in the August 18, 2005, *New England Journal of Medicine*.

The drug, misoprostol, has been used to reduce the risk of stomach ulcers that occur in people who take certain pain relievers for arthritis. Misoprostol is now more commonly used to induce labor, as it stimulates contractions of the uterus.

In recent years, physicians have begun prescribing misoprostol in place of surgery to women who have experienced a miscarriage. Until the current study, however, no large-scale studies have been undertaken to evaluate the safety and effectiveness of the drug in treating miscarriage.

"This is the first comprehensive study to show that misoprostol is an effective alternative to surgery in the treatment of miscarriage," said Duane Alexander, MD, Director of the National Institute of Child Health and Human Development (NICHD). "Unlike conventional surgery, which is usually conducted in an operating room, treatment with misoprostol can be done on an outpatient basis."

The study authors wrote that pregnancy failure, or miscarriage, occurs in 15 percent of pregnancies. With miscarriage, in some cases, a fetus dies in the womb, explained the study's first author, Jun Zhang, MD, PhD, an investigator in the Epidemiology Branch of NICHD's Division of Epidemiology, Statistics, and Prevention Research. In other cases, a fetus may no longer be present, and women may carry a placenta and sac of amniotic fluid.

In all of these cases, the standard treatment is a surgical procedure known as vacuum aspiration. In this procedure, the cervix is dilated, and a suction device is used to remove the uterine contents. As an alternative, women and their doctors may choose to wait for the uterus to expel the tissue without additional medical treatment. Such expulsion is by no means certain, and may take more than a month. Many women, grieving from the failed pregnancy, may prefer not to wait. Occasionally, the uterus may fail to expel the remaining fetal tissue, and in some of these cases, the uterus may become infected.

Within the last few years, physicians have used misoprostol to treat pregnancy failure, and some researchers have conducted a few small studies of the drug's effectiveness in treating that condition. However, no definitive evidence existed to determine whether the drug was safe and effective enough for routine medical practice.

For the current study, Dr. Zhang and colleagues at several institutions enrolled 652 women who experienced pregnancy failure. Of these, 491 were assigned at random to receive misoprostol. The rest of the women underwent vacuum aspiration. The women in the misoprostol group were treated with 4 vaginal doses of misoprostol, each containing 200 mcg of the drug. If the uterus had not expelled its contents by the end of three days, the women received a second misoprostol treatment. If, after 5 more days had passed, the uterine contents still had not been expelled, the women were offered vacuum aspiration.

By the end of the third day, 71 percent of the women receiving misoprostol experienced complete uterine expulsion. After 5 more days had passed, a total of 84 percent of the misoprostol group had complete uterine expulsion. The misoprostol treatment failed for 16 percent of the group, however. In contrast, 3 percent of the vacuum aspiration group experienced treatment failure, and needed to undergo the procedure a second time. Complications from either misoprostol or vacuum aspiration—uterine hemorrhage and infection of the uterine lining—were rare, occurring in less than 1 percent of each group.

Of the women in the misoprostol group, 78 percent said they would choose the drug again if they needed to, and 83 percent said they would recommend it to other women.

Dr. Zhang noted that, because misoprostol causes uterine contractions, treatment with the drug could bring about abdominal pain and cramping. The researchers treated minor pain caused by the treatment with ibuprofen and treated more intense pain with codeine.

He added that the misoprostol treatment provided an effective alternative for women who preferred to avoid the surgical procedure.

Moreover, because it could be performed on an outpatient basis, the misoprostol treatment was less expensive and could provide women more privacy and convenience than vacuum aspiration. Roughly one in four women experience miscarriage, so the availability of a non-surgical treatment may provide an effective alternative for many women, he added.

"Misoprostol is inexpensive and does not need to be refrigerated," Dr. Zhang said. "It could provide treatment for miscarriage in developing countries where safe surgical treatment may not be readily accessible."

Section 55.6

What Is a Stillbirth?

From "Stillbirth," by the National Institute of Child Health and Human Development (NICHD, www.nichd.nih.gov), part of the National Institutes of Health, September 10, 2006.

What is a stillbirth?

A stillbirth is the loss of pregnancy due to natural causes after the 20th week of pregnancy. It can occur before delivery or during delivery.

What are the signs of a stillbirth?

In some cases of stillbirth, the mother may notice a decrease in the movement or kicking of the fetus. In these cases, the health care provider uses an ultrasound, a machine that uses sound waves to create a picture of the fetus, to learn more about its health.

If the fetus has died, an autopsy and placental examination is performed to get information on why the baby died. But it is not always possible to tell why the baby died.

If you are pregnant and have concerns about stillbirth, ask your health care provider if there are ways he or she wants you to track movement.

What are the causes of a stillbirth?

Causes of a stillbirth may include:

• problems with the placenta, such an abruption in which the placenta peels away from the uterine wall;

• chromosomal abnormalities resulting from defects in the sperm or egg that make the fetus unable to develop properly;

• other physical problems in the fetus;

• fetuses that are small for their gestational age or not growing at an appropriate rate; or

• bacterial infections that can cause complications and death to the fetus.

In at least half of all cases, researchers can find no cause for the pregnancy loss.

What medical procedures are used when there is a stillbirth?

In some cases it is medically necessary for a woman to deliver the fetus immediately after the diagnosis of a stillbirth.

In other cases, the couple can decide when they want to deliver the fetus.

A health care provider can induce labor or perform a caesarean section to deliver the fetus. A woman will usually go into labor on her own within two weeks after the fetal death.

Section 55.7

Research on Miscarriage and Stillbirth

Excerpted from "Research on Miscarriage and Stillbirth," by the National Institute of Child Health and Human Development (NICHD, www.nichd .nih.gov), part of the National Institutes of Health, September 15, 2006.

Miscarriage

The NICHD supports and conducts research on the causes of miscarriage in hopes of finding ways to prevent women from having them. For instance, NICHD-supported researchers recently found that women with a disorder called polycystic ovary syndrome (PCOS) are three times more likely to miscarry during the early months of pregnancy than women who don't have PCOS. Women with PCOS often have great difficulty getting pregnant naturally.

Research has found that women with PCOS also tend to have a condition called insulin resistance, which means their bodies have trouble using the insulin they make to get energy from their cells. Insulin resistance often occurs before someone develops diabetes. To treat this insulin resistance, researchers had been prescribing a drug called metformin. What they found was that metformin not only reduced insulin resistance, but it also brought about changes to the uterine lining that could help women with PCOS get pregnant and reduce the risk of miscarriage during their first trimester (the first three months) of pregnancy.

Studies are now underway to confirm the positive effects of the using metformin in women with PCOS, and to evaluate the safety of taking the drug throughout pregnancy. The NICHD's Reproductive Sciences Branch, through its Reproductive Medicine Network (RMN) is currently conducting a clinical trial for the treatment of infertility related to PCOS, using metformin. The RMN website provides more information on this trial and on the RNM itself.

Other NICHD-supported research is trying to learn more about repeated miscarriage. Researchers estimate that between 1 percent and 2 percent of women in the United States has more than one miscarriage without a known cause. Women who experience repeated miscarriages may undergo expensive and lengthy tests to try to identify a cause, but often get no answers. NICHD researchers, examining the vulva of these women have found that many of them share a genetic mutation, or change. This mutation, on one of the X chromosomes, was found in nearly 15 percent of women who had a history of repeated, unexplained miscarriage. If this genetic mutation is confirmed as a cause of repeated miscarriages, researchers may be able to develop a simple blood test that could predict a woman's chances of having a miscarriage in future pregnancies.

Stillbirth

In spite of how often stillbirth occurs, and how emotionally painful it can be, little research has been done on this type of pregnancy loss. To encourage more research on stillbirth, the NICHD is supporting a new research initiative, Research on the Scope and Causes of Stillbirth in the United States. Through this effort, the NICHD will create a network of research sites whose sole focus will be on understanding stillbirth, its features, its causes, and its effects on a woman's uterus. Patients in this network will include women from a variety of ethnic and economic backgrounds to provide a clearer picture of this problem. Through this initiative, the NICHD hopes to support work that may some day be able to predict and prevent stillbirths.

Section 55.8

Coping with Pregnancy Loss

Pregnancy loss can happen anytime during a pregnancy. It may be a miscarriage, a tubal (ectopic) pregnancy, a stillbirth, or it may be the death of a baby shortly after birth (neonatal death).

When you have a pregnancy loss, you may feel both physical and emotional pain. Every woman reacts differently to the loss. There are no right or wrong feelings. You may have strong feelings of loss no matter how early or how late you were in the pregnancy.

At first you may feel a sense of shock and disbelief. Your emotions may range from guilt and sadness, to anger and feeling out of control. You may wonder if you or someone else could have prevented your loss. You may want to be with family and friends or you may want to spend time alone. All of this is normal. The length of time needed to grieve is different for everyone. More important than the length of time is just allowing yourself to grieve.

How the Father May Cope

The father may react differently to the loss. He may focus on your health and feel the need to protect you. He may feel helpless and not know what to do to "make it better." You and the father may not share the same feelings at the same time. The father may find other ways of grieving and coping. This does not mean he doesn't care or feel sad. Grieving will be different for each of you, and that's okay. It's important to talk and support each other.

Helping Children Cope

You may have other children who need help understanding and coping with the loss. Resources are available that can help you explain the pregnancy loss to your children.

For more information, call a women's and children's hospital to speak with a social worker.

How Others May Respond

Others may not respond in the ways you hope or expect. This can range from statements such as, "you can have another baby," to saying nothing at all. Allow your family and friends to provide the love and support you need at this difficult time.

Support

A pregnancy loss may leave you feeling alone. You may wonder, "Are there other women who feel the way I do?" or "Am I normal?" The answer is yes.

Helpful Tips

• Be patient and take care of yourself, emotionally and physically.

• Remember that everyone grieves in his or her own way. You and your loved ones may be at different points in the grief process.

• Let others know what you need. Family and friends may not know how to help.

• Remember that you are not alone. Consider attending a support group or ask your nurse, doctor, or midwife to help you find a social worker.

Chapter 56

Preterm and Postterm Labor and Birth

Chapter Contents

Section 56.1

What Is Preterm Labor?

From "Preterm Labor and Birth," by the National Institute of Child Health and Human Development (NICHD, www.nichd.nih.gov), part of the National Institutes of Health, April 6, 2009.

What are preterm labor and birth?

Preterm labor (also called premature labor) is labor that begins before 37 weeks of pregnancy. Because the fetus is not fully grown at this time, it may not be able to survive outside the womb. Health care providers will often take steps to try to stop labor if it occurs before this time.

A baby born before 37 weeks of pregnancy is considered a preterm birth (or premature birth). Preterm births occur in about 12 percent of all pregnancies in the United States. It is one of the top causes of infant death in this country.

Who is at risk for preterm labor and birth?

Health care providers currently have no way of knowing which women will experience preterm labor or deliver their babies preterm. But there are factors that place a woman at higher risk for preterm labor or birth:

- certain infections, such as bacterial vaginosis and trichomoniasis;
- shortened cervix;
- previously given birth preterm.

What are the challenges to a baby born preterm?

Premature infants may face a number of health challenges, including:

- low birth weight;
- breathing problems because of underdeveloped lungs;

- underdeveloped organs or organ systems;
- greater risk for life-threatening infections;
- greater risk for a serious lung condition, known as respiratory distress syndrome;
- greater risk for cerebral palsy (CP);
- greater risk for learning and developmental disabilities.

They may need to stay in the hospital for several weeks or more, often in a neonatal intensive care unit (NICU).

What methods are used to prevent preterm delivery?

Research supported by the National Institute of Child Health and Human Development (NICHD) found that treating high-risk pregnant women (those who have previously had a spontaneous preterm baby) with a certain type of progesterone reduces the risk of another preterm delivery. The treatment worked among all ethnic groups in the study and improved outcomes for the babies. Efforts to find out whether the treatment works for other at-risk women, such as those having twins and triplets, are ongoing.

Bed rest and medications that relax the muscles in the uterus are also commonly used to try to stop preterm labor.

Researchers have found that other methods of stopping preterm labor are not as effective as once thought. For instance, NICHD-supported researchers have found that home uterine monitors are not effective for predicting or preventing preterm labor.

In addition, NICHD-funded research found that screening women who don't show any symptoms of infection, but who have bacterial vaginosis, and treating them with antibiotics did not prevent preterm birth.

Section 56.2

Preventing Preterm Labor and Birth

This section contains text from "Preventing Preterm Labor and Premature Birth," by the National Institute of Child Health and Human Development (NICHD, www.nichd.nih.gov), part of the National Institutes of Health, August 13, 2007, and "Research on Preterm Labor and Premature Birth," by the NICHD, October 20, 2006.

Preventing Preterm Labor and Premature Birth

Preterm birth, defined as birth before the fetus is at 37 weeks' gestation, is a major public health priority for the United States and a major research priority for the NICHD. In 2003, one out of every eight infants born was preterm—accounting for more than $18.1 billion in hospital expenditures. Preterm infants are at high risk for a variety of disorders, including mental retardation, cerebral palsy, and vision impairment. These infants are also at high risk for long-term health issues, including cardiovascular disease (heart attack, stroke, and high blood pressure) and diabetes.

The NICHD supports and conducts a large portfolio on preterm birth. Among the main goals of this research is finding a way to prevent births from occurring before an infant is strong enough to survive outside the womb. Because women who have one preterm birth are considered to be at high risk for another preterm birth, investigators have focused their attention on trying to prevent preterm birth among these high-risk women.

Researchers have had success using a treatment of a specific type of progesterone—called 17P. Progesterone is a hormone that the body makes to support pregnancy. In fact, the word "progesterone" means "for pregnancy." An NICHD Maternal-Fetal Medicine Units (MFMU) Network study, which began in 2003, set out to determine whether injections of 17P could reduce the number of preterm births among women who had already had one preterm birth. The results were remarkable: for women carrying one baby and with a history of preterm delivery, injections of 17P reduced preterm birth by one third.

Women carrying two or more babies are also at risk for preterm delivery, so researchers in the MFMU Network studied whether or not injections of 17P could prevent preterm delivery among these women. Recently reported results from this study indicate that 17P is not effective at reducing preterm delivery among women carrying twins. However, the treatment is still a proven way to reduce preterm birth among women carrying a single baby who have had a preterm delivery before.

Studies are also underway to try and prevent preterm delivery among women with other risk factors for preterm delivery, including those who have a shortened cervix (the lower part of the uterus) and those who have certain infections.

The NICHD research portfolio on preterm birth includes not only preventing preterm labor and delivery, but also ways to care for infants who are born preterm. Research on the preterm infant ranges from ways to help the lungs mature to what types of facilities provide the best care for preterm infants. Some of the research extends beyond the infant period into childhood and adulthood, tracking developmental progress and cognitive features.

In this way, NICHD's preterm birth and infant portfolio embodies the Institute's mission of promoting healthy development through the lifespan.

Research on Preterm Labor and Premature Birth

Health care providers consider labor to be preterm if it starts before 37 weeks of pregnancy. Because a fetus is not fully grown at 37 weeks, and it may not be able to survive outside the womb, health care providers will often take steps to stop labor if it starts before this time. Common methods for trying to stop labor include bed rest and medications that relax the muscles in the uterus involved with labor and delivery.

However, the American College of Obstetricians and Gynecologists (ACOG) recently reported that many of the methods used to stop preterm labor are ineffective. The ACOG announcement confirms NICHD-supported research, which found that home uterine monitors were not effective for predicting or preventing preterm labor.

If efforts to stop labor fail, then the baby could be born prematurely. Premature infants face a number of health challenges, including low birth weight, breathing problems, and underdeveloped organs and organ systems. Many infants that are born prematurely need to stay in the hospital until their health is stable, sometimes several weeks or more.

Despite attempts to stop labor, many cases of preterm labor end in premature birth. Premature birth occurs in between 8 percent to 10 percent of all pregnancies in the United States; it remains one of the top causes of infant death in this country. Infants who survive being born prematurely are at increased risk for certain life-long health effects, such as cerebral palsy, blindness, lung diseases, learning disabilities, and developmental disabilities.

Current NICHD-supported research is trying to identify markers and predictors of preterm labor and premature birth. In one study, researchers are investigating premature rupture of membranes (PROM), a situation in which the membranes that support the fetus in the womb break (sometimes referred to as "when a woman's water breaks") before the fetus is fully developed. PROM can lead to preterm labor and premature birth. Researchers found that, in some cases, the womb and the fetus produce enzymes, proteins that speed up certain chemical reactions, which can cause the membranes to break apart. Further research is now underway to figure out whether other features may make some women more likely to experience PROM. The findings of this research may lead to new methods of preventing PROM and some premature births.

Past research revealed that certain infections can make a woman more likely to experience preterm labor and give birth early. For instance, women who have bacterial vaginosis, the most common vaginal infection for women of reproductive age, are more likely than other women to experience preterm labor and give birth prematurely.

Similarly, women who have trichomoniasis, a sexually transmitted infection, are also more likely to give birth prematurely than women who don't have the infection. It would stand to reason, then, that treating these infections would prevent premature births in these cases. But, NICHD-supported studies have shown that treating these infections is not an effective way to prevent premature birth. Further research is now underway to find other options for treating these infections that may reduce the risk of premature birth.

One effective way to understand preterm labor and premature delivery is to study the characteristics of women who have given birth prematurely. One group of NICHD-supported researchers found that, among women who had given birth prematurely in the past, a shortened cervix could be a warning sign in preterm labor for a current pregnancy. With this knowledge, scientists can work to develop ways of preventing this shortening of the cervix, which may help to prevent preterm labor and premature delivery.

In addition, research on preterm labor and premature birth is ongoing through the NICHD's Maternal-Fetal Medicine Units (MFMU) Network, a research program that uses 14 sites around the country to conduct studies related to the mechanisms of pregnancy and birth. Researchers in the MFMU Network recently completed a clinical trial, which showed that the hormone progesterone may prevent repeated premature birth in a specific group of women, those who were carrying a single fetus, and who previously gave birth prematurely, between 20 and 26 weeks of pregnancy. In this trial, the progesterone treatment started between the 16th and 20th week of pregnancy, and continued through the 36th week of pregnancy. This finding may help to reduce future premature births among women who have a history of preterm labor and premature delivery.

NICHD-supported researchers were also working to see whether having more uterine contractions during pregnancy could be a warning sign of premature birth. Many pregnant women have uterine contractions throughout their pregnancies. These contractions are often mild and usually occur after the mid-way point of pregnancy. But, this research showed that, even though how often a woman had contractions was significantly related to premature birth, it wasn't an effective way to predict which mothers would give birth prematurely.

Infant Problems Related to Premature Birth

Babies that are born prematurely face a number of problems, including low birth weight, respiratory and breathing difficulties, and underdeveloped organs and organ systems. Some research also suggests that babies born prematurely are at higher risk for certain health problems as they get older. To find ways to minimize the impact of premature birth on the health of infants, the NICHD supports and conducts observational and interventional studies on these topics.

Low Birth Weight (LBW) and Very Low Birth Weight (VLBW)

LBW refers to any baby that weighs less than 2,500 grams (about 5 pounds, 8 ounces). VLBW describes an infant that weighs less than 1,500 grams (about 3 pounds, 5 ounces). LBW and VLBW infants are at higher risk than other infants for a variety of problems, including cerebral palsy, sepsis (a type of blood infection), chronic lung disease, and death. These infants are also at higher risk for hypothermia, low body temperature, which can be dangerous.

Research is now underway to learn how to increase the level of nutrition for these infants, to improve their survival rates, and find out what, if any, long-term these conditions have on overall health.

Respiratory Distress Syndrome (RDS)

In RDS, the baby has trouble breathing. RDS can result from various situations, such as:

- The baby's lungs aren't fully developed. Health care professionals can give these infants certain types of steroids, called corticosteroids, to help the lungs mature more quickly. These steroids may also lower the risk of brain injury. Sometimes, giving the lungs a little extra push in their development can help the baby breathe easier, which allows the infant to get stronger. Health care providers may also give corticosteroids to a woman who is at risk of delivering her baby before 34 weeks of pregnancy, to try to prevent the infant from developing RDS.

- The lungs are missing an important material. For the lungs to work properly, their lining has to be completely covered with a slick, soapy coating called surfactant. A growing fetus doesn't make enough surfactant to breathe outside of the womb until a certain point in development. Babies born prematurely have about 5 percent of the total surfactant that they need, which puts them at high risk for RDS. Through research conducted and supported by the NICHD, premature babies can now receive replacement surfactant to coat their lungs and allow for easier breathing. In some cases, getting replacement surfactant can prevent RDS from occurring at all; in other cases, the replacement surfactant saves the baby's lungs from long-term damage.

In addition to the treatments for these situations, premature infants may also benefit from being placed on a respirator, a machine that helps them breathe by inflating and deflating their lungs. Oxygen treatments or treatments using nitric oxide may also improve the breathing.

Through this and other NICHD-supported research into the problems faced by premature infants, survival rates for premature infants with RDS are nearly 95 percent. The NICHD and other Institutes are also conducting clinical trials related to RDS.

The NICHD is currently conducting and sponsoring a number of clinical trials involving infants born prematurely. The Institute's Neonatal Research Network, established in 1986, strives to improve the care of and outcomes for infants, especially LBW and VLBW infants. The Neonatal Research Network follows thousands of infants, through its 16 clinical centers throughout the country, to conduct clinical trials and observational studies for preventing and treating problems related to pregnancy, premature birth, and the newborn period. The Institute's Maternal-Fetal Medicine Unit Network also conducts clinical trials on these topics. Among the trials currently underway are: the BEAM (Beneficial Effects of Antenatal Magnesium Sulfate) trial, to try and prevent cerebral palsy; and the FOX (Fetal pulse OXimetry) trial, to learn more about the effects of cesarean delivery.

Section 56.3

Common Treatment to Delay Labor Decreases Preterm Infants' Risk for Cerebral Palsy

From the National Institutes of Health (NIH, www.nih.gov), August 27, 2008.

Preterm infants born to mothers receiving intravenous magnesium sulfate—a common treatment to delay labor—are less likely to develop cerebral palsy than are preterm infants whose mothers do not receive it, report researchers in a large National Institutes of Health research network.

The study results appear in the August 28, 2008 *New England Journal of Medicine*.

"A third of all cases of cerebral palsy are associated with preterm birth," said National Institutes of Health (NIH) Director Elias A. Zerhouni, MD. "This study shows a significant reduction in cerebral palsy among preterm infants whose mothers were given magnesium sulfate."

The researchers theorized that magnesium sulfate protects against cerebral palsy because it can stabilize blood vessels, protect against damage from oxygen depletion, and protects against injury from swelling and inflammation.

Cerebral palsy refers to a group of neurological disorders affecting control of movement and posture and which limit activity. The brain may be injured or develop abnormally during pregnancy, birth, or in early childhood. The causes of cerebral palsy are not well understood.

The research was conducted by investigators in 20 participating research centers of the Maternal Fetal Medicine Units Network of NIH's Eunice Kennedy Shriver National Institute of Child Health and Human Development (NICHD). The study's first author was Dwight J. Rouse, MD, of the University of Alabama at Birmingham. Major funding was provided by NIH's National Institute of Neurological Disorders and Stroke (NINDS).

A 1995 study by NINDS researcher Karin Nelson, MD, and a researcher at the California Department of Health Services found that mothers of preterm infants who did not have cerebral palsy were more likely to have received magnesium sulfate than were mothers of infants who had cerebral palsy. Two larger randomized studies that subsequently were undertaken suggested that magnesium sulfate given to pregnant women delivering prematurely might protect their infants against cerebral palsy, but their results were inconclusive.

"Our study is the largest, most comprehensive effort to date that looked at using this inexpensive and commonly used treatment to reduce the occurrence of cerebral palsy after preterm birth," said Deborah Hirtz, MD, a pediatric neurologist at NINDS, and an author of the study. "Cerebral palsy can't always be prevented, but the data from our study and its predecessors will help obstetricians make informed treatment decisions for the women under their care."

Women at the 20 participating NICHD Maternal Fetal Medicine Unit Network sites were eligible to participate. The women were from 24 to 31 weeks pregnant and at risk for preterm delivery. When the women went into labor, they were assigned at random to receive intravenously a solution of either magnesium sulfate or a placebo. The women in the treatment group were given 6 grams of magnesium sulfate intravenously over 20 to 30 minutes, followed by 2 grams of magnesium sulfate every hour after that until either 12 hours had passed, labor had subsided, or they had given birth. If the women in either group did not deliver within 12 hours, they were treated again if they went into labor by the 34th week of pregnancy.

For purposes of their statistical analysis, the researchers calculated the rates of moderate cerebral palsy, severe cerebral palsy, and death among the infants in the study. The study authors did not include mild cerebral palsy in this calculation, as mild cerebral palsy will often disappear with time.

When the researchers considered only moderate and severe cerebral palsy together, cerebral palsy occurred less frequently in the magnesium sulfate group (1.9 percent) as compared to the placebo group (3.5 percent).

For their primary calculation, the researchers grouped the proportions of infants with moderate and severe cerebral palsy together with the proportion of infants who died. The researchers included the death rate in this primary calculation, because mortality among preterm infants is very high. The researchers found that a total of 11.3 percent of infants in the magnesium sulfate group had either moderate or severe cerebral palsy, or had died at birth or were stillborn. In contrast, a total of 11.7 percent of the infants in the placebo group had moderate to severe cerebral palsy or had died.

The proportion of deaths occurring in the magnesium sulfate group (9.5 percent) did not differ significantly from those in the placebo group (8.5 percent).

There was no difference in the average gestational age between the two groups of infants.

Cerebral palsy was diagnosed in 41 children from 942 magnesium sulfate-treated pregnancies, as compared to 74 children from 1,002 placebo-treated pregnancies. Of the children in the magnesium sulfate group, 2.2 percent had cerebral palsy classified as mild, 1.5 percent as moderate, and 0.5 percent as severe. A higher proportion of children in the placebo group than in the magnesium sulfate group had cerebral palsy. Of the children in the placebo group, 3.7 percent had mild cases of cerebral palsy, 2.0 percent had moderate cases, and 1.6 percent had severe cases.

"This is a major advance," said Catherine Y. Spong, MD, Chief of NICHD's Pregnancy and Perinatology Branch and an author of the study. "Our results show that obstetricians can use magnesium sulfate, which they have experience prescribing, to reduce the risk of a devastating condition, cerebral palsy, in preterm infants.

Section 56.4

Overdue Pregnancy

When is a pregnancy considered overdue?

A pregnancy is usually completed in 38 to 42 weeks. "Post-term pregnancy," "prolonged pregnancy," and "post-date pregnancy" are all words used to describe a pregnancy that lasts beyond 42 weeks. About 5% of pregnancies are post-term.

How is my due date determined?

Your due date is estimated on the basis of the first day of your last period and on the size of your uterus (womb) early in your pregnancy. An ultrasound (also called a sonogram) may also give your doctor information about how far along your pregnancy is.

A reliable way to know your due date is to count 40 weeks ahead from the first day of your last period. However, many women cannot remember the first day of their last period and are not exactly sure when they got pregnant. In addition, it's usually hard to figure an accurate due date if you get pregnant soon after you stop taking birth control pills.

An early pelvic exam to measure the size of the uterus can be helpful. If you're not sure about the date of your last period or your uterus is smaller or larger than expected, an early ultrasound exam is helpful.

What if my pregnancy goes one week past the due date?

If your pregnancy lasts one week or more past your expected due date, your doctor will usually begin checking your baby more closely. Your doctor may check your baby's heartbeat by using an electronic fetal monitor once or twice a week. In addition, an ultrasound exam might be done to look at the amniotic fluid around your baby. Ultrasound can also be used to see how much your baby is moving. You should continue to feel your baby move throughout your pregnancy. Decreased fetal movement may be a sign that you need to call your doctor.

In addition, your doctor may begin checking your cervix to see if it's dilated and thinned. Your doctor may also recommend inducing (starting) labor.

What if my pregnancy goes two weeks past the due date?

Many doctors induce labor if a woman is two weeks past her due date. This is done to avoid complications, such as fetal distress or a baby that grows too large to deliver easily. Fetal distress occurs when the baby doesn't get enough oxygen. Then the baby's heart rate drops, and the baby can't tolerate the stress of labor.

How will my doctor induce labor?

Labor can be induced in some women by using a medicine called oxytocin (brand name: Pitocin), which causes contractions to start. Oxytocin is given through your veins. It usually starts to work in one to two hours.

Labor can also be induced in some women by "breaking the water," or rupturing the membrane that holds the amniotic fluid. This is not painful, but you may feel the fluid leak out when the membrane is broken.

Part Six

Labor and Delivery

Chapter 57

All about Labor and Delivery

Prepare for Labor and Birth

Once you reach the third trimester, you should talk to your doctor or midwife about labor and delivery. Learn your options for pain relief. Find out how to reach her if you go into labor. And ask her at what point in labor should you call.

Before you reach the last few weeks of pregnancy, you and your partner should visit the hospital or birthing center. Make sure you know how to get there, where to park, and where to check-in. Find out if you can preregister so that your insurance information is already in the computer when you arrive.

Signs of Labor

Many women, especially with their first babies, think they are in labor when they're not. This is called false labor. So don't feel embarrassed if you go to the hospital thinking you're in labor, only to be sent home.

If you think labor has begun, you should call your doctor or midwife. They can decide if it's time to go to the hospital or if you should be seen at the office first. Learn the signs of labor so you will know when the time has come.

From "Labor and Birth," by the Office of Women's Health (www.womenshealth .gov), part of the U.S. Department of Health and Human Services, March 2007.

Call your doctor if you experience any of the following:

- You have contractions that come at regular and increasingly shorter intervals. Contractions should also become stronger over time.

- You have lower back pain that doesn't go away. You might also feel premenstrual and crampy.

- Your water breaks (can be a large gush or a continuous trickle).

- You have a bloody (brownish or red-tinged) mucous discharge. This is probably the mucous plug that blocks the cervix. Losing your mucous plug usually means your cervix is dilating (opening up) and becoming thinner and softer (effacing). Labor could start right away or may still be days away.

Choosing Where to Deliver

Many women carefully choose the kind of environment in which to deliver their babies. You will need to contact your health insurance to find out what options are available. Not all companies will cover care given at a birth center and fewer will cover planned homebirths. In general, women can choose to deliver at a hospital, birth center, or at home. Nowadays, most hospitals and birth centers offer birthing classes like Lamaze and breastfeeding support.

Hospital

Women with health problems, pregnancy complications, or those who are at risk for problems during labor and delivery should give birth in a hospital. Hospitals offer the most advanced medical equipment and highly trained doctors for pregnant women and their babies. In a hospital, doctors can do a cesarean section if you or your baby is in danger during labor. Women can get epidurals or many other pain relief options.

Only certain doctors and midwives have admitting privileges at each hospital. So before you choose your doctor or midwife learn about their affiliated hospital. When choosing a hospital you might consider:

- Is it close to your home?

- Is an anesthesiologist at the hospital 24 hours a day?

- Do you like the feel of the labor and delivery rooms?

- Are private rooms available?

- How many support people can you invite into the room with you?

- Does it have a neonatal intensive care unit (NICU) in case of serious problems with the baby?

- Can the baby stay in the room with you?

- Does it have an on-site birth center?

More and more hospitals are adding on-site birth centers. At these hospitals you can choose to deliver your baby in the comfortable, intimate setting of a birth center. If something goes wrong, you and your baby have the added security of already being in a hospital.

Birth Centers

Healthy women who are at low risk for problems during pregnancy, labor, and delivery may choose to deliver at a birth or birthing center. Birth centers give women a "homey" environment in which to labor and give birth. They try to make labor and delivery a special, warm, family-focused process. Usually certified nurse-midwives, not obstetricians, deliver babies at birth centers.

Birth centers do not do any "routine" medical procedures. So, you will not automatically be hooked up to an intravenous (IV) line. Likewise, you won't have an electronic fetal monitor around your belly the whole time. Instead, the midwife or nurse will check in on your baby from time to time with a handheld machine. Once the baby is born, all examinations and care will occur in your room. By doing away with most high-tech equipment and routine procedures, labor and birth remain a natural and personal process.

Women cannot receive epidurals at a birth center although some pain medicines may be available. If a cesarean section becomes necessary, women must be moved to a hospital for the procedure. Basic emergency care can be done on babies with problems while they are moved to a hospital.

Many birthing centers have showers or tubs in their rooms for laboring women. They also tend to have comforts of home like large beds and rocking chairs. In general, birth centers allow more people in the delivery room than do hospitals.

Birth centers can be inside of hospitals, affiliated with a hospital, or completely independent, separate facilities. If you are interested in delivering at a birth center, make sure it is accredited by the Commission for the Accreditation of Birth Centers. Accredited birth centers must have affiliated doctors at a nearby hospital in case of problems with the mom or baby.

Homebirth

Healthy pregnant women with no risk factors for complications during pregnancy, labor or delivery can consider a planned homebirth. Some certified nurse midwives and physicians will deliver babies at home. If you are considering this choice you should ask your insurance company about their policy on homebirths. Some health insurance companies cover the cost of care for home births and others don't.

Homebirths are common in many countries in Europe. But in the United States, planned homebirths are still a controversial issue. The American College of Obstetricians and Gynecologists (ACOG) is against homebirths. ACOG states that hospitals are the safest place to deliver a baby. In case of an emergency, says ACOG, a hospital's equipment and highly trained physicians can provide the best care for a woman and her baby.

If you are considering a homebirth, you need to weigh the pros and cons. The main advantage is that you will be able to experience labor and delivery in the privacy and comfort of your own home. Since there will be no routine medical procedures, you will have control of your experience.

The main disadvantage of a homebirth is that in case of a problem, you and the baby will not have immediate hospital/medical care. It will have to wait until you are transferred to the hospital. Plus, women who deliver at home have no options for pain relief.

To ensure your safety and that of your baby, you must have a highly trained and experienced midwife along with a fail-safe back-up plan. You will need fast, reliable transportation to a hospital. If you live far away from a hospital, homebirth may not be the best choice. Your midwife must be experienced and have the necessary skills and supplies to start emergency care for you and your baby if need be. Your midwife should also have access to a physician 24 hours a day.

Managing the Pain

Virtually all women worry about how they will cope with the pain of labor and delivery. Childbirth is different for everyone. So no one can predict how you will feel. The amount of pain a woman feels during labor depends partly on the size and position of her baby, the size of her pelvis, her emotions, and the strength of the contractions.

Natural Pain Relief

Many women choose to deliver their babies without using medicine for pain relief. Some of these women use other techniques to help them cope. Things women do to ease the pain include:

- use breathing and relaxation techniques;
- take warm showers or baths;
- receive massages;
- have the supportive care or a loved one, nurse, or doula;
- find comfortable positions while in labor (stand, crouch, sit, walk, etc.);
- use a labor ball; or
- listen to music.

Building a positive outlook on childbirth and managing fear may also help some women cope with the pain. It is important to realize that labor pain is not like pain due to illness or injury. Instead, it is caused by contractions of the uterus that are pushing your baby down and out of the birth canal. In other words, labor pain has a purpose.

Try the following to help you feel positive about childbirth:

- Take a childbirth class. Call the doctor, midwife, hospital, or birthing center for class information.
- Get information from your doctor or midwife. Write down your questions and talk about them at your regular visits.
- Share your fears and emotions with friends, family, and your partner.

Waterbirthing

More and more women in the United States are using water to find comfort during labor and delivery. In waterbirthing, laboring women get into a tub of water that is between 90 and 100 degrees. Some women get out of the tub to give birth. Others remain in the water for delivery.

The water helps women feel physically supported. It also keeps them warm and relaxed. This eases the pain of labor and delivery for many women. Plus, it is easier for laboring women to move and find comfortable positions in the water.

Waterbirthing is relatively new in this country. So there is very little research on its benefits. Even so, some women say giving birth in the water is faster and easier. Plus, women may tear less severely and need fewer episiotomies in the water.

Waterbirthing may be gentler for your baby, too. It may ease the baby's transition from the womb to the new world. The baby is born into an environment that is similar to the womb. Plus, the water dulls the lights, sound, and feel of the new world. Once the baby is born, it is brought to the surface of the water and wrapped in blankets.

Ask your doctor or midwife if you are a good candidate for waterbirthing. Water birth is not safe for women or babies who have health issues.

Medical Pain Relief

While you're in labor, your doctor, midwife, or nurse should ask if you need pain relief. It is her job to help you decide what option is the best for you. There are many different kinds of pain relief. Not all options are available at every hospital and birthing center. Plus your health history, allergies, and any problems with your pregnancy will make some options better than others.

Types of pain relief used for labor and delivery include the following.

Intravenous or Intramuscular Analgesic

A doctor gives you pain medicine through a tube inserted in a vein (intravenous) or by injecting the medicine into a muscle (intramuscular). These medicines go into your blood and help ease the pain. Opioids including morphine, fentanyl, and nalbuphine are usually used for this type of pain relief. This option does not get rid of all the pain. Instead it usually just makes the pain bearable. After getting this kind of pain relief, you can still get an epidural or spinal pain relief later.

Some disadvantages of getting intravenous or intramuscular analgesics include:

- They make you feel sleepy and drowsy.
- They can cause nausea and vomiting.
- They can make you feel very itchy.
- These medicines cross into the baby's bloodstream. So they can affect the baby's breathing, heart rate, and cause him/her to be very sleepy after birth.

466

Epidural Anesthesia

A doctor injects medicine into the lower part of your backbone or spine. The medicine blocks pain in the parts of the body below the shot. During a contraction, the feeling of pain travels from the uterus to the brain along nerves in the backbone. Epidurals block the pain of contractions by numbing these nerves.

Epidurals allow most women to be awake and alert with very little pain. Many women who get epidurals do not feel any pain during contractions and childbirth. Medicines used in epidurals include novocaine-like drugs that block the pain in that region combined with opioids like fentanyl.

Some disadvantages of getting an epidural include:

- It can make you shiver.
- It can lower your blood pressure.
- It can make you feel very itchy.
- It can cause headaches.
- It may not numb the entire painful area. So women continue to feel pain in an area of the abdomen and back.

Pudendal Block

A doctor injects numbing medicine into the vagina and a nearby nerve called the pudendal nerve. This nerve carries sensation to the lower part of your vagina and vulva. This is only used late in labor, usually right before the baby's head comes out. With a pudendal block, you have some pain relief but remain awake, alert, and able to push the baby out. The baby is not affected by this medicine and it has very few disadvantages.

Spinal Anesthesia

A doctor injects a medicine into the lower part of your backbone. This medicine numbs the body below where the medicine was injected. Spinal anesthesia gives immediate pain relief. So they are often used for women who need an emergency Cesarean section. Spinal anesthesia uses numbing medicines similar to novocaine combined with opioids like fentanyl.

Some disadvantages of spinal anesthesia include:

- It numbs the body from the chest down to the feet.

467

- It makes you feel short of breath.
- It can lower your blood pressure.
- It can cause headaches.

Cesarean Sections

Most healthy pregnant women with no risk factors for problems during labor or delivery have their babies vaginally. Still, the rate of babies born by cesarean section (c-section) in the United States is on the rise. In 2004, 29.1 percent of babies were born by c-section in this country. This is an increase of more than 40 percent since 1996.

Many experts think that up to half of all c-sections are unnecessary. Thus, the U.S. government is trying to reduce the rate. So it is important for pregnant women to get the facts about c-sections before they deliver. Women should find out what c-sections are, why they are performed, and the pros and cons of this surgery.

What Is a C-Section?

During a c-section, the doctor makes a cut in the mother's abdomen and uterus and removes the baby. So, the baby is delivered through surgery instead of coming out of the vagina. Most women get spinal or epidural anesthesia during a c-section. This allows her to stay awake without feeling pain. But sometimes general anesthesia is needed. With general anesthesia the woman is asleep during the procedure.

A c-section can save the life of a baby or mother. If health problems come up before or during labor and delivery, a c-section can get the baby out very quickly. Most c-sections result in a healthy mother and baby.

Still, a c-section is major surgery. And all surgeries have risks. These include infection, dangerous bleeding, blood transfusions, and blood clots. Women who have c-sections stay at the hospital for longer than women who have vaginal births. Plus, recovery from this surgery takes longer and is often more painful than that after a vaginal birth. So, c-sections should only be done when the health or the mother of baby is in danger.

When Do Doctors Recommend C-Sections?

Doctors recommend c-sections when the health of the baby or mother is in danger. Even so, there are risks of delivering by c-sections. Limited studies show that the benefits of having a c-section may outweigh the risks when:

- the mother is carrying more than one baby (twins, triplets, etc.);
- the mother has health problems including HIV [human immunodeficiency] infection, herpes infection, and heart disease;
- the mother has dangerously high blood pressure;
- the mother has problems with the shape of her pelvis;
- there are problems with the placenta;
- there are problems with the umbilical cord;
- there are problems with the position of the baby (e.g., breech presentation);
- the baby shows signs of distress (e.g., slowed heart rate); or
- the mother has had a previous c-section.

Elective C-Sections: Can Women Choose?

A growing number of women are asking their doctors for c-sections when there is no medical reason. Some women want a c-section because they fear the pain of childbirth. Others like the convenience of being able to decide when and how to deliver their baby. Still others fear the risks of vaginal delivery including tearing and sexual problems.

But is it safe and ethical for doctors to allow women to make medical decisions? The answer is unclear. Only more research on both types of deliveries will provide the answer. In the meantime, many obstetricians feel it is their ethical obligation to talk women out of elective c-sections. Others believe that women should be able to choose a c-section if they understand the risks and benefits.

Experts who believe c-sections should only be performed for medical reasons point to the risks. C-sections can be dangerous for the mother and baby. This major surgery increases the risk of infection, bleeding, and pain in the mother. C-sections also increase the risk of problems in future pregnancies. Women who have had c-sections have a higher risk of uterine rupture. If the uterus ruptures, the life of the baby and mother is in danger. Babies born by c-section have more breathing problems right after birth and are very rarely cut during the surgery.

Supporters of elective c-sections say that this surgery may protect a woman's pelvic organs, reduces the risk of bowel and bladder problems, and is as safe for the baby as vaginal delivery. The American College of Obstetricians (ACOG) is not opposed to elective c-sections. ACOG states that "if the physician believes that (cesarean) delivery promotes the overall health and welfare of the woman and her fetus more than vaginal birth, he or she is ethically justified in performing" a c-section.

Can I Try a Vaginal Birth If I've Had a C-Section (VBAC)?

Some women who have delivered previous babies by c-section would like to have their next baby vaginally. This is called vaginal delivery after c-section or VBAC. Women give many reasons for wanting a VBAC. Some want to avoid the risks and long recovery of surgery. Others want to experience vaginal delivery.

Studies show that VBACs are more risky for the woman and baby than a repeat c-section. The most serious danger of VBACs is the chance that the c-section scar on the uterus will open up during labor and delivery. This is called uterine rupture. While very rare, uterine rupture is very dangerous for the mother and baby. Less than 1 percent of VBACs lead to uterine rupture. Even so, uterine rupture can lead to life-threatening bleeding for the mother and brain damage or even death for the baby.

The biggest and best study on VBACs was published in the *New England Journal of Medicine* in 2004. The researchers studied more than 30,000 women who had had a c-section and were pregnant again. Some of these women chose to have a VBAC. Others decided on a repeat c-section. The doctors compared the health of the women and babies after both types of delivery.

Almost three-quarters (73%) of women had a successful VBAC. The other 27% of women who tried to deliver vaginally ended up having another c-section. While rare, problems with the woman and baby were more common among VBACs compared with repeat c-sections. Only 0.8 % of women had a uterine rupture. Women who tried VBACs had more blood transfusions and a greater risk of endometriosis than those who had repeat c-sections. Babies born by VBAC had a higher risk of brain damage than those born by repeat c-section.

The percent of VBACs is dropping in the United States for many reasons. Women, doctors, and hospitals are worried about the rare, yet possible problems of VBACs. A growing number of doctors and hospitals are banning VBACs. They are afraid of lawsuits that might follow VBACs that go wrong. In 2004 the American College of Obstetricians and Gynecologists recommended that hospitals have a surgical team "immediately available" whenever a woman is having a

VBAC. In other words, ACOG suggests that a surgeon, nurses, and an anesthesiologist be standing by in case an emergency c-section is needed. Guaranteeing this stand-by team is just too expensive for many hospitals.

Doctors are also discouraging or flat out refusing to perform VBACs. Sometimes this is because their affiliated hospital does not allow them. In other cases, doctors can not get malpractice insurance to cover claims related to VBACs. And some doctors admit they are afraid of getting sued if a VBAC goes wrong.

Choosing to try a VBAC is a difficult decision for many women. If you are interested in a VBAC, talk to your doctor and read up on the subject. Only you and your doctor can decide what is best for you. VBACs and planned c-sections both have their benefits and risks. Learn the pros and cons and be aware of possible problems before you make your decision.

The American College of Obstetricians and Gynecologists (ACOG) recommends that doctors consider VBACs when:

- a woman has had one previous planned c-sections done with a low, horizontal cut or incision ("bikini" incision);

- a woman has no other uterine scars (aside from the prior c-section) or problems;

- a woman has no known problems with her pelvis;

- a doctor is present during all of labor and delivery and can perform an emergency c-section if needed; and

- an anesthesiologist and other members of a surgical team are standing by in case an emergency c-section is needed.

Chapter 58

Birthing Centers and Hospital Maternity Services

You'll make plenty of decisions during pregnancy, and choosing where to give birth—whether in a hospital or in a birth center setting—is one of the most important.

Hospitals

Many women fear that a hospital setting will be cold and clinical, but that's not necessarily true. A hospital setting can accommodate a variety of birth experiences.

Traditional hospital births (in which the mother-to-be moves from a labor room to a delivery room and then, after the birth, to a semi-private room) are still the most common option. Doctors "manage" the delivery with their patients. In many cases, women in labor are not allowed to eat or drink (possibly due to anesthesia or for other medical reasons), and they may be required to deliver in a certain position.

Pain medications are available during labor and delivery (if the woman chooses); labor may be induced, if necessary; and the fetus is usually electronically monitored throughout the labor. A birth plan can help a woman communicate her preferences about these issues, and doctors will abide by these as much possible.

In response to a push for more "natural" birth events, many hospitals now offer more modern options for low-risk births, often known as family-centered care. These may include private rooms with baths (birthing suites) where women can labor, deliver, and recover in one place without having to be moved.

Although a doctor and medical staff are still present, the rooms are usually set up to create a nurturing environment, with warm, soothing colors and features that try to simulate a home-like atmosphere that can be very comforting for new moms. Rooming in—when the baby stays with the mother most of the time instead of in the infant nursery—also may be available.

In addition, many hospitals offer a variety of childbirth and prenatal education classes to prepare parents for the birth experience and parenting classes after birth.

The number of people allowed to attend the birth varies from hospital to hospital. In more traditional settings, as many as three support people are permitted to be with the mother during a vaginal birth. In a family-centered approach, more family members, friends, and sometimes even kids may be allowed. During a routine or nonemergency C-section [cesarean section], usually just one support person allowed.

If you decide to give birth in a hospital, you will encounter a variety of health professionals.

Obstetrician/gynecologists (OB/GYNs) are doctors with at least four additional years of training after medical school in women's health and reproduction, including both surgical and medical care. They can handle complicated pregnancies and also perform C-sections.

Look for obstetricians who are board-certified, meaning they have passed an examination by the American Board of Obstetrics and Gynecology (ACOG). Board-certified obstetricians who go on to receive further training in high-risk pregnancies are called maternal-fetal specialists or perinatologists.

If you deliver in a hospital, you also might be able to use a certified nurse-midwife (CNM). CNMs are registered nurses who have a graduate degree in midwifery, meaning they're trained to handle normal, low-risk pregnancies and deliveries. Most CNMs deliver babies in hospitals or birth centers, although some do home births.

In addition to obstetricians and CNMs, registered nurses (RNs) attend births to take care of the mother and baby. If you give birth in a teaching hospital, medical students or residents might be present during the birth. Some family doctors also offer prenatal care and deliver babies.

While you're in the hospital, if you choose or if it's necessary for you to receive anesthesia, it will be administered by a trained anesthesiologist. A variety of pain-control measures, including pain medication and local, epidural, and general anesthesia, are available in the hospital setting.

Birth Centers

Women who experience delivery in a birth center are usually those who have already given birth without any problems and whose current pregnancies are considered low risk (meaning they are in good health and are the least likely to develop complications).Women giving birth to multiples, who have certain medical conditions (such as gestational diabetes or high blood pressure), or whose baby is in the breech position are considered higher risk and should not deliver in a birth center. Women are carefully screened early in pregnancy and given prenatal care at the birth center to monitor their health throughout their pregnancy.

Natural childbirth is the focus in a birth center. Since epidural anesthesia usually isn't offered, women are free to move around in labor, get in the positions most comfortable to them, spend time in the Jacuzzi, etc. The baby is monitored frequently in labor typically with a handheld Doppler. Comfort measures such as hydrotherapy, massage, warm and cold compresses, and visualization and relaxation techniques are often used. The woman is free to eat and drink as she chooses.

A variety of health care professionals operate in the birth center setting. A birth center may employ registered nurses, CNMs, and doulas (professionally trained providers of labor support and/or postpartum care). Although a doctor is seldom present and medical interventions are rarely done, birth centers may work with a variety of obstetric and pediatric consultants. The professionals affiliated with a birth center work closely together as a team, with the nurse-midwives present and the OB/GYN consultants available if a woman develops a complication during pregnancy or labor that puts her into a higher risk category.

Birth centers do have medical equipment available, including intravenous (IV) lines and fluids, oxygen for the mother and the infant, infant resuscitators, infant warmers, local anesthesia to repair tears and episiotomies (although these are seldom performed), and oxytocin to control postpartum bleeding.

A birth center can provide natural pain control and pain control with mild narcotic medications, but if a woman decides she wants an epidural, or if complications develop, she must be taken to a hospital.

Birth centers often provide a homey birth experience for the mother, baby, and extended family. In most cases, birth centers are freestanding buildings, although they may be attached to a hospital. Birth centers may be located in residential areas and generally include amenities such as private rooms with soft lighting, showers, and whirlpool tubs. A kitchen may be available for the family to use.

Look for a birth center that is accredited by the Commission for the Accreditation of Birth Centers (CABC). Some states regulate birth centers, so find out if the birth center you choose has all the proper credentials.

Which One Is Right for You?

How do you decide whether a hospital or a birth center is the right choice for you? If you've chosen a particular health care provider, he or she may only practice at a particular hospital or birth center, so you should discuss your decision. You should also verify your choice with your health insurance carrier to make sure it's covered. In many cases, accredited birth centers as well as hospitals are covered by major insurance companies.

If you have any conditions that would classify your pregnancy as higher risk (such as being older than 35, carrying multiple fetuses, or having gestational diabetes or high blood pressure, to name a few), your health care provider may advise you to have your child in a hospital where you and your baby can receive the required medical treatment, if necessary. In fact, you may be ineligible to deliver in a birth center because of your risk factors.

If you desire interventions such as an epidural or continuous fetal monitoring, a hospital is probably the better choice for you.

For a woman without significant problems in her medical history and whose pregnancy has been classified as low risk, a birth center might be an option. Someone who desires a natural birth with minimal medical intervention or pain control may feel more comfortable in a birth center. Because the number of labor and support people you can choose to be present is less limited, if you want to have your entire family participate in the birthing experience, you might consider a birth center.

Once you've decided on either a hospital or a birth center, you may still have to choose which hospital or which birth center. Before you make a choice, you'll have to verify if your health care provider, whether he or she is a doctor or a CNM, will only deliver at certain facilities. In addition, try to get a tour of the hospital or birth center so you can determine for yourself if the staff is friendly and the atmosphere is one in which you'll feel relaxed.

Choosing a Hospital: Questions to Ask

Before your labor pains start, get answers to the following questions.

- Is the hospital easy to get to?

- How is it equipped to handle emergencies?

- What level nursery is available? (Nurseries are rated I, II, or III—a level III neonatal intensive care unit [NICU] is equipped to handle any neonatal emergency. A lower rating may require transportation to a level III NICU.)

- How many deliveries take place at the hospital each year? (A higher number means the hospital has more experience with various birth scenarios.)

- What is the nurse-to-patient ratio? (A ratio of 1:2 is considered good during low-risk labor; a 1:1 ratio is best in complicated cases or during the pushing stage.)

- What are the hospital's statistics for cesarean sections, episiotomies, and mortality? (Keep in mind, though, that these numbers include high-risk and complicated deliveries.)

- How many labor and support people may be present for the birth?

- What procedures are followed after your baby's birth? Can you breastfeed immediately if desired? Is rooming in available?

- How long is the typical postpartum stay for vaginal deliveries? For C-sections?

- Can the baby and the father stay with you in your room around the clock, if you desire?

Choosing a Birth Center: Questions to Ask

- Is the birth center accredited by the Commission for the Accreditation of Birth Centers?

- Is the birth center easy to get to?

- What situations during labor would lead to a transfer to a hospital? How are transfers handled? What emergencies are the transfer facilities able to handle?

- What professionals (such as midwives, doctors, and nurses) are available on staff? On a consulting basis? Are they licensed?

- What childbirth and prenatal education classes are offered?

- What are the center's statistics for hospital transfers, episiotomies, and mortality?

- What procedures are followed after your baby's birth? How long is the typical postpartum stay and how will your baby be examined?

It's wise to choose where to deliver your baby as early in your pregnancy as possible. That way, if complications do arise, you'll be well informed and can concentrate on your health and the health of your baby.

Chapter 59

Birth Partners

Chapter Contents

Section 59.1

Labor Tips for Fathers and Birth Partners

"A Birth Partner Cheat Sheet,"
© 2009 Lamaze International. All Rights Reserved.
Reprinted with permission.

Uncertain about your role as a birth partner? Follow these nine easy guidelines.

1. Support is a key element to a woman having a positive birth and postpartum experience. As a birth partner, identify the resources you have for informational, emotional, and physical backup early on.

2. As you learn more about the process of birth, you will discover your strengths in offering support, and you can decide how you want to contribute to the birth of this child. Will you be the primary support, work more with the other team members, or be by the mother's side with your full love and support while others do the hands-on work? A birth partner can serve in any manner that helps the laboring woman, so be comfortable, even joyful, in whatever role you both agree upon.

3. Whether you decide to actively work with the mother or just shower her with love, simply being present makes a difference. The birth partner is usually the one member of the team who best knows her desires and can interpret her cues and express her wishes to others. Your personal history with the laboring woman is something the rest of the team doesn't have.

4. In order to care for a mother in labor, you must also care for yourself. Eating and drinking during labor will give you the energy you need. Wear comfortable clothes and let the doula or nurse care for your partner while you take an occasional break.

5. Ask questions. Unless you are birthing at home, you are in an unfamiliar setting surrounded by unfamiliar people. A doula can

help you get the attention of the health-care provider so that you are heard.

6. Be prepared to experience some strong emotions. Often, a birth partner is so absorbed in supporting the mother and remaining strong that he or she is surprised by the powerful feelings of love and awe that accompany seeing this incredible woman go through birth.

7. You and the mother may have the most familiar voices to the infant. When you talk to the baby, he experiences a feeling of calmness that has a positive effect on his transition to the outside world. Stroking him will also reduce stress hormones and improve his breathing and temperature regulation.

8. The postpartum period is a mix of joyous and difficult moments. The unpredictability of each day and getting to know your baby can sometimes make for a challenging situation.

9. After the excitement of birth dies down a bit, enjoy quiet time with the mother and baby, and delight in the miracle of birth and the part you played.

Section 59.2

Having a Doula:
Is It Right for You?

"Frequently Asked Questions About Birth Doulas,"
© 2005 DONA International (www.dona.org).
Reprinted with permission.

What is a birth doula?

A birth doula is a person trained and experienced in childbirth who provides continuous physical, emotional, and informational support to the mother before, during, and just after childbirth.

Where does the word "doula" come from?

The word "doula" comes from ancient Greek, meaning "Woman's servant." Throughout history and in much of the world today, a cadre of women support a woman through labor and birth, giving back rubs and providing continuous emotional support. Like their historical counterparts, DONA International birth doulas know how to help a woman in labor feel better. However, today's doulas are much more diverse than their predecessors. DONA International membership includes men and women from a wide range of ages and cultural backgrounds.

What effects does the presence of a doula have on birth outcomes?

Numerous clinical studies have found that a doula's presence at birth:

- tends to result in shorter labors with fewer complications;

- reduces negative feelings about one's childbirth experience;

- reduces the need for Pitocin (a labor-inducing drug), forceps, or vacuum extraction;

- reduces the requests for pain medication and epidurals, as well as the incidence of cesareans.

What effects does the presence of a doula have on the mother?

When a doula is present during and after childbirth, women report greater satisfaction with their birth experience, make more positive assessments of their babies, have fewer cesareans and requests for medical intervention, and less postpartum depression.

What effects do the presence of doulas have on babies?

Studies have shown that babies born with doulas present tend to have shorter hospital stays with fewer admissions to special care nurseries, breastfeed more easily, and have more affectionate mothers in the postpartum period.

How can I find a doula in my area?

Use DONA International's online doula locator [http://www.dona .org/mothers/find_a_doula.php].

How do doulas practice?

Doulas practice in three ways: privately hired directly by clients, as hospital employees, and as volunteers in community or hospital programs.

Does a doula replace nursing staff?

No. Doulas do not replace nurses or other medical staff. Doulas do not perform clinical or medical tasks such as taking blood pressure or temperature, monitoring fetal heart rate, doing vaginal examinations, or providing postpartum clinical care. They are there to comfort and support the mother and to enhance communication between the mother and medical professionals.

Does a doula make decisions on my behalf?

A doula does not make decisions for clients or intervene in their clinical care. She provides informational and emotional support, while respecting a woman's decisions.

Will a doula make my partner feel unnecessary?

No, a doula is supportive to both the mother and her partner, and plays a crucial role in helping a partner become involved in the birth to the extent he/she feels comfortable.

Chapter 60

Birth Plans

In the happy haze of early pregnancy, you're probably already thinking of baby names and planning to shop for baby clothes. The reality of labor and birth may seem extremely far off—which makes this the perfect time to start planning for the arrival of your baby by creating a birth plan that details your wishes.

What's a Birth Plan?

The term birth plan can actually be misleading—it's less an exact plan than a list of preferences. In fact, the goal of a birth plan isn't for you and your partner to determine exactly how the birth of your child will occur—because labor involves so many variables, you can't predict exactly what will happen. A birth plan does, however, help you to realize what's most important to you in the birth of your baby.

While completing a birth plan, you'll be learning about, exploring, and understanding your labor and birthing options well before the birth of your child. Not only will this improve your communication with the people who'll be helping during your delivery, it also means you won't have to explain your preferences right at the moment when you're least in the mood for conversation—during labor itself.

A birth plan isn't a binding agreement—it's just a guideline. Your doctor or health care provider may know, from having seen you throughout the pregnancy, what you do and don't want. Also, if you go into labor when there's an on-call doctor who you don't know well, a well thought-out birth plan can help you communicate your goals and wishes to the people helping you with the labor and delivery.

What Questions Does a Birth Plan Answer?

A birth plan typically covers three major areas:

1. What are your wishes during a normal labor and delivery?

These range from how you want to handle pain relief to enemas and fetal monitoring. Think about the environment in which you want to have your baby, who you want to have there, and what birthing positions you plan to use.

2. How are you hoping for your baby to be treated immediately after and for the first few days after birth?

Do you want the baby's cord to be cut by your partner? If possible, do you want your baby placed on your stomach immediately after birth? Do you want to feed the baby immediately? Will you breastfeed or bottle-feed? Where will the baby sleep—next to you or in the nursery? Hospitals have widely varying policies for the care of newborns—if you choose to have your baby in a hospital, you'll want to know what these are and how they match what you're looking for.

3. What do you want to happen in the case of unexpected events?

No one wants to think about something going wrong, but if it does, it's better to have thought about your options in advance. Since some women need cesarean sections (C-sections), your birth plan should probably cover your wishes in the event that your labor takes an unexpected turn. You might also want to think about other possible complications, such as premature birth.

Factors to Consider

Before you make decisions about each of your birthing options, you'll want to talk with your health care provider and tour the hospital or birthing center where you plan to have your baby.

486

You may find that your obstetrician, nurse-midwife, or the facility where they admit patients already has birth-plan forms that you can fill out. If this is the case, you can use the form as a guideline for asking questions about how women in their care are routinely treated. If their responses are not what you're hoping for, you might want to look for a health provider or facility that better matches your goals.

And it's important to be flexible—if you know one aspect of your birthing plan won't be met, be sure to weigh that aspect against your other wishes. If your options are limited because of insurance, cost, or geography, focus on one or two areas that are really important to you. In the areas where your thinking doesn't agree with that of your doctor or nurse-midwife, ask why he or she usually does things a certain way and listen to the answers before you make up your mind. There may be important reasons why a doctor believes some birth options are better than others.

Finally, you should find out if there are things about your pregnancy that might prevent certain choices. For example, if your pregnancy is considered high risk because of your age, health, or problems during previous pregnancies, your health care provider may advise against some of your birthing wishes. You'll want to discuss, and consider, this information when thinking about your options.

What Are Your Birthing Options?

In creating your plan, you're likely to have choices in the following areas:

Where to have the baby: Most women still give birth in the hospital. However, most are no longer confined to a cold, sterile maternity ward. Find out if your hospital practices family-centered care. This usually means the patient rooms will have a door, furnishings, a private bathroom, and enough space to accommodate a family, including the baby's crib and supplies.

Additionally, many hospitals now offer birthing rooms that allow a woman to stay in the same bed for labor, delivery, and sometimes, postpartum care (care after the birth). These rooms are fully equipped for uncomplicated deliveries. They're often attractive and have gentle lighting.

But some women believe that the most comfortable environment is their own home. Advocates of home birth believe that labor and delivery can and should occur at home, but they also stress that a certified nurse-midwife or doctor should attend the birth. An important thing to remember about home birth is that if something goes wrong, you don't have the amenities and technology of a hospital. It can take a while to get to the hospital, and during a complicated birth those minutes can be invaluable.

For women with low-risk pregnancies who want something in between the hospital and home, birthing centers are a good option. These provide a more homey, relaxed environment with some of the medical amenities of a hospital. Some birthing centers are associated with hospitals and can transfer patients if necessary.

Who will assist at the birth: Most women choose an obstetrician (OB/GYN), a specialist who's trained to handle pregnancies (including those with complications), labor, and delivery. If your pregnancy is considered high risk, you may be referred to an obstetrician who subspecializes in maternal-fetal medicine. These doctors have specialized training to care for pregnant women with medical conditions or complications, as well as their fetuses.

Another medical choice is a family practitioner who has had training and has maintained expertise in managing non-high-risk pregnancies and deliveries. In some areas of the United States, especially rural areas where obstetricians are less available, family practitioners handle most of the deliveries. As your family doctor, a family practitioner can continue to treat both you and your baby after birth.

And doctors aren't the only health care providers a pregnant woman can choose to deliver her baby. You might decide that you want your delivery to be performed by a certified nurse-midwife, a health professional who's medically trained and licensed to handle low-risk births and whose philosophy emphasizes educating expectant parents about the natural aspects of childbirth.

Increasing numbers of women are choosing to have a doula, or birth assistant, present in addition to the medical personnel. This is someone who's trained in childbirth and is there to provide support to the mother. The doula can meet with the mother before the birth and can help communicate her wishes to the medical staff, should it be necessary.

Your birth plan can also indicate who else you'd like to have with you before, during, and immediately after the birth. In a routine birth, this may be your partner, your other children, a friend, or other family member. You can also make it clear at what points you want no one to be there but your partner.

Atmosphere during labor and delivery: Many hospitals and birthing centers now allow women to make some choices about the atmosphere in which they give birth. Do you want music and low lighting? How about the freedom to walk around during labor? Is a hot tub something you'd like access to? If possible, would you like to eat or drink during labor? You might be able to request things that may make you the most comfortable—from what clothes you'll wear to whether you'll have a VCR or DVD player in your room.

Procedures during labor: Hospitals used to perform the same procedures on all women in labor, but many now show increased flexibility in how they handle their patients. Some examples include:

- **Enemas:** Used to clean out the bowels, enemas used to be routinely administered when women were admitted. Now, you may choose to give yourself an enema or to skip it entirely.

- **Induction of labor:** At times, labor may need to be induced or sped up for medical reasons. But sometimes, practitioners will give women the option of getting some help to move things along, or giving labor a little more time to progress on its own.

- **Shaving the pubic area:** Once routine, shaving is no longer done unless a woman requests it.

Other procedures that you can include in your birth plan are requests about fetal monitoring, extra birthing equipment you'd like in the room, and how often you have internal exams during labor.

Pain management: This is important for most women and is certainly something you have a lot of control over. It's also something you'll want to discuss carefully with your health care provider. Some women change their minds about pain relief during labor only to discover that they're too far along in their labor to use certain methods, such as an epidural. You'll also want to be aware of the alternative forms of pain relief, including massage, relaxation, breathing, and hot tubs. Know your options and make your wishes known to your health provider.

Position during delivery: You can try a variety of positions during labor, including the classic semi-recline with the feet in stirrups that you've seen in the movies. Other choices include lying on your side, squatting, standing, or simply using whatever stance feels right at the time.

Episiotomies: When necessary, doctors perform episiotomies (when the perineum—the area of skin between the vagina and the anus—is partially cut to ease the delivery). You may have one if you risk tearing or in the case of a medical emergency, but if there is an option, you can discuss your preference with your provider.

Assisted birth: If the baby becomes stuck in the birth canal, an assisted birth (i.e., using forceps or vacuum extraction) may be necessary.

Cesarean section (C-section): You might not want to think about this, but if you have to have a cesarean, you'll need to consider a few things. Do you want your partner to be present, if possible? If you have a choice, would you like to be conscious or unconscious? What about viewing the birth—do you want to see the baby coming out?

Post-birth: Decisions to be made about the time immediately after birth include:

- Would your partner like to cut the umbilical cord?

- Does your partner want to hold the baby when the baby emerges?

- Do you want immediate contact with the baby, or would you like the baby to be cleaned off first?

- How would you like to handle the delivery of the placenta? Would you like to keep the placenta?

- Do you want to feed the baby right away?

Communicating Your Wishes

Birth plans are relatively new inventions, and your doctor or nurse-midwife may not be completely comfortable with them. For this reason, make sure you communicate clearly that you intend to create a birth plan.

Give your health care provider your reasons for doing so—not because you don't trust him or her, but to help ensure cooperation and to cover the possibilities if something should go wrong. If your caregiver seems offended or is resistant to the idea of a birth plan, you might want to reconsider whether this is the right caregiver for you.

Also, think about the language of your plan. You can use many online resources to create one or you can make one yourself. Here are some tips:

- Make your birth plan read like a list of requests or best-case scenarios, not like a set of demands. Phrases such as "I would prefer" and "if medically necessary" will help your health care provider and caregivers know that you understand that they might have to alter the plan.

- Think about the other personnel who'll be using it—hospital staffers might feel more comfortable if you call it your "birth preferences" rather than your "birth plan," which could seem as though you're trying to tell them how to do their jobs.

- Try to be positive ("we hope to") as opposed to negative ("under no circumstances").

Once you've made your birth plan, schedule a time to go over it with your doctor or nurse-midwife. Find out and discuss where you agree or disagree. During your pregnancy, review the birth plan with your partner periodically to make sure that it's still in line with both of your wishes.

Strive to keep the plan as simple as possible—preferably less than two pages—and list them in order of importance. Focusing on your priorities will help ensure that the most important of your wishes are met.

You may also want to make several copies of the plan: one for you, one for your chart, one for your doctor or nurse-midwife, and one for your birthing coach or partner. And bringing a few extra copies in your labor bag is a good idea, especially if your doctor ends up not being on call when your baby is born.

Although you might not be able to control everything that happens to you during your baby's birth, you can play a role in the decisions that are made about your body and your baby. A well thought-out birth plan can help you to do that.

Chapter 61

Banking Your Newborn's Cord Blood

What is cord blood?

After your baby is born and the umbilical cord is cut, the placenta—along with the rest of the cord—is usually thrown away. But there is still blood in the cord. Blood from the cord has lots of stem cells. Stem cells from the cord can be used to treat some serious illnesses that may occur later in the baby's life. For this reason, some people think it is a good idea to save the cord blood stem cells—or "bank" them.

What illnesses can be treated with stem cells?

Stem cells can be used to treat leukemia and other diseases that attack the immune system. Research is being done on using stem cells to treat illnesses like Parkinson's disease, diabetes, or Alzheimer disease, but these uses are still unproven.

How are the stem cells collected from the cord?

After the cord has been cut, a member of the health care team will insert a needle into the part of the cord that is still attached to the placenta which has not been delivered yet. Blood from the cord is collected in a tube just like when you have blood taken from your arm.

"Cord Blood Banking: What's It All About?" *Journal of Midwifery and Women's Health,* March/April 2008. © 2008 American College of Nurse-Midwives (www .midwife.org). Reprinted with permission.

This process does not cause you or your baby any pain, because there are no nerves in the umbilical cord. The blood that is collected has thousands of stem cells in it. The stem cells in the cord blood are packaged, frozen, and sent to be stored in a cord blood bank.

Are there reasons I wouldn't want to bank my baby's cord blood?

If you choose to bank your baby's cord blood, the cord will be clamped and cut right after the baby is born so the cord blood does not flow back from the placenta to your baby. Many health care providers think that it is best for your baby if you allow most of the cord blood to flow into your baby before cutting the cord. This can prevent anemia and may help your baby fight illness later.

The chance that your baby will develop a disease that might be treated with cord blood stem cells is very low. Another concern is that if your child develops a disease that can be treated with stem cells, the cells collected and stored from birth may have the same disease and therefore they might not be recommended for use.

If my child needs stem cells, can I donate some of mine— like donating a kidney?

Stem cells can be taken from the umbilical cord, from embryos, and also from adult tissues and organs, such as bone. There has been a lot of research done on adult stem cells and they are used to treat many diseases. If you or your child needs stem cells to treat a disease, the National Marrow Donor Program will help you find a donor if there is one available.

What is the difference between public and private cord blood banks?

Public cord blood banks like the National Marrow Donor Program offer stored stem cells to anyone who needs them. These banks have stored cord blood donated by parents who want their baby's stem cells to be available to anyone who needs them. There is no fee to donate cord blood to a public bank.

Private cord blood banks store your baby's cord blood for possible future use for your baby or members of your immediate family. Private banks charge between $1000 and $2000 to collect the blood and about $100 a year to keep stem cells frozen in the "bank."

How do I decide?

The following are some questions to ask yourself as you decide whether to bank your baby's stem cells in the cord blood bank.

Things to Consider about Banking Cord Blood Stem Cells

At this time, the American Academy of Pediatrics does not recommend cord blood banking for everyone. There isn't a large enough chance that your baby will have an illness that can be treated with stem cells to justify the cost for every family. Below, you'll find some things to consider as you make your decision.

Is it very likely that your child will need his stem cells in the future?

Some families have illnesses that "run in the family"—inherited illnesses that can only be cured with stem cells. If you already know that your child is at risk for such an illness, you may want to bank the cord blood stem cells.

Do you have another child who already needs treatment with stem cells?

If you have a child who needs a stem cell treatment but does not have his own stem cells available, you may want to bank cord blood stem cells from your next child. This child's stem cells may be a match for the child who needs them.

Do you want to be sure your baby's stem cells will always be available only for her?

Private cord blood banks will store stem cells for future use in your family only. The charges vary from one cord bank to another cord bank. The services provided vary, too. You will want to shop around for the best service and best price.

Are you willing to donate your baby's stem cells for someone else?

You can donate your baby's cord blood stem cells to one of the public cord blood banks for free if there is one in your area. Another person who matches your baby might use the cells. If your child needs to be treated using stem cells someday, he might be able to get his own cells from the bank, but you run the risk that he might not.

Would you like to make your own stem cells available to someone who might need them for treatment of illness?

If you would like to donate your own stem cells to help save someone's life, consider signing up as a potential donor with the National Marrow Donor Program. In order to sign up, you will need to get your cells typed. Your type will then be kept in a registry of types. When someone needs a stem cell or bone marrow transplant, his or her type will be checked against the registry. If you are a match, you may be asked to donate. You could save a life!

Chapter 62

Natural Childbirth

Some women choose to give birth using no medications at all, relying instead on relaxation techniques and controlled breathing for pain. With natural childbirth, the mother is in charge, usually with a labor assistant gently guiding and supporting her through the stages of labor.

For many moms-to-be, having a natural childbirth isn't about being "brave" or a "martyr"—it's about treating labor and delivery as a natural event, not a medical problem. Many women find the experience, despite the pain, extremely empowering and rewarding.

What is natural childbirth?

Natural childbirth is a "low-tech" way of giving birth by letting nature take its course. This may include:

- going through labor and delivery without the help of medications, including pain relievers such as epidurals;

- using few or no artificial medical interventions such as continuous fetal monitoring, cesareans (C-sections), or episiotomies (when the area between the vagina and anus, called the perineum, is cut to make room for the baby during delivery);

- allowing the woman to lead the labor and delivery process, dealing with it in any way she is comfortable.

Many women with low-risk pregnancies choose to go au natural to avoid the risks that medications may pose for the mother or baby. Pain medications can affect your labor—your blood pressure may drop, your labor may slow down or speed up, you may become nauseous, and you may feel a sense of confusion and lack of control.

But many women choose natural childbirth to feel more in touch with the birth experience and to deal with labor in a proactive manner.

Where is it done?

Many women who opt for natural childbirth choose to deliver in a non-hospital setting such as a birth center, where natural childbirth is the focus. Women are free to move around in labor, get in positions that are most comfortable to them, and spend time in the Jacuzzi. The baby is monitored frequently, typically with a handheld Doppler. Comfort measures such as hydrotherapy, massage, warm and cold compresses, and visualization and relaxation techniques are often used. The woman is free to eat and drink as she chooses.

A variety of health care professionals may work in the birth center setting—registered nurses, certified nurse midwives, and doulas (professionally trained providers of labor support and/or postpartum care) that act as labor assistants.

Studies indicate that getting continuous support during labor from a trained and experienced woman, such as a midwife or doula, can mean shorter labor, less (or no) medications, less chance of needing a cesarean, and a more positive feeling about the labor when it's over.

These days, it's also possible to have a more natural childbirth in some hospitals. Many have modified their approach for low-risk births. They may have rooms with homelike settings where women can labor, deliver, and recover without being moved. They may take their cues from the laboring woman, allowing labor to proceed more slowly and without intervention if it all seems to be going well. They may use alternative pain medications if requested and welcome the assistance of labor assistants like midwives or doulas.

In addition to the father, children, grandparents, and friends may be allowed to attend the births (which is also common practice at birth centers). After birth, babies may remain with the mother longer. In its fullest form, this approach is sometimes called family-centered care.

If you're having a high-risk pregnancy, it's usually best to give birth in a hospital, where you can receive any necessary medical care (especially in the event of an emergency).

How is it done?

How you choose to work through the pain is up to you. Different women find that different methods work best for them. Many are able to control the pain by channeling their energy and focusing their minds on something else. The two most common childbirth philosophies in the United States are the Lamaze technique and the Bradley method.

The Lamaze technique teaches that birth is a normal, natural, and healthy process but takes a neutral position toward pain medication, encouraging women to make an informed decision about whether it's right for them.

The Bradley method (also called Husband-Coached Birth) emphasizes a natural approach to birth and the active participation of the baby's father as birth coach. A major goal of this method is the avoidance of medications unless absolutely necessary. The Bradley method also focuses on good nutrition and exercise during pregnancy and relaxation and deep-breathing techniques as a method of coping with labor. Although the Bradley method advocates a medication-free birth experience, the classes do prepare parents for unexpected complications or situations, like emergency C-sections.

Some other ways you can handle pain during labor include:

- hypnosis (also called "hypnobirthing");
- yoga;
- meditation;
- walking;
- massage or counterpressure;
- changing position (such as walking around, showering, rocking, or leaning on birthing balls);
- taking a bath or shower;
- immersing yourself in warm water or a Jacuzzi;
- distracting yourself by performing an activity that keeps your mind otherwise occupied;

- listening to soothing music;
- visual imagery.

What will it feel like?

Although labor is often thought of as one of the more painful events in human experience, it varies widely from woman to woman and even from pregnancy to pregnancy. Women experience labor pain differently—for some, it resembles menstrual cramps; for others, severe pressure; and for others, extremely strong waves that feel like diarrheal cramps. First-time mothers are more likely to give their pain a higher rating than women who've had babies before.

How long will it take?

There's no magic timetable when you're giving birth. For some women, the baby comes in a few hours; for many others it may take all day (or longer). Whether you opt for medications or not, every woman's body reacts to labor differently.

What are the risks?

Natural childbirth is, in general, very safe. It only becomes risky when a woman ignores her health care provider's recommendations, or when she refuses medical intervention if everything doesn't go as planned.

It's important for the well-being of you and your baby to be open to other options if there are complications. In an emergency situation, refusing medical help could put your life and your baby's at serious risk.

What will I feel like afterward?

Like any woman who's given birth, you'll probably feel:

- exhausted—both you and your baby will probably want to sleep as much as possible;
- shaky or cold—many women shiver after delivery—this is a natural reaction;
- sore—you'll probably feel cramping in your uterus, especially if you breastfeed, and you'll have some pain and discomfort in and around your vagina;

- elated and empowered—you may feel an overwhelming sense of accomplishment knowing that you did it on your own.

What if I can't handle the pain?

Labor may hurt more than you had anticipated. Some women who had previously said they want no pain medicine whatsoever end up changing their minds once they're actually in labor. This is very common and completely understandable.

You should be applauded for your willingness and enthusiasm to try to deliver naturally. But if it turns out that the pain is just too much to bear, don't feel bad about requesting medications. And if something doesn't go according to plan, you may need to be flexible as circumstances change. That doesn't make you any less brave or committed to your baby or the labor process. Giving birth is a beautiful and rewarding experience, with or without medical intervention.

Chapter 63

Pain Relief during Labor

Each Woman's Labor Is Unique

The amount of pain a woman feels during labor may differ from that felt by another woman. Pain depends on many factors, such as the size and position of the baby and the strength of contractions.

Some women take classes to learn breathing and relaxation techniques to help cope with pain during childbirth. Others may find it helpful to use these techniques along with pain medications. Some women need little or no pain relief, and others find that pain relief gives them better control over their labor and delivery. Talk with your doctor about your options.

This text explains:

- types of pain medications for labor and delivery;
- how they are given;
- how pain relief methods work.

Types of Pain Relief

There are two types of pain-relieving drugs—analgesics and anesthetics. Analgesia is the relief of pain without total loss of feeling

"Planning Your Childbirth: Pain Relief During Labor and Delivery" © 2008, is reprinted with permission of the American Society of Anesthesiologists, 520 N. Northwest Highway, Park Ridge, Illinois 60068-2573.

or muscle movement. Analgesics do not always stop pain completely, but they do lessen it.

Anesthesia is blockage of all feeling, including pain. Some forms of anesthesia, such as general anesthesia, cause you to lose consciousness. Other forms, such as regional anesthesia, remove all feeling of pain from parts of the body while you stay conscious. In most cases, analgesia is offered to women in labor or after surgery or delivery, whereas anesthesia is used during a surgical procedure such as cesarean delivery.

Not all hospitals are able to offer all types of pain relief medications. However, at most hospitals, an anesthesiologist will work with your health care team to pick the best method for you.

Systemic Analgesics

Systemic analgesics are often given as injections into a muscle or vein. They lessen pain but will not cause you to lose consciousness. They act on the whole nervous system rather than a specific area. Sometimes other drugs are given with analgesics to relieve the tension or nausea that may be caused by these types of pain relief.

Like other types of drugs, this pain medicine can have side effects. Most are minor, such as nausea, feeling drowsy or having trouble concentrating. Systemic analgesics are not given right before delivery because they may slow the baby's reflexes and breathing at birth.

Local Anesthesia

Local anesthesia provides numbness or loss of sensation in a small area. It does not, however, lessen the pain of contractions.

A procedure called an episiotomy may be done by your doctor before delivery. Local anesthesia is helpful when an episiotomy needs to be done or when any vaginal tears that happened during birth are repaired.

Local anesthesia rarely affects the baby. There usually are no side effects after the local anesthetic has worn off.

Regional Analgesia

Regional analgesia tends to be the most effective method of pain relief during labor and causes few side effects. Epidural analgesia, spinal blocks, and combined spinal–epidural blocks are all types of regional analgesia that are used to decrease labor pain.

Epidural analgesia: Epidural analgesia, sometimes called an epidural block, causes some loss of feeling in the lower areas of your body, yet you remain awake and alert. An epidural block may be given soon after your contractions start, or later as your labor progresses. An epidural block with more or stronger medications (anesthetics, not analgesics) can be used for a cesarean delivery or if vaginal birth requires the help of forceps or vacuum extraction. Your doctors will work with you to determine the proper time to give the epidural.

An epidural block is given in the lower back into a small area (the epidural space) below the spinal cord. You will be asked to sit or lie on your side with your back curved outward and to stay this way until the procedure is completed. You can move when it's done, but you may not be allowed to walk around.

Before the block is performed, your skin will be cleaned and local anesthesia will be used to numb an area of your lower back. After the epidural needle is placed, a small tube (catheter) is usually inserted through it, and the needle is withdrawn. Small doses of the medication can then be given through the tube to reduce the discomfort of labor. The medication also can be given continuously without another injection. Low doses are used because they are less likely to cause side effects for you and the baby. In some cases, the catheter may touch a nerve. This may cause a brief tingling sensation down one leg.

Because the medication needs to be absorbed into several nerves, it may take a short while for it to take effect. Pain relief will begin within 10–20 minutes after the medication has been injected.

Although an epidural block will make you more comfortable, you still may be aware of your contractions. You also may feel your doctor's exams as labor progresses. Your anesthesiologist will adjust the degree of numbness for your comfort and to assist labor and delivery. You might notice a bit of temporary numbness, heaviness, or weakness in your legs.

Although rare, complications or side effects, such as decreased blood pressure or headaches, can occur. To help prevent a decrease in blood pressure, fluids will be given through a vein by a tube in the arm. This may increase the risk of shivering. However, a woman may shiver during labor and delivery even if an epidural is not given. Keeping a woman warm often helps to stop the shivering.

Some women (less than 1 out of 100) may get a headache after the procedure. A woman can help decrease the risk of a headache by holding as still as possible while the needle is placed. If a headache does occur, it often subsides within a few days. If the headache does not stop or if it becomes severe, a simple treatment may be needed to help the headache go away.

The veins located in the epidural space become swollen during pregnancy. Because of this, there is a risk that the anesthetic medication could be injected into one of them. If this occurs, you may notice dizziness, rapid heartbeat, a funny taste, or numbness around the mouth when the epidural is placed. If this happens, let your doctor know right away.

Spinal block: A spinal block—like an epidural block—is an injection in the lower back. While you sit or lie on your side in bed, a small amount of medication is injected into the spinal fluid to numb the lower half of the body. It brings good relief from pain and starts working fast, but it lasts only an hour or two. A spinal block can be given using a much thinner needle in the same place on the back where an epidural block is placed. The spinal block uses a much smaller dose of the drug, and it is injected into the sac of spinal fluid below the level of the spinal cord. Once this drug is injected, pain relief occurs right away.

A spinal block usually is given only once during labor, so it is best suited for pain relief during delivery. A spinal block with a much stronger medication (anesthetic, not analgesic) is often used for a cesarean delivery. It also can be used in a vaginal birth if the baby needs to be helped out of the birth canal with forceps or by vacuum extraction. Spinal block can cause the same side effects as epidural block, and these side effects are treated in the same way.

Combined spinal–epidural block: A combined spinal–epidural block has the benefits of both types of pain relief. The spinal part helps provide pain relief right away. Drugs given through the epidural provide pain relief throughout labor. This type of pain relief is injected into the spinal fluid and into the space below the spinal cord. Some women may be able to walk around after the block is in place. For this reason this method sometimes is called the "walking epidural." In some cases, other methods, such as an epidural or a spinal block, also can be used to allow a woman to walk during labor.

General Anesthesia

General anesthetics are medications that put you to sleep (make you lose consciousness). If you have general anesthesia, you are not awake and you feel no pain. General anesthesia often is used when a regional block anesthetic is not possible or is not the best choice for medical or other reasons. It can be started quickly and causes a rapid loss of consciousness. Therefore, it is often used when an urgent cesarean delivery is needed.

A major risk during general anesthesia is caused by food or liquids in the woman's stomach. Labor usually causes undigested food to stay in the stomach. During unconsciousness, this food could come back into the mouth and go into the lungs where it can cause damage. To avoid this, you may be told not to eat or drink once labor has started. If you need general anesthesia, your anesthesiologist will place a breathing tube into your mouth and windpipe after you are asleep. If you are having a cesarean delivery, you also will be given an antacid to reduce stomach acid. In some cases, ice chips or small sips of water are allowed during labor. Talk to your doctor about what is best for you.

Anesthesia for Cesarean Births

Whether you have general, spinal, or epidural anesthesia for a cesarean birth will depend on your health and that of your baby. It also depends on why the cesarean delivery is being done. In emergencies or when bleeding occurs, general anesthesia may be needed.

If you already have an epidural catheter in place and then need a cesarean delivery, most of the time your anesthesiologist will be able to inject a much stronger drug through the same catheter to increase your pain relief. This will numb the entire abdomen for the surgery. Although there is no pain, there may be a feeling of pressure.

Finally

Many women worry that receiving pain relief during labor will somehow make the experience less "natural." The fact is, no two labors are the same, and no two women have the same amount of pain. Some women need little or no pain relief, and others find that pain relief gives them better control over their labor and delivery. Talk with your doctor about your options. In some cases, he or she may arrange for you to meet with an anesthesiologist before your labor and delivery. Be prepared to be flexible. Don't be afraid to ask for pain relief if you need it.

Easing Discomforts

Following are some ways to ease discomfort you may feel during labor:

- Do relaxation and breathing techniques taught in childbirth class.
- Have your partner massage or firmly press on your lower back.

- Change positions often.

- Take a shower or bath, if permitted.

- Place an ice pack on your back.

- Use tennis balls for massage.

- When contractions are closer together and stronger, rest in between and take slow, deep breaths.

- If you become warm or perspire, soothe yourself with cool, moist cloths.

Side Effects and Risks

Although most women have epidurals with no problems, there may be some drawbacks to using this pain relief method:

- An epidural can cause your blood pressure to decrease. This, in turn, may slow your baby's heartbeat. To decrease this risk, you'll be given fluids through an intravenous line before the drug is injected. You also may need to lie on your side to improve blood flow.

- After delivery, your back may be sore from the injection for a few days. However, an epidural should not cause long-term back pain.

- If the covering of the spinal cord is pierced, you can get a bad headache. If it's not treated, this headache may last for days. This is rare.

- When an epidural is given late in labor or a lot of anesthetic is used, it may be hard to bear down and push your baby through the birth canal. If you cannot feel enough when it is time to push, your anesthesiologist can adjust the dosage.

Serious complications are very rare:

- If the drug enters a vein, you could get dizzy or, rarely, have a seizure.

- If anesthetic enters your spinal fluid, it can affect your chest muscles and make it hard for you to breathe.

As long as your analgesia or anesthesia is given by a trained and experienced anesthesiologist, there's little chance you'll run into trouble. If you are thinking regional block may be the choice for you, bring up any concerns or questions you have with your doctor.

Chapter 64

Is It Labor?

Chapter Contents

Section 64.1

True Labor and False Labor

"How will I know when it is real labor?" This is a question you may have as you near the end of your pregnancy.

Many women have periods of "false" labor late in their pregnancy. During false labor, you have contractions that seem to come and go. False labor pains are called "Braxton Hicks" contractions. These contractions help soften and thin your cervix. They tend to happen more often as you get closer to your due date (two to four weeks before birth).

Sometimes it is hard to tell the difference between false labor and true labor. Don't be upset or embarrassed if you think labor is beginning when it is actually a false alarm.

Differences between False Labor and True Labor

There are several ways to tell the difference between true and false labor.

Timing of Contractions

- False labor: Contractions are often irregular. They don't get closer together over time.

- True labor: Contractions come regularly and get closer together. Each contraction lasts about 30 to 60 seconds.

Strength of Contractions

- False labor: Contractions are often weak and do not get stronger.

- True labor: Contractions get stronger as time goes on.

Change with Movement

- False labor: Contractions may stop or slow down when you walk, lie down, or change positions.

- True labor: Contractions continue no matter what you do.

Pain with Contractions

- False labor: Discomfort is usually felt in the front, like menstrual cramps.

- True labor: Discomfort or pressure starts in the back and moves to the front.

If Your Water Breaks

Sometimes labor begins when the bag of waters, or membranes, breaks. This may happen with your early contractions. Or your water may not break until later into your labor. If your water breaks, you may notice a near constant trickle of fluid from the vagina or a sudden gush of fluid.

If you think your bag of waters is leaking or broken, call your doctor right away.

Other Physical Changes

You also may have physical changes that occur as your body gets ready for labor. It is normal to have a slight increase of thin, white discharge at the end of pregnancy. Activities like coughing, sneezing, or laughing may cause leaking of urine.

You also may notice a change in appetite, nausea, diarrhea, or constipation. The loss of your mucus plug often precedes labor by a few days. Mucus may be present 2 to 14 days before true labor begins.

Everyone experiences labor in a different way. Call your doctor if you think you are in labor.

Section 64.2

When Does the Bag of Waters Break?

"When Does the Bag of Waters Break?" *Journal of Midwifery and Women's Health,* September/October 2004. © 2004 American College of Nurse-Midwives (www.midwife.org). Reprinted with permission. Reviewed by David A. Cooke, MD, FACP, April 12, 2009. Dr. Cooke is not affiliated with the American College of Nurse-Midwives.

What is my bag of waters?

The bag of waters—or amniotic sac—is a bag or membrane filled with fluid that surrounds your baby in your uterus during pregnancy. The bag of waters is very important to your baby's health. The fluid protects your baby and gives your baby room to move around. The bag itself protects your baby from infections that may get into your vagina.

When does the bag of waters usually break?

Usually the bag of waters breaks just before you go into labor or during the early part of labor. It happens most often when you are in bed sleeping. You may wake up and think you have wet the bed. Sometimes women feel or even hear a small "pop" when the bag breaks. Sometimes there is a gush of fluid from the vagina that makes your underwear wet; or maybe just a trickle that makes you feel damp. Sometimes the bag does not break until the baby is being born. In about one in every 10 women, the bag of waters breaks several hours before labor starts. Although rare, the bag of waters can break days before labor starts.

Is it a problem if the bag breaks and the labor does not start right away?

If your bag of waters breaks more than three weeks before your due date, your health care provider may try to stop labor if the baby would be too premature. Because the bag of waters protects against infection, you will be checked to make sure there is no infection in your uterus.

If your bag of waters breaks within three weeks of your due date, your health care provider will recommend either waiting to let your labor start on its own or inducing your labor right away. You can discuss the pros and cons of each of these options with your health care provider. If you have a bacteria, such as Group B strep [streptococcus] in your vagina, your health care provider may want to give you antibiotics or get your labor started (induction). The longer the bag of waters is broken before birth, the more chance there is that infection will get to the baby.

What should I do if my bag does break?

Information at the end of this text gives instructions on what to do if your bag of waters breaks. If you think your bag of waters has broken, your health care provider might check in your vagina with a sterile speculum to find out for sure. Except for that one examination, it is very important that nothing is put in your vagina.

Every time you have a vaginal examination after the bag of waters is broken, your risk of getting an infection gets higher. You can help protect yourself and your baby by asking your care providers to only do vaginal examinations when absolutely necessary.

What should I do if I feel wet but am not sure the bag of waters has broken?

Your health care provider can do a simple test using a sterile speculum to see inside your vagina. A sample of the fluid in the vagina will be collected and placed on special paper that turns very dark blue if it touches amniotic fluid.

What if your bag of waters breaks, and you are not in labor yet?

Labor contractions can start any time from right away to many hours or a few days after your water breaks. If you think your bag of waters has broken, call your health care provider.

Call your health care provider right away if:

- your due date is more than three weeks away from today;

- the water is green, or yellow, or brown, or has a bad smell;

- you have a history of genital herpes, whether or not you have any herpes sores right now;

- you have a history of Group B strep infection ("GBS positive");
- you don't know if you have GBS or not;
- your baby is not in the head-down position, or you've been told it is very high in your pelvis;
- you have had a very quick labor in the past, or feel rectal pressure now;
- you are worried or discouraged.

Call your health care provider within a few hours if:

- your due date is within the next three weeks and;
- you are not in labor and;
- the fluid is clear, pink, or has white flecks in it and;
- your baby is in the head-down position.

Some health care providers will want you to come in to the office to confirm that the bag of waters has broken and listen to the baby's heartbeat as soon as you notice that the bag of waters has broken. Others will suggest you stay home for several hours to wait for labor to start.

What do I do until labor starts?

Most women will go into labor within 48 hours. If you are waiting for labor to start and your bag of waters has broken:

- put on a clean pad;
- do not put anything in your vagina;
- drink plenty of liquids—a cup of water or juice each hour you are awake;
- get some rest;
- take a shower or bath;
- if there is any change in your baby's movements, call your health care provider right away;
- check your temperature with a thermometer every four hours— call right away if your temperature goes above 99.6.

Chapter 65

Inducing Labor

It's common for many women, especially first-time mothers, to watch their baby's due date come and go without so much as a contraction. The farther away from the expected delivery date (called the EDD) you get, the more anxious you may become. You may start to feel like a ticking time bomb. You may wonder—is this baby ever going to come?

Late pregnancy can be challenging—you may feel large all over, your feet and back may hurt, you might not have the energy to do much of anything, and you're beyond ready to meet the little one you've nurtured all this time. Which is why waiting a little longer than you'd expected can be particularly hard.

Still, being past your due date doesn't guarantee that your doctor (or other health care provider) will do anything to induce (or artificially start) labor—at least not right away.

What is it?

Labor induction is what doctors use to try to help labor along using medications or other medical techniques. Years ago, some doctors routinely induced labor. But now it's not usually done unless there's a true

---

medical need for it. Labor is typically allowed to take its natural course, with less medical intervention, in most birthing settings today.

Why is it done?

Your doctor may suggest an induction if:

- your water broke;

- your baby still hasn't arrived by 2 weeks after the due date (when you're considered post-term—more than 42 weeks into your pregnancy);

- you have an infection in the uterus called chorioamnionitis;

- you're having a pregnancy with certain risks (i.e., if you have gestational diabetes or high blood pressure, or your baby has growth problems).

Some doctors will perform "elective inductions"—in other words, they will induce labor if the mother wants it for nonmedical reasons. However, this isn't always the best option because inductions do come with risks.

Doctors try to avoid inducing labor early because the due date may be wrong and/or the woman's cervix may not be ready yet.

How is it done?

Some methods of induction are less invasive and carry fewer risks than others. Ways that doctors may try to induce labor by getting contractions started include:

- **Stripping the membranes:** The doctor puts on a glove and inserts a finger into your vagina and through your cervix (the opening that connects the vagina to the uterus). He or she moves the finger back and forth to separate the thin membrane connecting the amniotic sac (which houses the baby and amniotic fluid) to the wall of your uterus. When the membranes are stripped, the body releases hormones called prostaglandins, which help prepare the cervix for delivery and may bring on contractions. This method works for some women, but not all.

- **Breaking your water (also called an amniotomy):** The doctor ruptures the amniotic sac. During a vaginal exam, he or she uses a little plastic hook to break the membranes. This usually brings on labor in a matter of hours.

- **Giving the hormone prostaglandin to help ripen the cervix:** A gel or vaginal insert of prostaglandin (often the drug Cervidil) is inserted into the vagina or a tablet is given by mouth. This is typically done overnight in the hospital to make the cervix "ripe" (soft, thinned out, or dilated) for delivery. Administered alone, prostaglandin may induce labor or may be used before giving oxytocin.

- **Giving the hormone oxytocin to stimulate contractions:** Given continuously through an IV [intravenous line], the drug (often Pitocin) is started in a small dose and then increased until labor is progressing well. After it's administered, the fetus and uterus need to be closely monitored. Oxytocin is also frequently used to spur labor that's going slowly or has stalled.

What will it feel like?

Stripping the membranes can be a little painful or uncomfortable, although it usually only takes a minute or so. You may also have some intense cramps and spotting for the next day or two.

It may also be a little uncomfortable to have your water broken. You may feel a tug followed by a warm trickle or gush of fluid.

With prostaglandin, you may have some strong cramping as well. With oxytocin, contractions are usually more frequent and regular than in a labor that starts naturally.

What are the risks?

Inducing labor is not like turning on a faucet. If the body isn't ready, an induction may fail and, after hours or days of trying, a woman may end up having a cesarean delivery (or C-section). This appears to be more likely if the cervix is not yet ripe.

If rupturing the amniotic sac doesn't work, your doctor may need to induce labor a different way. Why? Because there's a risk of infection to both you and your baby if the membranes are ruptured for a long time before the baby is born.

When prostaglandin and/or oxytocin are used, there is a risk of abnormal contractions developing. In that case, the doctor may remove the vaginal insert and turn the oxytocin dose down. While it is rare, there is an increase in the risk of developing a tear in the uterus (uterine rupture) when these medications are used. Some other complications associated with oxytocin use are low blood pressure and low blood sodium (which can cause problems such as seizures).

Another potential risk of inducing labor is giving birth to a late pre-term baby (born between 34 and 36 weeks). Why? Because the due date (also called the expected delivery date, or EDD) may be wrong. Your due date is 40 weeks from the first day of your last menstrual period (LMP).

If you deliver on your due date, your baby is actually only about 38 weeks old—that's because your egg didn't become fertilized until about 2 weeks after the start of your last menstrual period. Women who have irregular periods or first trimester bleeding may be mistaken regarding when their last menstrual period was. Although ultrasounds can help to narrow it down, the estimated date of conception may still be off by a couple of weeks.

Babies born late pre-term are generally healthy but may have temporary problems such as jaundice, trouble feeding, problems with breathing, or difficulty maintaining body temperature.

Even though inductions do come with risks, going beyond 42 weeks of pregnancy can be risky, too. Many babies are born "post-term" without any complications, but concerns include:

- a vaginal delivery may become harder as the baby gets bigger;
- the placenta that helps to provide the baby with nourishment is deteriorating;
- the amniotic fluid can become low or contain meconium—the baby's first feces.

Old wives' tales abound about ways to induce labor. One of the oldest involves the use of castor oil. It is not safe to try to artificially start labor yourself by taking castor oil, which can lead to nausea, diarrhea, and dehydration. Breast stimulation can cause uterine contractions by causing the release of oxytocin. However, the safety of this practice has not been well studied. Earlier studies had suggested that the baby might have abnormal heartbeats after breast stimulation. Several recent studies looked at whether having sex in late pregnancy can induce labor, but there is no conclusion on this yet.

Talk to your doctor before doing anything to try to encourage your little one to come out. Inducing labor is best left to medical professionals—you may cause more harm than good.

As frustrating as it can be waiting for your baby to finally decide to arrive, letting nature take its course is often best, unless your doctor tells you otherwise. Before you know it, you'll be too busy to remember your baby was ever late at all!

Chapter 66

Vaginal and Cesarean Childbirth

Chapter Contents

Section 66.1

The Stages of Vaginal Childbirth

This section contains text from "Stages of Childbirth: Stage 1," © 2007 American Pregnancy Association (www.americanpregnancy.org); "Stages of Childbirth: Stage 2," © 2007 American Pregnancy Association; and "Stages of Childbirth: Stage 3," © 2006 American Pregnancy Association. Reprinted with permission.

Stages of Childbirth: Stage 1

Going through the birth of your child is a wonderful and unique experience. No two deliveries are alike and there is no way to tell how your delivery is going to be. What we can tell you is the stages you will go through during this process and what you can generally expect. Childbirth can be broken into three stages:

- **First stage:** Begins from the onset of true labor and lasts until the cervix is completely dilated to 10 cm.

- **Second stage:** Continues after the cervix is dilated to 10 cm until the delivery of your baby.

- **Third stage:** Delivery of your placenta.

First Stage

The first stage of labor is the longest and is broken down into three phases:

- **Early labor phase:** Starts from the onset of labor until the cervix is dilated to 3 cm.

- **Active labor phase:** Continues until the cervix is dilated to 7 cm.

- **Transition phase:** Continues until the cervix is fully dilated to 10 cm.

Each phase is full of different emotions and physical challenges. It is one big adventure you are about to take and we would like to give you a guide for it.

Early Labor Phase

What to do: During this phase you should just relax. It is not necessary for you to rush to the hospital or birth center. It will be more comfortable for you to spend this time at home, in familiar territory. If early labor is during the day you should do simple routines around the house. Keep yourself occupied but still conserve some of your energy. Drink plenty of water and eat small snacks. Keep track of the time of your contractions.

If early labor begins during the night it is a good idea to try and get some sleep. If you can't fall asleep, do things that will distract you like cleaning out your closet, packing your bag, or making sack lunches for the next day.

What to expect:

- Duration will last approximately 8–12 hours.

- Your cervix will efface and dilate to 3 cm.

- Contractions will last about 30–45 seconds, giving you 5–30 minutes of rest in between contractions.

- Contractions are typically mild, somewhat irregular, but progressively stronger and closer together.

- Contractions may feel like aching in your lower back, menstrual cramps, and pressure or tightening in the pelvis area.

- Your water may break; also known as amniotic sac rupture (this can happen any time within the first stage).

When monitoring contractions observe the following:

- Growing more intense
- Following a regular pattern
- Lasting longer
- Becoming closer together

When your water breaks (amniotic sac ruptures) note the following:

- Color of fluid
- Odor of fluid
- Time rupture occurred

Tips for the support person:

- Practice timing contractions.

- Be a calming influence.

- Offer comfort, reassurance, and support.

- Suggest activities that will distract her.

- Keep up your own strength; you will need it!

Active Labor Phase

What to do: It is about time for you to head to the hospital or birth center. Your contractions will be stronger, longer, and closer together. It is very important that you have all the support you can get. Now is also a good time for you to start your breathing techniques and try some relaxation exercises for you to use in between contractions. You should switch positions often during this time. You may want to try walking or taking a nice bath. Continue to drink water and remember to urinate periodically.

What to expect:

- Duration will last about 3–5 hours.

- Your cervix will dilate from 4 cm to 7 cm.

- Contractions during this phase will last about 45–60 seconds with 3–5 minutes rest in between.

- Contractions will feel stronger and longer.

- This is usually the time that you head to the hospital or birth center.

Tips for the support person:

- Give your undivided attention.

- Offer verbal reassurance and encouragement.

- Massage her abdomen and lower back.

- Keep track of contractions (if she is being monitored, ask how the machine works).

- Go through the breathing techniques with her.

- Help make her comfortable (prop pillows, get her water, apply touch).

- Remind her to change positions frequently (take her for a walk or offer her a bath).
- Continue with distractions (music, reading a book, playing a simple card game).
- Don't feel badly if she is not responding to you.

Transition Phase

What to do: During this phase you will rely heavily on your support person. This is the hardest phase but it is also the shortest. Think "one contraction at a time." This may be hard to do if the contractions are very close together, but just think about how far you have come. When you feel an urge to push, tell your health care provider.

What to expect:

- Duration will last about 30 minutes–2 hours.
- Your cervix will dilate from 8 cm to 10 cm.
- Contractions during this phase will last about 60–90 seconds with a 30-second–2-minute rest in between.
- Contractions are long, strong, intense, and may overlap.
- This is the hardest phase but thankfully the shortest.
- You may experience hot flashes, chills, nausea, vomiting, or gas.

Tips for the support person:

- Offer lots of encouragement and praise.
- Avoid small talk.
- Continue breathing with her.
- Help guide her through her contractions with encouragement.
- Encourage her to relax in between contractions.
- Don't feel hurt if she seems to be angry; it's just part of transition!

Stages of Childbirth: Stage 2

The second stage of childbirth is pushing and delivery of your baby. Up until this point your body has been doing all the work for you. Now that your cervix has fully dilated to 10 cm it is time for your help. Time to push!

Pushing and What to Expect

- The entire process of the second stage lasts anywhere from 20 minutes to 2 hours.
- Contractions will last about 45–90 seconds with a 3–5 minute rest in between.
- You will have a strong natural urge to push.
- You will feel strong pressure at your rectum.
- You will likely have a slight bowel or urination accident.
- Your baby's head will eventually crown (become visible).
- You will feel a burning, stinging sensation during crowning.
- During crowning you will be instructed by your health care provider not to push.

Pushing and What to Do

- Get into a pushing position (one that uses gravity to your advantage).
- Push when you feel the urge.
- Relax your pelvic floor and anal area (Kegel exercises can help).
- Rest between contractions so you can regain your strength.
- Use a mirror so you can see your progress (this can be very encouraging).
- Use all your energy to push.
- Do not feel discouraged if your baby's head emerges and then slips back into the vagina (this process can take two steps forward and one step back).

Tips for the Support Person

- Help her to be relaxed and comfortable (give her ice chips if you can and support her in her position).
- Encourage, encourage, encourage.
- Be her guide through her contractions.
- Affirm what a great job she has done and is doing.
- Don't feel bad if she becomes angry or emotional with you.

What Your Baby Is Doing

While you are in labor your baby is taking steps to enter this world.

1. Your baby's head will turn to one side and the chin will automatically rest on the chest so the back of the head can lead the way.

2. Once you are fully dilated, your baby's head leads the way and the head and torso begin to turn to face your back as they enter your vagina.

3. Next your baby's head will begin to emerge or "crown" through the vaginal opening.

4. Once your baby's head is out, the head and shoulders again turn to face your side. This position allows your baby to easily slip out.

Delivery and What to Expect

Keep in mind your baby has been soaking in a sac full of amniotic fluid for nine months. He/she has been through contractions, and your very narrow birth canal.

The results of this journey include:

- cone-shaped head;
- vernix coating (cheesy substance that coats the fetus in the uterus);
- puffy eyes;
- lanugo (fine downy hair that cover the shoulders, back, forehead, and temple);
- enlarged genitals.

Stages of Childbirth: Stage 3

The third stage is the delivery of the placenta and is the shortest stage. The time it takes to deliver your placenta is anywhere from 5 to 30 minutes.

What to Expect and What to Do

After the delivery of your baby, your health care provider will be waiting for small contractions to begin again. This is the signal that your placenta is separating from the uterine wall and ready to be delivered. Pressure may be applied by massage to your uterus; and the umbilical cord may be gently pulled.

The result will be the delivery of your placenta, also known as afterbirth. You may experience some severe shaking and shivering after your placenta is delivered. This is common and nothing to be alarmed about.

You have now completed all the stages of childbirth and will be monitored for the next few hours to make sure that the uterus continues to contract and bleeding is not excessive.

Now you can relax and enjoy your little bundle of joy. Congratulations!

Section 66.2

Vaginal Birth after a Previous Cesarean Delivery or Repeat Cesarean Section

"Vaginal Birth after a Previous Cesarean Delivery or Repeat Cesarean Delivery," © 2009 Childbirth Connection. Accessed May 6, 2009 at www.childbirthconnection.org and reproduced with permission.

This text presents results of recent systematic reviews that can help women compare risks of planned vaginal birth after cesarean (VBAC) and of planned C-section. While more high-quality studies are needed, a large body of research already exists and sheds light on these questions for those who need guidance now.

When deciding whether to plan a VBAC or a repeat cesarean, it is important to understand the full range of risks to you and your baby. This means comparing the short- and long-term risks of cesarean surgery and risks of accumulating cesarean surgery scars to mothers and babies on the one hand, to the risk that the uterine scar will give way (uterine rupture) and lead to problems and a few risks that are worse for vaginal birth generally.

Even if you do not plan to have more children, you should be aware of risks of multiple cesarean scars to future pregnancies and babies. Many women change their mind and decide to become pregnant again or continue with unplanned pregnancies.

What is the bottom line?

If you do not have a clear and compelling need for a cesarean in the present pregnancy, having a VBAC rather than a repeat C-section is likely to be:

- safer for you in this pregnancy;
- far safer for you and your babies in any future pregnancies.

When thinking about the welfare of your baby in the present pregnancy, there are trade-offs to consider: VBAC has some advantages, and a repeat C-section has others. You can learn more in the following text.

What are key messages about VBAC vs. repeat cesarean section?

Despite limitations of the best available research, the following conclusions seem clear:

- **Scar giving way:** The scar is more likely to give way during a VBAC labor than in a repeat C-section; for most women (exceptions noted below), the added risk of the scar giving way is about 27 in every 10,000 VBAC labors. In other words, nearly 400 women would need to experience the risks involved with repeat C-section to prevent one uterine rupture during a VBAC labor.

- **Death of baby:** While the scar giving way poses a threat to the baby, the added risk that the baby will die from a problem with the scar during a VBAC labor, compared with women planning repeat C-sections, is about 1.4 in every 10,000 VBAC labors. In other words, over 7,100 women would need to experience the risks involved with repeat C-sections to prevent the death of one baby due to uterine rupture.

- **Hysterectomy in mother:** If the scar gives way, some women have a hysterectomy (removal of the uterus). The added risk of needing a hysterectomy from this cause is about 3.4 in every 10,000 VBAC labors, when compared with women planning repeat C-sections. However, considering risk for hysterectomy from all causes, women who plan a VBAC are not more likely to experience an unplanned hysterectomy than women planning repeat C-section.

527

- **Concerns about specific risks:** The following factors do not increase risk of the scar giving way during labor:

  - Type of uterine scar not known

  - Low vertical uterine incision for prior C-section (may have been used if C-section was performed earlier in pregnancy before growth in lower part of the uterus)

  - Baby estimated to be large, and to weigh more than 4,000 grams (8 pounds, 13 ounces)

  - Pregnancy goes past 40 weeks

- **Concerns about other risks:** The following factors have not been shown to increase the risk of the scar giving way, but too few cases have been studied to be confident:

  - Twin pregnancy

  - Use of external cephalic version: turning a baby who is positioned buttocks- or feet-first (breech) to head-first position by manipulating the woman's belly

- **Infection:** Women planning C-sections are more likely to develop infections than women planning VBACs.

- **Multiple scars in uterus:** Accumulating C-section scars increase risk for experiencing a number of serious problems relating to future pregnancies and births. These include:

  - scar rupture in a subsequent labor;

  - ectopic pregnancy: the embryo develops outside the uterus;

  - placenta previa: the placenta grows over the cervix, the opening to the uterus;

  - placental abruption: the placenta separates from the uterus before the baby is born;

  - placenta accreta: the placenta growing abnormally into or even through the uterus.

What are some concerns about risks of C-section compared with vaginal birth?

When weighing planned VBAC versus planned C-section, the focus is often on potential problems with the uterine scar in labor or on problems associated with accumulating scars. But this results in an incomplete picture because it overlooks other risks that also differ between vaginal birth and cesarean section. Summarized here are some of the many extra risks associated with cesarean surgery as well as the few advantages.

Most of what we know about these risks comes from studies of cesarean in general, not planned C-section. Available research suggests that some of these risks may be lessened when the C-section is planned. The next question: What are some ways that a planned C-section may differ from an unplanned C-section? points to adverse effects where research finds differences in risk.

As you consider these, keep in mind that on average, 3 out of 4 women who labor after a C-section will give birth vaginally with care that encourages and supports VBAC (and fewer than 1 in 100 will experience the scar giving way). Even in cases where women scored 0 to 2 on a scale where 10 indicated greatest likelihood of vaginal birth, half gave birth vaginally

- **Physical problems for mothers:** Compared with vaginal birth, cesarean section increases a woman's risk for a number of physical problems. These range from less common but potentially life-threatening problems, including hemorrhage (severe bleeding), blood clots, and bowel obstruction (due to scarring and adhesions from the surgery), to much more common problems such as longer-lasting and more severe pain and infection. Even after recovery from surgery, scarring and adhesion tissue increase risk for ongoing pelvic pain and for twisted bowel.

- **Hospital stays:** If a woman has a C-section, she is more likely to stay in the hospital longer and to be re-hospitalized.

- **Emotional well-being:** A woman who has a C-section may be at greater risk for poorer overall mental health and some emotional problems. She is also more likely to rate her birth experience poorer than a woman who has had a vaginal birth.

- **Mother-baby relationship:** A woman who has a C-section is more likely to have less early contact with her baby and initial negative feelings about her baby.

- **Breastfeeding:** Recovery from surgery poses challenges for getting breastfeeding under way, and a baby who was born by C-section is less likely to be breastfed and get the benefits of breastfeeding.

- **Impact on babies:** Babies born by C-section are more likely to:
  - be cut during the surgery (usually minor);
  - have breathing difficulties around the time of birth;
  - experience asthma in childhood and in adulthood.
- **Impact on any future babies:** A cesarean section in this pregnancy increases risk for babies in future pregnancies. Some research finds that babies who develop in a scarred uterus are more likely to:
  - be born too early (preterm);
  - weigh less than they should (low birth weight);
  - have a physical abnormality or injury to their brain or spinal cord;
  - die before or shortly after the birth.

What are some concerns about risks of vaginal birth compared with C-section?

C-section offers advantages in a few areas, primarily during the recovery period after birth. (Some practices used with vaginal birth, such as episiotomy, are associated with pelvic floor problems. It is wrong to conclude at this time that vaginal birth itself causes such problems.)

A woman who has a vaginal birth is more likely to:

- have a painful vaginal area in the weeks after birth;
- leak urine (urinary incontinence) (about 3 women per hundred still have a problem 1 year after birth);
- leak gas, or more rarely, feces (bowel incontinence) (about 3 women per hundred still have a problem 1 year after birth).

Babies born vaginally have been shown to be at higher risk for a nerve injury affecting the shoulder, arm, or hand (brachial plexus injury) (usually temporary).

What are some ways that a planned C-section may differ from an unplanned C-section?

A planned C-section offers some advantages over an unplanned C-section that occurs after labor is under way. For example, there is a lower risk of surgical injuries and of infections. The emotional impact of a cesarean that is planned in advance appears to be similar to or somewhat worse than a vaginal birth. By contrast, unplanned cesareans can take a greater emotional toll. In addition, a woman planning repeat cesarean surgery would almost certainly be less likely to experience difficulty breastfeeding if she had breastfed before or to have negative feelings for her baby compared with a first-time mother having an unplanned cesarean. Nonetheless, a planned cesarean still involves the risks associated with major surgery. And both planned and unplanned cesareans result in a uterine scar, which increases risk for serious concerns for mothers and babies in future pregnancies, and for adhesion-relation problems in mothers at any time.

To learn more about these differences, see:

- Best Evidence: C-Section [http://www.childbirthconnection.org/article.asp?ck=10166] for a summary of research comparing cesarean and vaginal birth;

- Preventing Pelvic Floor Dysfunction [http://www.childbirth connection.org/article.asp?ck=10206] for in depth information about the relationship between giving birth and a woman's pelvic floor health;

- details in the following text about effects of giving birth when a woman's uterus has a scar from a previous cesarean.

What is the added likelihood that the scar will give way (uterine rupture) during a VBAC labor?

Best research suggests that an extra 27 women experience a ruptured uterus in every 10,000 VBAC labors, compared with planned C-section deliveries. Thus, nearly 400 women would need to experience surgical birth to prevent one instance of uterine rupture during VBAC labors. While the scar giving way usually requires an urgent cesarean, loss of the baby is much less common. Added likelihood for a woman with a known low-transverse (horizontal) scar: moderate for scar rupture compared with planned repeat C-section.

What is the added likelihood that the baby will die as a result of the scar giving way (uterine rupture) during a VBAC labor?

Best research suggests that about 1.4 extra babies die due to problems with the scar in every 10,000 VBAC labors, compared with planned C-section deliveries. Thus, over 7,000 women would need to experience risks of surgical birth to prevent the death of one baby from scar problems during VBAC.

Added likelihood for a woman with a known low-transverse (horizontal) scar: low for death of the baby around the time of birth compared with repeat C-section.

What is the added likelihood of the scar giving way (uterine rupture) with any of these factors?

• Type of uterine scar not known

• Low vertical uterine incision at prior C-section (may have been used if C-section took place earlier in pregnancy before growth in lower part of the uterus)

• Baby estimated to be large, weighing over 4,000 grams (8 lb 13 oz) or pregnancy extends past 40 weeks

Some caregivers recommend planned repeat C-section with these factors on the grounds that VBAC is riskier, but the research does not support that belief.

No added likelihood for scar rupture in a woman with unknown type of uterine scar, prior low vertical uterine incision, baby estimated to weigh more than 4,000 grams, or pregnancy extending past 40 weeks, in comparison with women planning VBAC without these factors.

What is the added likelihood of the scar giving way (uterine rupture) with twin pregnancy or the use of external cephalic version (turning a baby in a buttocks- or feet-first (breech) position to a head-first position by manipulating the woman's belly)?

While studies have not found an excess incidence of scar rupture in these situations, not enough women have been studied to rule out an increase. No currently known added likelihood for scar rupture in a woman with a twin pregnancy or a woman experiencing external version, in comparison with women planning VBAC without these factors.

What is the added likelihood that a woman planning VBAC will require a hysterectomy compared with a woman planning repeat C-section?

Most studies find an excess of hysterectomies (surgical removal of the uterus) among women planning repeat C-section. However, this could be because those studies may have included cases where the C-section was planned for reasons that could increase the risk of complications during surgery such as the placenta overlaying the cervix (placenta previa). A study that took care to exclude women having planned repeat cesareans for medical reasons found no difference in the percentages of women having hysterectomies.

No apparent added likelihood for hysterectomy for a woman planning VBAC compared with a woman planning repeat C-section.

What is the added likelihood that a woman will require a hysterectomy as a result of the scar giving way (uterine rupture) during a VBAC labor?

Best research suggests that about 3.4 extra women have a scar-related hysterectomy (surgical removal of uterus) occur in every 10,000 VBAC labors, compared with planned C-section deliveries. Thus, nearly 3,000 women would need to experience surgical birth to prevent one instance of hysterectomy due to scar problems during VBAC labors.

Added likelihood for a woman with a known low-transverse (horizontal) scar: low for hysterectomy as a result of uterine rupture compared with repeat cesarean.

What is the added likelihood that a woman will develop an infection after a planned cesarean?

Surgery always introduces the risk of infection. Even though some women who plan VBAC will have repeat C-sections, most will not. This puts women planning VBAC at lower risk of having an infection than women planning repeat C-sections.

Added likelihood for a woman planning repeat cesarean: moderate for developing a wound or internal infection compared with planned VBAC.

What are some concerns about effects of accumulating uterine scars on future pregnancies and births?

The likelihood of the following problems grows as the number of previous cesareans (and C-section scars) grows:

- **Placenta previa:** A woman whose uterus has a cesarean scar is more likely than a woman with an unscarred uterus to have a future placenta attach near or over the opening to her cervix; this increases her risk for serious bleeding, shock, blood transfusion, blood clots, planned or emergency delivery, emergency removal of her uterus (hysterectomy), placenta accreta, and other complications. Added likelihood for a woman with a previous cesarean: moderate for placenta previa in a future pregnancy after having one cesarean; high for placenta previa in a future pregnancy after having more than one cesarean.

- **Placenta accreta:** A woman whose uterus has a cesarean scar is more likely than a woman with an unscarred uterus to have a future placenta grow through the uterine lining and into or through the muscle of the uterus; this increases her risk for uterine rupture, serious bleeding, shock, blood transfusion, emergency surgery, emergency removal of her uterus (hysterectomy), and other complications. Added likelihood for a woman with at least one previous cesarean: moderate for placenta accreta in a future pregnancy, with increasing risk as the number of previous cesareans grows.

- **Rupture of the uterus:** A woman whose uterus has a cesarean scar is more likely than a woman with an unscarred uterus to have the uterine wall give way in a future pregnancy or labor, especially at the site of the scar; this increases her risk for severe bleeding, shock, blood transfusion, blood clots, planned or emergency cesarean delivery, emergency removal of the uterus (hysterectomy), and other complications; whether a woman plans a repeat cesarean or a VBAC (vaginal birth after cesarean), she is at greater risk for a ruptured uterus than a woman with no previous cesarean. Added likelihood for a woman with a previous cesarean: moderate for rupture of the uterus, with increasing risk for two or more cesareans.

Questions about Impact of Repeated Cesareans

We did not find research to clarify whether some scar-related risks in future pregnancies increase as the number of previous cesareans increases. The following risks for mothers are worse after one cesarean and may or may not grow as the number of C-section scars grow: fertility problems, ectopic pregnancy (not within the uterus), and placental abruption (placenta detaches before birth). The following risks for babies are worse after one cesarean and may or may not grow as the number of C-section scars grows: being born too early (preterm), being born too small (low birthweight), having a physical abnormality or injury to the brain or spinal cord, and dying before birth (stillbirth) or shortly after birth.

Scarring and adhesion tissue often increase as the number of cesareans increases, creating greater and greater challenges for any future surgical procedures in the area. We did not find information to clarify whether the likelihood of the following adhesion-related problems grows as the number of cesareans grows: ongoing pelvic pain and risk for twisted and blocked bowel in women.

References

Guise J-M, Berlin M, McDonagh M, Osterweil P, Chan B, Helfand M. Safety of vaginal birth after cesarean: a systematic review. *Obstet Gynecol* 2004;103:420–9.

Guise J-M, McDonagh MS, Osterweil P, Nygren P, Chan BKS, Helfand M. Systematic review of the incidence and consequences of uterine rupture in women with previous caesarean section. *BMJ* 2004;329: 159–65.

Hashima JN, Eden KB, Osterweil P, Nygren P, Guise J-M. Predicting vaginal birth after cesarean delivery: a review of prognostic factors and screening tools. *Am J Obstet Gynecol* 2004;190:547–55.

Lieberman E. Risk factors for uterine rupture during a trial of labor after cesarean. *Clin Obstet Gynecol* 2001;44:609–21. [Alone among references, this article is not a systematic review; it is included, however, as a well done review that addresses important questions for women facing the VBAC/repeat c-section decision.]

Childbirth Connection. Comparing risks of cesarean and vaginal birth to mothers, babies, and future reproductive capacity: a systematic review. New York: Childbirth Connection, April 2004.

Section 66.3

Cesarean Sections

"Should I Have a Cesarean Section?" *Journal of Midwifery and Women's Health,* March/April 2004. © 2004 American College of Nurse-Midwives (www.midwife.org). Reprinted with permission. Reviewed by David A. Cooke, MD, FACP, April 12, 2009. Dr. Cooke is not affiliated with the American College of Nurse-Midwives.

What is a cesarean section?

A cesarean section, or C-section, is major surgery that is done to deliver a baby through the abdomen. A doctor makes a 6- to 7-inch-long cut through the skin and muscle of the abdomen. Then the doctor makes a 5- to 6-inch cut in the uterus. The doctor puts his or her hand into the uterus through the cut and pulls the baby out. Usually the cut is made across the lower abdomen between the hip bones. This is called a low-transverse C-section. If the cut goes up and down, it is called a classic C-section.

Why are C-sections done?

Most of the time, C-sections are done when labor is not proceeding normally. If you or your baby has severe trouble during labor, your health care provider will talk with you and your family about the possibility of a C-section. Then, together, you will decide on the best plan: continue labor or have a C-section. Sometimes, problems develop so quickly a C-section needs to be done as an emergency operation. In that case, there will not be time to allow labor to continue, and a C-section will be done immediately. Occasionally, a C-section is planned ahead and done before you go into labor. Most women do not need a C-section.

Will I need a C-section?

If you have had a C-section before, you should talk with your health care provider during your pregnancy about the safest way to give birth this time. Your health care provider may offer you the choice of a C-section or vaginal birth (vaginal birth after C-section, or VBAC).

Can I choose to have a C-section?

Unless you have one of the problems listed on the flip side of this page, vaginal birth is safer than a C-section for both you and your baby.

Isn't a C-section safe?

C-sections are often considered a "safe surgery" because women having babies are usually healthy and able to recover easily. However, any surgery has some risk. Women who have C-sections have a higher risk of heavy bleeding and infection after the birth of the baby. There is also some added risk from having anesthesia. The major risk to you from having a C-section occurs the next time you are pregnant. In the next pregnancy, there is a higher chance of placenta previa (a placenta that partly or completely covers the cervix, which is the mouth of the uterus) or placenta accreta (a placenta that grows too deeply into the wall of the uterus). Either of these placenta problems can cause severe bleeding that is very dangerous for you and your baby. New studies also show a higher chance of stillbirth in women who are pregnant again after having a C-section. If you need a C-section, your health care provider will talk to you about the risks in more detail.

I've heard that some women have a C-section to avoid problems with leaking urine later in life. Is this a good reason to have a C-section?

There have been many studies trying to find out which is the safest way to have a baby. At this time, there is no proof that having a C-section is safer or protects against future problems with leaking urine or stool, or uterine prolapse. Because there are more medical risks for women who have a C-section compared to women who have a vaginal birth, vaginal birth is safer.

Chapter 67

Problems during Childbirth

Chapter Contents

Section 67.1

Cephalopelvic Disproportion

The accurate definition of cephalopelvic disproportion (CPD) is when a baby's head or body is too large to fit through the mother's pelvis. It is believed that true CPD is rare, but many cases of "failure to progress" during labor are given a diagnosis of CPD. When an accurate diagnosis of CPD has been made, the safest type of delivery for mother and baby is a cesarean delivery.

What causes cephalopelvic disproportion (CPD)?

The possible causes of cephalopelvic disproportion (CPD) include:

- large baby due to:
  - hereditary factors;
  - diabetes;
  - postmaturity (still pregnant after due date has passed);
  - multiparity (not the first pregnancy);
- abnormal fetal positions;
- small pelvis;
- abnormally shaped pelvis.

How is cephalopelvic disproportion diagnosed (CPD)?

The diagnosis of cephalopelvic disproportion is often used when labor progress is not sufficient and medical therapy such as use of oxytocin is not successful or attempted. CPD can rarely be diagnosed before labor begins even if the baby is thought to be large or the mom's pelvis is known to be small. During labor, the baby's head molds and the pelvis joints spread, creating more room for the baby to pass through the pelvis. Ultrasounds are used to estimate fetal size, however they are not 100% accurate in determining fetal weight. A physical examination that measures pelvic size can often be the most accurate at determining a diagnosis of CPD. If a true diagnosis of CPD cannot be made, the use of oxytocin is often administered to see if this aides in labor progression or change in fetal positioning.

What about future pregnancies?

Cephalopelvic disproportion is a rare occurrence. According to the American College of Nurse Midwives (ACNM), CPD occurs in 1 out of 250 pregnancies. If you have been diagnosed with CPD, this does not automatically mean that you will have this problem in future deliveries. According to a study published by the *American Journal of Public Health,* over 65% of women who had been diagnosed with CPD in previous pregnancies were able to deliver vaginally in subsequent pregnancies.

Section 67.2

Episiotomy

From "What You Need To Know About Episiotomy," by the Agency for Healthcare Research and Quality (AHRQ, www.ahrq.gov), AHRQ Publication No. 06-0005, December 2005.

Research shows that routine use of episiotomies (surgical cuts in the area between the vagina and anus) does not keep the mother's skin from tearing during birth. It does not speed up a normal birth. It does not help avoid the bladder control problems women sometimes get after having a baby.

What do I need to know?

An episiotomy is a surgical cut in the perineum. (That is the area between the vagina and the anus.) When a woman has a baby, the doctor, nurse-midwife, or midwife may make this cut.

If you are pregnant, you should talk to your doctor, nurse-midwife, or midwife about episiotomies, just as you talk about whether you want pain medicine during childbirth. Do it before you get to the delivery room.

Should I have or not have an episiotomy?

Some doctors perform episiotomies for every birth. Researchers looked at the evidence for this routine use of episiotomies. They did not look at special cases, such as when a baby's shoulders get stuck during birth.

The research shows that routine use of episiotomies does not keep the mother's skin from tearing during birth. It does not speed up a normal birth. It does not help avoid the bladder control problems women sometimes get after having a baby.

You should know that:

- Both episiotomies and tears that occur when giving birth may be painful. They may be slow to heal. They can become infected.

- If you do not have an episiotomy, your skin may tear during delivery. But the tear is likely to be smaller than an episiotomy and to heal with less pain.

Women who do not have episiotomies:

- are likely to start having sex sooner after childbirth than women who have them.

- have less pain the first time they have sexual intercourse after childbirth.

What should I do?

- Talk with your doctor, nurse-midwife, or midwife. Ask the reasons they might perform an episiotomy. Ask how often they perform them.

- Tell your doctor, nurse-midwife, or midwife any questions or concerns you have about having an episiotomy.

- Tell them what you prefer. Your voice counts.

Section 67.3

Birth Injuries

What is a birth injury?

Occasionally during the birth process, the baby may suffer a physical injury that is simply the result of being born. This is sometimes called birth trauma or birth injury.

What causes birth injury?

A difficult birth or injury to the baby can occur because of the baby's size or the position of the baby during labor and delivery. Conditions that may be associated with a difficult birth include, but are not limited to, the following:

- Large babies— birthweight over about 4,000 grams (8 pounds, 13 ounces)
- Prematurity—babies born before 37 weeks (premature babies have more fragile bodies and may be more easily injured)
- Cephalopelvic disproportion—the size and shape of the mother's pelvis is not adequate for the baby to be born vaginally
- Dystocia—difficult labor or childbirth
- Prolonged labor
- Abnormal birthing presentation—such as breech (buttocks first) delivery

What are some of the more common birth injuries?

The following are common birth injuries:

- **Caput succedaneum:** Caput is a severe swelling of the soft tissues of the baby's scalp that develops as the baby travels through the birth canal. Some babies have some bruising of the area. The swelling usually disappears in a few days without problems. Babies delivered by vacuum extraction are more likely to have this condition.

- **Cephalohematoma:** Cephalohematoma is an area of bleeding between the bone and its fibrous covering. It often appears several hours after birth as a raised lump on the baby's head. The body reabsorbs the blood. Depending on the size, most cephalohematomas take two weeks to three months to disappear completely. If the area of bleeding is large, some babies may develop jaundice as the red blood cells break down.

- **Bruising/forceps marks:** Some babies may show signs of bruising on the face or head simply as a result of the trauma of passing though the birth canal and contact with the mother's pelvic bones and tissues. Forceps used with delivery can leave temporary marks or bruises on the baby's face and head. Babies delivered by vacuum extraction may have some scalp bruising or a scalp laceration (cut).

- **Subconjunctival hemorrhage:** Subconjunctival hemorrhage is the breakage of small blood vessels in the eyes of a baby. One or both of the eyes may have a bright red band around the iris. This is very common and does not cause damage to the eyes. The redness is usually absorbed in a week to 10 days.

- **Facial paralysis:** During labor or birth, pressure on a baby's face may cause the facial nerve to be injured. This may also occur with the use of forceps for delivery. The injury is often seen when the baby cries. There is no movement on the side of the face with the injury and the eye cannot be closed. If the nerve was only bruised, the paralysis usually improves in a few weeks. If the nerve was torn, surgery may be needed.

- **brachial palsy:** Brachial palsy occurs when the brachial plexus (the group of nerves that supplies the arms and hands) is injured. It is most common when there is difficulty delivering the baby's shoulder, called shoulder dystocia. The baby loses the ability to flex and rotate the arm. If the injury caused bruising and swelling around the nerves, movement should return within a few months. Tearing of the nerve may result in permanent nerve damage. Special exercises are used to help maintain the range of motion of the arm while healing occurs.

- **Fractures:** Fracture of the clavicle or collarbone is the most common fracture during labor and delivery. The clavicle may break when there is difficulty delivering the baby's shoulder or during a breech delivery. The baby with a fractured clavicle rarely moves the arm on the side of the break. However, healing occurs quickly. As new bone forms, a firm lump on the clavicle often develops in the first 10 days. If the fracture is painful, limiting movement of the arm and shoulder with a soft bandage or splint may be helpful.

Chapter 68

How to Perform an Emergency Delivery

Although most women do not go into labor during emergencies and most of those who do can get to a hospital or birth center, recent events have raised concerns about what to do if travel is not possible. Being prepared can help. The information here includes a list of supplies and directions for managing a normal labor and delivery while taking shelter in place.

This is not a "do it-yourself" guide for a planned home birth, nor is it all the information you need for every emergency. It is not meant to replace the knowledge and skills of a doctor or midwife. The information is a basic guide for parents-to-be who want to be ready in case they have to give birth before they can get to a hospital or birth center.

Supplies for Giving Birth in Place

The following list is not a "do-it-yourself" list of supplies for a planned home birth, nor is it all the information you need for every emergency.

The following supplies can be found at most drugstores, cost about $70, and should be kept in a waterproof bag away from children and pets. Keep them in a tote bag in case you leave home.

"Giving Birth 'In Place': A Guide to Emergency Preparedness for Childbirth," *Journal of Midwifery and Women's Health,* July/August 2004. © 2004 American College of Nurse-Midwives (www.midwife.org). Reprinted with permission.

- Baby size bulb syringe (made of soft plastic, often called an ear syringe; should not be a nasal syringe as the plastic tip does not fit into a baby-sized nose)
- A bag of large-sized under pads with plastic backing to protect sheets from messy fluids
- Small bottle of isopropyl alcohol
- Package of large cotton balls
- Box of disposable plastic or latex gloves
- White shoe laces (to tie umbilical cord)
- Sharp scissors (to cut umbilical cord)
- 12 large sanitary pads
- Chemical cold pack (the kind you squeeze to get it cold)
- Hot water bottle (to help keep baby warm)
- Six disposable diapers
- Pain pills such as Tylenol or Advil
- Small bar of antibacterial soap or liquid antibacterial hand sanitizer

Additional items you will use:

- Shower curtain
- Four cotton baby blankets
- Newborn cap
- Medium-sized mixing bowl
- Four towels
- Wash cloth
- Blankets to keep mom warm
- Pillows
- Five large trash bags for dirty laundry
- Two medium-sized trash bags for the placenta
- Instructions for CPR [cardiopulmonary resuscitation] for adults and babies
- Emergency contact information

If you think you are going to have to give birth at home, put the scissors and shoe laces in a pan of boiling water for 20 minutes.

When done, pour off the water but do not touch the items until needed. If there is no way to boil water, wash the scissors and laces with soap and water and soak them in alcohol during the labor.

Call for Help

If you think you are in labor, try to get to a hospital, birth center, or clinic. If you are alone or travel seems unwise, call the emergency number in your community and ask for help. After you have called for help, keep your front door unlocked so that rescue workers can get in if you are unable to come to the door. Call a neighbor to come and help the family. If the phones are working, keep talking to emergency services or your health care provider who can "talk you through" a labor and birth.

If your labor is going fast and birth seems near, stay at home and have your baby in a safe place rather than in the back seat of the car. Fast labors are usually very normal, and the mothers and babies can both do well. Slow labors will give you time to get to a hospital or birth center, or for a health care provider to get to you. Get out your supply kit and put the supplies where you can easily reach them.

As the helper, your job is to:

- Keep mom comfortable. It is good for her to walk, take a shower, get a massage, and move even if she is in bed.

- Be sure she drinks lots of fluids. Water, tea, and juice are the best.

- Be sure she goes to the bathroom every hour.

- Say and do things that create a calm feeling, even if you are very nervous.

- Wear gloves if you are going to be touching blood.

- Wash your hands or gloves often.

- Do not let pets into the labor and birth room.

- Talk to mom about the sounds of childbirth. Making groaning or crying noise during labor is okay and can help the mom-to-be. It can scare the helpers. So mom has to try to not scream and lose control, and the helpers have to let mom make the noise that helps her cope.

- Decide how to help other members of the family. Will they be present for the birth? What do they need to feel safe?

Prepare the Bed

To keep the mattress from getting wet, cover it and the sheets with a shower curtain and then cover the shower curtain with another clean sheet, plastic-backed under pads and lots of pillows for comfort. The mother may want to spend a lot of time in bed, or she may prefer to be on her feet or in a chair. Whatever feels best is okay.

When the Baby's Head Is Coming First

If you know your baby has been head down during the last weeks of pregnancy, chances are good that the baby will be head first at birth. This is the most common position for a baby. First labors can last for 12 hours or more, whereas the next babies can come much faster.

The Urge to Push

The longest part of labor is the time it takes for the cervix to open wide enough for the baby to pass into the birth canal or vagina (first stage). You can tell the cervix has opened all the way (fully dilated) when the mother has a very strong need to push (second stage). She cannot hold back that urge and may make sounds like she is going to the bathroom. Once she starts pushing, the baby can be born in a few minutes or a couple of hours. As birth gets closer, the area around the vagina begins to bulge out until the top of the baby's head can be seen at the vaginal opening. The mother should be encouraged to push the baby's head out gently in any position that is comfortable for her. She does not have to lie on her back in bed, but you will feel safer if she is lying down or squatting so the baby can slip gently onto a soft surface.

Put on your gloves and get in a place where you can see the baby come out. Remind mom to push gently even when she wants to push hard. As the baby comes out, mom will feel a lot of burning around the vagina and this is when she may make a lot of noise. After the head is born, look and feel with your fingers to find out if the cord is around the baby's neck. If you find a cord around the neck, this is not an emergency. Gently lift the cord over the baby's head, or loosen it so there is room for the body to slip through the loop of cord.

The baby's head will turn to one side and with the next contraction the mother should push to deliver the body. If the body does not come out, push on the side of the baby's head to move the head toward the mother's back. The shoulder will be born. The rest of the body slips out easily followed by a lot of blood-colored water.

If the Head Is Born But the Body Does Not Come out after Three Pushes

The mom must lie down on her back, put two pillows under her bottom, bring her knees up to her chest, grab her knees, and push hard with each contraction. After the baby is born, place her or him on the mother's chest and tummy, skin to skin, and cover both with towels. If the baby is not crying, rub her back firmly. If she still does not cry, lay her down so that she is looking up at the ceiling, tilt her head back to straighten her airway, and keep rubbing. Not every baby has to cry, but this is the best way to be sure the baby is getting the air she needs.

If the Baby Is Gagging on Fluids in Her Mouth and Turning Blue

Use the baby blanket to wipe the fluids out of her mouth and nose. If this does not help, use the bulb syringe to help clear things out. Just squeeze the bulb, place the tip in the nose or mouth, and release the squeeze. This will suck fluid into the bulb. Move the bulb away from the baby and squeeze again to empty the bulb. Repeat until the fluid is removed.

If the baby is still not breathing, follow the CPR directions.

The Umbilical Cord

There is no rush to cut the cord. All you have to do is keep the baby close to the mom so the cord is not pulled tight. If you pick the cord up between your fingers, you can feel the baby's pulse. Within about 10 minutes the pulse will stop. At that time you can tie and cut the cord. Remember the cord is connected to the placenta (afterbirth) which is still inside the mother.

The Baby

At the time of birth, most babies are blue or dusky. Some cry right away and others do not. Do not spank the baby, but rub up and down her back until you know she is taking deep breaths. Once the baby starts to cry, her color will be more like her mom, but her hands and feet will still be blue. Now is the time to keep the baby warm. Remove the wet towel that is over the baby and put another dry towel and blanket over the mother and baby. Put a hat on the baby. The mother can help keep the baby warm with her body heat.

Put the baby to breast. Even if you did not plan to breastfeed, one of the safest things you can do for mom and baby is put the baby to breast. A breastfeeding baby helps keep the mother from bleeding too much and gets the food it needs right away. If the cord is too short to allow the baby to reach the breast, it is okay to wait until you cut the cord.

Cutting the Cord

There are no nerve endings in the cord so it does not hurt either the baby or the mother when it is cut. It is very slippery so take your time because there is no rush. Wash your hands, put on gloves, and then get the container with the scissors and shoelace. Tie one of the laces around the cord very tightly with a double knot about 3 inches from the baby's tummy. The baby will cry when she is uncovered because she is cold, not because it hurts. Tie the other shoelace around the cord about 2 inches from the first knot.

Pick up the scissors by the handle without touching the blades. Cut between the knots you have tied. It is rubbery and tough to cut especially if you have dull scissors. After it is cut, place the end of the cord that is still connected to the mother's placenta into the mixing bowl. Cover the baby again to keep her warm.

The Placenta or Afterbirth (Third Stage)

The placenta looks like a big piece of raw meat with a shiny film on one side. On the other side it has membranes that are attached to the placenta (the membranes look like skin that has been peeled off). When the placenta is ready to come, you will see a gush of blood from the vagina and the cord will get a little longer. Put the bowl close to the mother's vagina and put more waterproof pads under her bottom. Ask the mother to sit up and push out the placenta into the bowl.

There will be a lot of blood and water coming after the placenta. Firmly rub the mother's stomach below her belly button until most of the bleeding stops. This will hurt but needs to be done. The heaviest bleeding should stop in a minute and then the bleeding will be more like a heavy period. If the bleeding increases again, very firmly rub the mother's lower belly until the bleeding slows. When it is firm, you will be able to feel the uterus (womb), which is the size of a large grapefruit, in the lower belly. A firm uterus is a good thing because it will stop the mom from bleeding too much.

Mom's bottom and her uterus may be sore. You may see places where the mother's skin has torn around her vagina. Most of these tears will heal without any problems. Mom will feel better when you put an ice pack on her bottom where the baby came out and then put the sanitary pad on top of the ice pack. She may want to take a couple of pain pills at this time.

Put the placenta in a medium-sized trash bag and wipe off any blood on the outside of the bag. Put this bag into a second trash bag. Take the placenta with you to the hospital or birth center. If you cannot leave the house for more than 4 hours, put the bagged placenta in a container with a lid and put it in the freezer.

Clean Up

After the mother has delivered the placenta and the bleeding has slowed down, give her a drink of juice, soup, or milk and something to eat like crackers and cheese or a peanut butter and jelly sandwich. Put on gloves to clean up the bed. Roll up the sheet and pads inside the shower curtain and put in a large plastic bag. Have clean under pads ready to cover the sheets and a sanitary pad for the mother.

The dirty sheets and towels can be washed in cold water with bleach or ammonia added. Wear gloves when touching items that are bloody. Put a diaper on the baby or you will be sorry.

Breastfeeding

It is important for the mother to breastfeed the baby in the first hour after birth and at least every 2 hours until her milk comes in.

- Breastfeeding will keep the uterus firm and decrease bleeding.
- Colostrum, the liquid that is in the breasts right after birth until the milk comes in, will give the baby all of the food she needs and it will help prevent infection.
- Even if the emergency situation continues for days, weeks, or months, there will always be a ready supply of safe and perfect food for the baby.

Getting Started with Breastfeeding

A newborn will nurse best in the first hour after birth when she is awake and alert. The mother may be more comfortable if she lies on her side with pillows under her head. The mother and baby should be face-to-face and belly-to-belly.

The baby will also nurse better if they are skin-to-skin. The mother should place her nipple and breast against the baby's lips. The baby will lick and try to nurse. The mother needs to help out by placing her nipple into the baby's open mouth. It may take a few tries before the baby can start sucking. If the baby is sleepy, rub her belly and back firmly to wake her up. If the baby is too sleepy, try uncovering her for a short time and rubbing the mother's nipple against the baby's lips. If the mother gets tired, take short breaks and start again. Once the baby nurses for the first time it gets easier.

If the baby sucks a few times and then lets go and the mom has large breasts, mom may need to help the baby breathe by using her finger to hold some breast tissue away from the baby's nose.

What to Avoid

- Don't use a pacifier or a bottle to start the baby sucking. It confuses some babies because they do not suck the same on the mother's breast and a bottle or pacifier.

- Do not separate the mother and baby for very long. The more they stay together, including when they sleep, the sooner breast-feeding will be well established.

Care of the Mother

If you still cannot get to the hospital or birth center to be checked, the mother should go to the bathroom within an hour after the baby is born.

If the room is cold, you can use the hot water bottle to help keep the baby warm. Just wrap the warm bottle in a blanket and place it next to the baby's back.

After birth in a hospital, women are usually offered Tylenol or Advil for pain every 3 to 4 hours as needed. This would be a good choice at home if the mother does not have an allergy to this medication.

When a new mother gets out of bed for the first time, she may feel dizzy. It is important to have her leave the baby on the center of the bed and get up slowly:

- Sit up on the side of the bed to see how she feels.

- Have an adult take her to the bathroom and wait to be sure that she is not feeling faint.

- If she says she is going to faint, believe her and have her lie down on the floor. Do not attempt to walk her back to bed. You have about 10 seconds to get her down on the floor before she passes out and bangs her head on the way down. Once she is down flat, she will wake up and feel better. Just wait a few minutes and then carefully help her back to bed.

In a couple of hours the mom may want to take a shower. Be sure she has had something to eat and is not dizzy when she gets up. It is good to have someone close by because dizziness can return quickly.

What to Do for the Mother and Baby in the First 2 to 3 Days

If you still are unable to get professional health care for several days, you can take care of yourself and your baby during this time by remembering the basic needs: eat, drink fluids, rest, and feed and care for the baby.

Keep someone with you as a helper so you can rest most of the time. The helper should see that you always have plenty of fluids at your bedside and something to eat each time you breastfeed the baby.

Keep ice on the vagina where the baby came out for the first 24 hours. To keep the area extra clean, pour warm water over the vagina every time you go to the bathroom.

Check the uterus for firmness every few hours until the gushes of blood and/or clots stop and the baby is breastfeeding every 2 to 3 hours.

Change the baby's diaper every few hours. The baby's first bowel movements will be black and sticky (meconium), so be sure that the diaper is snug. The baby needs to wet at least once every 24 hours until the mother's milk comes in. After the milk is in, the baby will wet six to eight diapers a day. If the baby is not wetting, nurse the baby more often.

Each time you change the diaper, clean off the umbilical cord with cotton balls soaked with alcohol. The diaper should be placed below the umbilical cord to help keep it clean and dry (it turns dark as it dries). If the cord has a bad smell, a sign of infection, clean it with alcohol until the smell is gone.

What If the Baby Is Coming Bottom First?

A few babies are born bottom first. You will probably not know this is the case until mom pushes and you see a bottom or feet and not a head coming out. At that time you must:

555

- Bring the mom's bottom to the edge of the bed and have her legs pulled up to her chest.

- Prepare a soft landing spot for the baby on the floor.

- Let the baby's body (arms too) come out without touching the baby. You will be looking at the baby's back. Yes, you have to let her little bottom hang down toward the floor even if you are afraid she will fall. If you have to touch something, grab another pillow for the landing zone.

- When the head slips out, grab the baby under the arms and bring her up to the mom.

- If the baby's arms are out but the head does not come with the next contraction, you should have the mother get out of bed, squat, and push.

Key Points

All parents-to-be should go to:

- childbirth education classes;
- infant/child CPR (cardiopulmonary resuscitation) classes;
- breastfeeding classes.

Parents-to-be should keep the family car:

- in good repair;
- filled with gas.

If you have to labor at home during a terrorist attack or other emergency:

- Call your midwife or physician.
- Call for an ambulance.
- Call a neighbor to help you.
- Unlock the front door.
- Keep these instructions and the birth supplies handy.

Women in labor need lots of encouragement and need helpers who are calm, positive, and caring. No matter what is happening in the rest of the world, it is important to keep the room peaceful and to focus on the mother's needs. She needs support and reassurance to do the hard work of labor. Be there for her and her baby.

Disclaimer

The information provided in this chapter is not a do-it-yourself guide for a planned home birth, nor is it all the information you need for every emergency. Following these directions will not replace the knowledge and skills of a doctor or midwife and cannot ensure a safe outcome. The information is a basic guide for parents-to-be who want to be ready in case they have to give birth before they can get to a hospital or birth center. In all cases, it is critical that you attempt to make contact with a trained health care professional.

Part Seven

Postpartum and Newborn Care

Chapter 69

Recovering from Delivery: Physical and Emotional Concerns

Your baby's finally here, and you're thrilled—but you're also exhausted, uncomfortable, on an emotional roller-coaster, and wondering whether you'll ever fit into your jeans again. Childbirth classes helped prepare you for giving birth, but you weren't prepared for all of this!

What to Expect in the First Few Weeks

After your baby arrives, you'll notice some changes—both physical and emotional.

Physically, you might experience:

- **Sore breasts:** Your breasts may be painfully engorged for several days when your milk comes in and your nipples may be sore.

- **Constipation:** The first postpartum bowel movement may be a few days after delivery, and sensitive hemorrhoids, healing episiotomies, and sore muscles can make it painful.

- **Episiotomy:** If your perineum (the area of skin between the vagina and the anus) was cut by your doctor or if it was torn during

"Recovering From Delivery," June 2008, reprinted with permission from www.kidshealth.org. Copyright © 2008 The Nemours Foundation. This information was provided by KidsHealth, one of the largest resources online for medically reviewed health information written for parents, kids, and teens. For more articles like this one, visit www.KidsHealth.org, or www.TeensHealth.org.

the birth, the stitches may make it painful to sit or walk for a little while during healing. It also can be painful when you cough or sneeze during the healing time.

- **Hemorrhoids:** Although common, hemorrhoids (swollen anal tissues) are frequently unexpected.

- **Hot and cold flashes:** Your body's adjustment to new hormone and blood flow levels can wreak havoc on your internal thermostat.

- **Urinary or fecal incontinence:** The stretching of your muscles during delivery can cause you to inadvertently pass urine when you cough, laugh, or strain or may make it difficult to control your bowel movements, especially if a lengthy labor preceded a vaginal delivery.

- **"After pains":** After giving birth, your uterus will continue to have contractions for a few days. These are most noticeable when your baby nurses or when you are given medication to reduce bleeding.

- **Vaginal discharge (lochia):** Initially heavier than your period and often containing clots, vaginal discharge gradually fades to white or yellow and then stops within 2 months.

- **Weight:** Your postpartum weight will probably be about 13 pounds (the weight of the baby, placenta, and amniotic fluid) below your full-term weight, before additional water weight drops off within the first week as your body regains its sodium balance.

Emotionally, you may be feeling:

- **"Baby blues":** Up to 80% of new moms experience irritability, sadness, crying, or anxiety, beginning within days or weeks postpartum. These baby blues are very common and may be related to physical changes (including hormonal changes, exhaustion, and unexpected birth experiences) and the emotional transition as you adjust to changing roles and your new baby.

- **Postpartum depression (PPD):** More serious than the baby blues, this condition is evident in 10%–25% of new moms and may cause mood swings, anxiety, guilt, and persistent sadness. Your baby may be several months old before PPD is diagnosed, and it's more common in women with a history of depression, multiple life stressors, and a family history of depression.

In addition, when it comes to sexual relations, you and your partner may be on completely different pages. He may be ready to pick up where you left off before baby's arrival, whereas you may not feel comfortable enough—physically or emotionally—and may be craving nothing more than a good night's sleep. Doctors often ask women to wait several weeks before having sex in order to allow healing to occur.

The Healing Process

It took your body months to prepare to give birth, and it takes time to recover. If you've had a cesarean section (C-section), it can take even longer because surgery requires a longer healing time. If unexpected, it may have also raised emotional issues.

Pain is greatest the day (or two days) after the surgery and should gradually subside. Your doctor will advise you on precautions to take after surgery, and give you directions for bathing and how to begin gentle exercises to speed recovery and help avoid constipation.

Things to know:

- Drink 8–10 glasses of water daily.

- Expect vaginal discharge.

- Avoid stairs and lifting until you've healed.

- Don't drive until you can make sudden movements and wear a safety belt properly without discomfort.

- If the incision becomes red or swollen, call your doctor.

Some other things to consider during the healing process include:

- **Birth control:** You can become pregnant again before your first postpartum period. Even though this is less likely if you are exclusively breastfeeding (day and night, no solids, at least 8 times a day, never going more than 6 hours without feeding), have not had a period, and your baby is younger than 6 months old, it is still possible. If you want to protect against pregnancy, discuss your options with your doctor. This may include barrier methods (condoms, diaphragms, spermicidal jellies, and foams), IUDs [intrauterine devices], pills, or shots.

- **Breastfeeding:** You need adequate sleep, fluids, and nutrition. An easy way to stay on top of drinking enough fluids is to have a glass of water whenever your baby nurses. Until your milk supply is well established, try to avoid caffeine, which causes loss of fluid through urine and sometimes makes babies wakeful and fussy. If you have any breastfeeding problems, talk to your doctor or a lactation specialist. Your clinic or hospital lactation specialist can advise you on how to deal with any breastfeeding problems. Relieve clogged milk ducts with breast massage, frequent nursing, feeding after a warm shower, and warm moist packs applied throughout the day. If you develop a fever or chills or your breast becomes tender or red, you may have an infection (mastitis) and need antibiotics. Continue nursing or pumping from both breasts. Drink plenty of fluids.

- **Engorged breasts:** They resolve as your breastfeeding pattern becomes established or, if you're not breastfeeding, when your body stops producing milk—usually within a few days.

- **Episiotomy care:** Continue sitz baths (sitting in just a few inches of water and covering the buttocks, up to the hips, in the bathtub) using cool water for the first few days, then warm water after that. Squeeze the cheeks of your bottom together when you sit to avoid pulling painfully on the stitches. Use a squirt bottle to wash the area with water when you use the toilet; pat dry. After a bowel movement, wipe from front to back to avoid infection. Reduce swelling with ice packs or chilled witch hazel pads. Talk to your doctor about taking an anti-inflammatory drug like ibuprofen to help with the pain and swelling.

- **Exercise:** Resume as soon as you've been cleared by your doctor to help restore your strength and pre-pregnancy body, increase your energy and sense of well-being, and reduce constipation. Begin slowly and increase gradually. Walking and swimming are excellent choices.

- **Hemorrhoids and constipation:** Alternating warm sitz baths and cold packs can help. Ask your doctor about a stool softener. Don't use laxatives, suppositories, or enemas without your doctor's OK. Increase your intake of fluids and fiber-rich fruits and vegetables.

- **Sexual relations:** Your body needs time to heal. Doctors usually recommend waiting 4–6 weeks to have sex to reduce the risk of infection, increased bleeding, or re-opening healing tissue. Begin slowly, with kissing, cuddling, and other intimate activities. You'll probably notice reduced vaginal lubrication (this is due to hormones and usually is temporary), so a water-based lubricant might be useful. Try to find positions that put less pressure on sore areas and are most comfortable for you. Tell your partner if you're sore or frightened about pain during sexual activity—talking it over can help both of you to feel less anxious and more secure about resuming your sex life.

- **Urinary or fecal incontinence:** This often resolves gradually as your body returns to its normal prepregnancy state. Encourage the process with Kegel exercises, which help strengthen the pelvic floor muscles. To find the correct muscles, pretend you're trying to stop urinating. Squeeze those muscles for a few seconds, then relax (your doctor can check to be sure you're doing them correctly). Wear a sanitary pad for protection. Let the doctor know about any incontinence you experience.

What Else You Can Do to Help Yourself

You'll get greater enjoyment in your new role as mom—and it will be much easier—if you care for both yourself and your new baby. For example:

- When your baby sleeps, take a nap. Get some extra rest for yourself!
- Set aside time each day to relax with a book or listen to music.
- Shower daily.
- Get plenty of exercise and fresh air—either with or without your baby, if you have someone who can babysit.
- Schedule regular time—even just 15 minutes a day—for you and your partner to be alone and talk.
- Make time each day to enjoy your baby, and encourage your partner to do so, too.
- Lower your housekeeping and gourmet meal standards—there's time for that later. If visitors stress you, restrict them temporarily.
- Talk with other new moms (perhaps from your birthing class) and create your own informal support group.

Getting Help from Others

Remember, Wonder Woman is fiction. Ask your partner, friends, and family for help. Jot down small, helpful things people can do as they occur to you. When people offer to help, check the list. For example:

- Ask friends or relatives to pick things up for you at the market, stop by and hold your baby while you take a walk or a bath, or just give you an extra hand.

- Hire a neighborhood teen—or a cleaning service—to clean once a week, if possible.

- Investigate hiring a doula, a supportive companion professionally trained to provide postpartum care.

When to Call the Doctor

You should call your doctor about your postpartum health if you:

- experience an unexplained fever of 100.4 degrees Fahrenheit (38 degrees Celsius) or above;

- soak more than one sanitary napkin an hour, pass large clots, or if the bleeding level increases;

- had a C-section or episiotomy and the incision becomes more red or swollen or drains pus;

- have new pain, swelling, or tenderness in your legs;

- have hot-to-the-touch, reddened, sore breasts or any cracking or bleeding from the nipple or areola (the dark-colored area of the breast);

- find your vaginal discharge has become foul-smelling;

- have painful urination or a sudden urge to urinate or inability to control urination;

- have increasing pain in the vaginal area;

- develop a cough or chest pain, nausea, or vomiting;

- become depressed or experience hallucinations, suicidal thoughts, or any thoughts of harming your baby.

Chapter 70

Your Baby's First Hours and Newborn Screening Tests

After months of waiting, finally, your new baby has arrived. Mothers-to-be often spend so much time in anticipation of labor, they don't think about or even know what to expect during the first hours after delivery. Read on so you will be ready to bond with your new bundle of joy.

What Newborns Look Like

You might be surprised by how your newborn looks at birth. If you had a vaginal delivery, your baby entered this world through a narrow and bony passage. It's not uncommon for newborns to be born bluish, bruised, and with a misshapen head. An ear might be folded over. Your baby may have a complete head of hair or be bald. Your baby also will have a thick, pasty, whitish coating, which protected the skin in the womb. This will wash away during the first bathing.

Once your baby is placed into your arms, your gaze will go right to his or her eyes. Most newborns open their eyes soon after birth. Eyes will be brown or bluish-gray at first. Looking over your baby, you might notice that the face is a little puffy. You might notice small white bumps inside your baby's mouth or on his or her tongue. Your baby might be very wrinkly. Some babies, especially those born early, are covered in soft, fine hair, which will come off in a couple of weeks. Your

Excerpted from "Your Baby's First Hours of Life," by the Office of Women's Health (www.womenshealth.gov), part of the U.S. Department of Health and Human Services, March 2009.

baby's skin might have various colored marks, blotches, or rashes, and fingernails could be long. You might also notice that your baby's breasts and penis or vulva are a bit swollen.

How your baby looks will change from day to day, and many of the early marks of childbirth go away with time. If you have any concerns about something you see, talk to your doctor. After a few weeks, your newborn will look more and more like the baby you pictured in your dreams.

Medical Care for Your Newborn

Right after birth babies need many important tests and procedures to ensure their health. Some of these are even required by law. But as long as the baby is healthy, everything but the Apgar test can wait for at least an hour. Delaying further medical care will preserve the precious first moments of life for you, your partner, and the baby. A baby who has not been poked and prodded may be more willing to nurse and cuddle. So before delivery, talk to your doctor or midwife about delaying shots, medicine, and tests.

The following tests and procedures are recommended or required in most hospitals in the United States.

Apgar Evaluation

The Apgar test is a quick way for doctors to figure out if the baby is healthy or needs extra medical care. Apgar tests are usually done twice: one minute after birth and again five minutes after birth. Doctors and nurses measure five signs of the baby's condition. These are:

- heart rate;
- breathing;
- activity and muscle tone;
- reflexes;
- skin color.

Apgar scores range from 0 to 10. A baby who scores 7 or more is considered very healthy. But a lower score doesn't always mean there is something wrong. Perfectly healthy babies often have low Apgar scores in the first minute of life.

In more than 98 percent of cases, the Apgar score reaches 7 after 5 minutes of life. When it does not, the baby needs medical care and close monitoring.

Eye Care

Your baby may receive eye drops or ointment to prevent eye infections he or she can get during delivery. Sexually transmitted infections (STIs) including gonorrhea and chlamydia are a main cause of newborn eye infections. These infections can cause blindness if not treated.

Medicines used can sting and/or blur the baby's vision. So you may want to postpone this treatment for a little while. Some parents question whether this treatment is really necessary.

Many women at low risk for STIs do not want their newborns to receive eye medicine. But there is no evidence to suggest that this medicine harms the baby.

It is important to note that even pregnant women who test negative for STIs may get an infection by the time of delivery. Plus, most women with gonorrhea and/or chlamydia don't know it because they have no symptoms.

Vitamin K Shot

The American Academy of Pediatrics recommends that all newborns receive a shot of vitamin K in the upper leg. Newborns usually have low levels of vitamin K in their bodies. This vitamin is needed for the blood to clot. Low levels of vitamin K can cause a rare but serious bleeding problem. Research shows that vitamin K shots prevent dangerous bleeding in newborns.

Newborns probably feel pain when the shot is given. But afterwards babies don't seem to have any discomfort. Since it may be uncomfortable for the baby, you may want to postpone this shot for a little while.

Newborn Metabolic Screening

Doctors or nurses prick your baby's heel to take a tiny sample of blood. They use this blood to test for many diseases. All babies should be tested because a few babies may look healthy but have a rare health problem. A blood test is the only way to find out about these problems. If found right away, serious problems like developmental disabilities, organ damage, blindness, and even death might be prevented.

All 50 states and U.S. territories screen newborns for phenylketonuria (PKU), hypothyroidism, galactosemia, and sickle cell disease. But many states routinely test for up to 30 different diseases. The

March of Dimes recommends that all newborns be tested for at least 29 diseases.

You can find out what tests are offered in your state by contacting your state's health department or newborn screening program.

Hearing Test

Most babies have a hearing screening soon after birth, usually before they leave the hospital. Tiny earphones or microphones are used to see how the baby reacts to sounds. All newborns need a hearing screening because hearing defects are not uncommon and hearing loss can be hard to detect in babies and young children.

When problems are found early, children can get the services they need at an early age. This might prevent delays in speech, language, and thinking. Ask your hospital or your baby's doctor about newborn hearing screening.

Hepatitis B Vaccine

All newborns should get a vaccine to protect against the hepatitis B virus (HBV) before leaving the hospital. HBV can cause a lifelong infection, serious liver damage, and even death.

The hepatitis B vaccine (HepB) is a series of three different shots. The American Academy of Pediatrics and the Centers for Disease Control (CDC) recommend that all newborns get the first HepB shot before leaving the hospital. If the mother has HBV, her baby should also get a HBIG (hepatitis B immune globulin) shot within 12 hours of birth. The second HepB shot should be given 1 to 2 months after birth. The third HepB shot should be given no earlier than 24 weeks of age, but before 18 months of age.

Complete Checkup

Soon after delivery most doctors or nurses also:

- measure the newborn's weight, length, and head;
- take the baby's temperature;
- measure that baby's breathing and heart rate;
- give the baby a bath and clean the umbilical cord stump.

Chapter 71

Newborn Health Concerns

What is infancy?

Infancy is generally the period from birth until age two years. It is a time of a lot of growth and change for children and families.

This information is provided with full-term infants specifically in mind. It is not meant to provide all the information you need to care for your infant. Preterm infants (those born before the mother has been pregnant about 38 weeks) often have special needs.

What is jaundice?

Jaundice is an illness that can cause a baby's skin, eyes, and mouth to turn a yellowish color. The yellow color is caused by a buildup of bilirubin, a substance that is produced in body during the normal process of breaking down old red blood cells and forming new ones.

What causes jaundice?

Normally the liver removes bilirubin from the body. But for many babies, in the first few days after birth the liver is not yet working at its full power. As a result, bilirubin level in the blood gets too high, causing the baby's color to become slightly yellow. This is called jaundice.

Excerpted from "Infant Health," by the National Institute of Child Health and Human Development (NICHD, www.nichd.nih.gov), part of the National Institutes of Health, July 20, 2008.

If your baby has jaundice, it usually does not mean that your baby has liver problems or a "bad liver." In most cases, it just means that the baby's liver is slower in removing bilirubin from the blood during the first few days after birth.

How is jaundice treated?

Although jaundice is common and is often not serious, all babies with jaundice need to be seen by a health care provider.

Many babies need no treatment for jaundice. Their livers start to catch up quickly, usually within a few days after birth, and begin to remove bilirubin normally.

For some babies, however, doctors prescribe photo-therapy—treatment using a special lamp—to help break down the bilirubin in their bodies. In some cases, high levels of bilirubin could cause brain injury.

If your baby has jaundice, ask your health care provider how long his or her jaundice will last after leaving the hospital, and schedule a followup appointment as directed. If your baby's jaundice lasts longer than expected, or an infant who did not have jaundice before starts to turn yellowish after going home, contact your health care provider right away.

How can I help my child with sleep?

Helping a child learn to fall asleep and stay asleep is one of the more challenging parts of infant care. Newborns tend to sleep or drowse for 16 to 20 hours a day. Their "internal clocks" are not yet set, so they sleep a lot both during the day and night. Newborns also have small stomachs, so they need to be awake for regular feedings.

After a few months, babies usually begin to sleep in longer stretches at night and are awake for longer periods during the day. Practicing bedtime routines and putting your baby into the crib before he or she falls asleep can help build better sleep patterns.

What is sudden infant death syndrome (SIDS)?

SIDS is the sudden, unexplained death of an infant younger than one year old. It is the leading cause of death in children between one month and one year of age. Health care providers don't know exactly what causes SIDS, but they do know certain things can help reduce the risk of SIDS.

How can parents reduce the risk of SIDS?

The best way to reduce the risk of SIDS is to always place babies on their backs to sleep for naps and at night. Babies who sleep on their backs are less likely to die of SIDS than babies who sleep on their stomachs or sides. Placing your baby on his or her back to sleep, for naps and at night, is the number one way to reduce the risk of SIDS.

What are some ways to keep my baby safe?

Keeping your baby safe is one of the most important jobs for parents. The U.S. Consumer Product Safety Commission publishes a booklet called The Safe Nursery that provides information on a variety of potential hazards and ways to help keep your infant safe.

What about safety for my infant in the car?

In addition to safety at home, car seat safety is an important part of taking care of your child. Each car seat is different so it is important to carefully review and follow the manufacturer's instructions.

What about child care for infants?

For many parents and families, child care comes from someone other than the child's mother. To understand how this type of care influences child development, the NICHD started the Study of Early Child Care and Youth Development (SECCYD) in 1991.

The major goal of the study was to examine how differences in child care experiences relate to children's social, emotional, intellectual, and language development, and to their physical growth and health. The study examined how quality, quantity, and type of child care setting affect children's development.

Specific findings from the study include the following:

- Higher quality care was associated with better child outcomes.

- The number of hours in care mattered in terms of child outcomes to some degree.

- The child care type or setting (child care home, child care center, etc.) had different effects on children at different ages.

- Parent and family characteristics were more strongly linked to child development and child outcomes than any aspect of child care.

The study also developed a positive caregiving checklist that parents can use to examine the quality of care their child is receiving.

Do preterm infants have special care needs?

Preterm infants, also known as preemies, are babies born before the mother has completed 37 weeks of pregnancy (or on or before 259 days from the first day of the last menstrual period). Preterm infants often have special needs, even after they leave the hospital. Infants born only a few weeks preterm (between 34 and 37 weeks, or "late preterm") often have special needs during the first two years of age.

Preterm infants may need to spend time in a neonatal intensive care unit (NICU) at the hospital until they are big and strong enough to go home. Preterm babies may also need special care even after leaving the NICU.

You should talk to your health care provider about your infant's specific care needs.

Chapter 72

Infant Feeding

Chapter Contents

Section 72.1

Breastfeeding

Excerpted from "Breastfeeding: Frequently Asked Questions,"
by the Office of Women's Health (www.womenshealth.gov), part of the
U.S. Department of Health and Human Services, March 2009.

Why should I breastfeed?

Breastfeeding is normal and healthy for infants and moms. Breast milk has disease-fighting cells called antibodies that help protect infants from germs, illness, and even sudden infant death syndrome (SIDS). Breastfeeding is linked to a lower risk of various health problems for babies, including:

- ear infections;
- stomach viruses;
- respiratory infections;
- atopic dermatitis;
- asthma;
- obesity;
- type 1 and type 2 diabetes;
- childhood leukemia;
- necrotizing enterocolitis, a gastrointestinal disease in preterm infants.

In moms, breastfeeding is linked to a lower risk of type 2 diabetes, breast cancer, ovarian cancer, and postpartum depression. Infant formula cannot match the exact chemical makeup of human milk, especially the cells, hormones, and antibodies that fight disease.

For most babies, breast milk is easier to digest than formula. It takes time for their stomachs to adjust to digesting proteins in formula because they are made from cow's milk.

How long should I breastfeed?

It is best to give your baby only breast milk for the first six months of life. This means not giving your baby any other food or drink—not even water—during this time. Drops of liquid vitamins, minerals, and medicines are, of course, fine, as advised by your baby's doctor. It is even better if you can breastfeed for your baby's first year or longer, for as long as you both wish. Solid iron-rich foods, such as iron-fortified cereals and pureed vegetables and meats, can be started when your baby is around six months old. Before that time, a baby's stomach cannot digest them properly. Solids do not replace breastfeeding. Breast milk stays the baby's main source of nutrients during the first year. Beyond one year, breast milk can still be an important part of your child's diet.

How can I find support for breastfeeding when I go back to work?

Before you deliver, talk to your employer about taking as much time off as you can. This will help you and your baby get into a good breast-feeding routine and help you make plenty of milk. Also, talk with your employer about why breastfeeding is important, why pumping is necessary, and how you plan to fit pumping into your workday, such as during lunch or other breaks. You could suggest making up work time for time spent pumping milk. If your day care is near your workplace, try to arrange to go there to breastfeed your baby during work time. If you can't breastfeed your baby directly during your work breaks, plan to leave your expressed or pumped milk for your baby. The milk can be given to your baby by the caregiver with a bottle or cup.

Do I still need birth control if I am breastfeeding?

Breastfeeding can delay the return of normal ovulation and menstrual cycles. But, like other forms of birth control, breastfeeding is not a sure way to prevent pregnancy. You should still talk with your doctor or nurse about birth control choices that are compatible with breastfeeding.

Section 72.2

Formula Feeding

Excerpted from "Infant Formula," by the U.S. Food and
Drug Administration (FDA, www.fda.gov), April 3, 2006.

What is an infant formula?

The Federal Food, Drug, and Cosmetic Act (FFDCA) defines infant
formula as "a food which purports to be or is represented for special
dietary use solely as a food for infants by reason of its simulation of
human milk or its suitability as a complete or partial substitute for
human milk."

How is infant formula regulated in the United States?

Because infant formula is a food, the laws and regulations govern-
ing foods apply to infant formula. Additional statutory and regula-
tory requirements apply to infant formula, which is often used as the
sole source of nutrition by a vulnerable population during a critical
period of growth and development.

Does FDA have nutrient specifications for infant formulas?

Yes, FDA has requirements for nutrients in infant formulas. These
nutrient specifications include minimum amounts for 29 nutrients and
maximum amounts for 9 of those nutrients. If an infant formula does
not contain these nutrients at or above the minimum level or within
the specified range, it is an adulterated product unless the formula
is "exempt" from certain nutrient requirements. An "exempt infant
formula" is "any infant formula which is represented and labeled for
use by an infant who has an inborn error of metabolism or low birth
weight, or who otherwise has an unusual medical or dietary problem."

How do parents know what formula to feed to their infant?

A wide selection of different types of infant formulas is available
on the market. Parents should ask their infant's health care provider
if they have questions about selecting a formula for their infant.

Do infants fed infant formulas need to take additional vitamins and minerals?

Infants fed infant formulas do not need additional nutrients unless a low-iron formula is fed. If infants are fed a low-iron formula, a health care professional may recommend a supplemental source of iron, particularly after 4 months of age.

FDA's nutrient specifications for infant formulas are set at levels to meet the nutritional needs of infants. In addition, manufacturers set nutrient levels for their label claims that are generally above the FDA minimum specifications and they add nutrients at levels that will ensure that their formulas meet their label claims over the entire shelf-life of the product.

Do "house brand" or generic infant formulas differ nutritionally from name brand formulas?

All infant formulas marketed in the United States must meet the nutrient specifications listed in FDA regulations. Infant formula manufacturers may have their own proprietary formulations but they must contain at least the minimum levels of all nutrients specified in FDA regulations without going over the maximum levels, when maximum levels are specified.

Chapter 73

Bonding with Your Baby

Bonding is the intense attachment that develops between parents and their baby. It makes parents want to shower their baby with love and affection and to protect and nourish their little one. Bonding gets parents up in the middle of the night to feed their hungry baby and makes them attentive to the baby's wide range of cries.

Scientists are still learning a lot about bonding. They know that the strong ties between parents and their child provide the baby's first model for intimate relationships and foster a sense of security and positive self-esteem. And parents' responsiveness to an infant's signals can affect the child's social and cognitive development.

Why Is Bonding Important?

Bonding is essential for a baby. Studies of newborn monkeys who were given mannequin mothers at birth showed that, even when the mannequins were made of soft material and provided formula to the baby monkeys, the babies were better socialized when they had live mothers to interact with. The baby monkeys with mannequin mothers were more likely to suffer from despair, as well as failure to thrive.

581

Scientists suspect that lack of bonding in human babies can cause similar problems.

Most infants are ready to bond immediately. Parents, on the other hand, may have a mixture of feelings about it. Some parents feel an intense attachment within the first minutes or days after their baby's birth. For others—especially if the baby is adopted or has been placed in intensive care—it may take a bit longer.

But bonding is a process, not something that takes place within minutes and not something that has to be limited to happening within a certain time period after birth. For many parents, bonding is a byproduct of everyday caregiving. You may not even know it's happening until you observe your baby's first smile and suddenly realize that you're filled with love and joy.

The Ways Babies Bond

When you're a new parent, it often takes a while to understand your newborn's true capabilities and all the ways you can interact:

- Touch becomes an early language as babies respond to skin-to-skin contact. It's soothing for both you and your baby while promoting your baby's healthy growth and development.

- Eye-to-eye contact provides meaningful communication at close range.

- Babies can follow moving objects with their eyes.

- Your baby tries—early on—to imitate your facial expressions and gestures.

- Babies prefer human voices and enjoy vocalizing in their first efforts at communication. Babies often enjoy just listening to your conversations, as well as your descriptions of their activities and environments.

Making an Attachment

Bonding with your baby is probably one of the most pleasurable aspects of infant care. You can begin by cradling your baby and gently stroking him or her in different patterns. If you and your partner both hold and touch your infant frequently, your little one will soon come to know the difference between your touches. Each of you should also take the opportunity to be "skin to skin" with your newborn by holding him or her against your own skin when feeding or cradling.

Babies, especially premature babies and those with medical problems, may respond to infant massage. Because babies aren't as strong as adults, you'll need to massage your baby gently. Before trying out infant massage, be sure to educate yourself on proper techniques by checking out the many books, videos, and websites on the subject. You can also contact your local hospital to find out if there are classes in infant massage in your area.

Bonding also often occurs naturally almost immediately for a breastfeeding or bottle-feeding mother. Infants respond to the smell and touch of their mothers, as well as the responsiveness of the parents to their needs. In an uncomplicated birth, caregivers try to take advantage of the infant's alert period immediately after birth and encourage feeding and holding of the baby. However, this isn't always possible and, though ideal, immediate contact isn't necessary for the future bonding of the child and parent.

Adoptive parents may be concerned about bonding with their baby. Although it might happen sooner for some than others, adopted babies and their parents have the opportunity to bond just as well as biological parents and their children.

Bonding with Daddy

Men these days spend more time with their infants than dads of past generations did. Although dads frequently yearn for closer contact with their babies, bonding frequently occurs on a different timetable, partially because they don't have the early contact of breastfeeding that many moms have.

But dads should realize, early on, that bonding with their child isn't a matter of being another mom. In many cases, dads share special activities with their infants. And both parents benefit greatly when they can support and encourage one another.

Early bonding activities that both mom and dad can experience together include:

- participating together in labor and delivery;
- feeding (breast or bottle); sometimes dad forms a special bond with baby when handling a middle-of-the-night feeding and diaper change;
- reading or singing to baby;
- sharing a bath with baby;
- mirroring baby's movements;

- mimicking baby's cooing and other vocalizations—the first efforts at communication;

- using a front baby carrier during routine activities;

- letting baby feel the different textures of dad's face.

Building a Support System

Of course, it's easier to bond with your baby if the people around you are supportive and help you develop confidence in your parenting abilities. That's one reason experts recommend having your baby stay in your room at the hospital. While taking care of a baby is overwhelming at first, you can benefit from the emotional support provided by the staff and start becoming more confident in your abilities as a parent. Although rooming-in often is not possible for parents of premature babies or babies with special needs, the support from the hospital staff can make bonding with the infant easier.

At first, caring for a newborn can take nearly all of your attention and energy—especially for a breastfeeding mom. Bonding will be much easier if you aren't exhausted by all of the other things going on at home, such as housework, meals, and laundry. It's helpful if dads can give an extra boost with these everyday chores, as well as offer plenty of general emotional support.

And it's OK to ask family members and friends for help in the days—even weeks—after you bring your baby home. But because having others around during such a transitional period can be uncomfortable, overwhelming, or stressful, you might want to ask people to drop off meals, walk the dog, or watch any of the new baby's siblings outside the home.

Factors That May Affect Bonding

Bonding may be delayed for various reasons. Parents-to-be may form a picture of their baby having certain physical and emotional traits. When, at birth or after an adoption, you meet your baby, reality might make you adjust your mental picture. Because a baby's face is the primary tool of communication, it plays a critical role in bonding and attachment.

Hormones can also significantly affect bonding. While nursing a baby in the first hours of life can help with bonding, it also causes the outpouring of many different hormones in mothers. Sometimes mothers have difficulty bonding with their babies if their hormones are raging or they have postpartum depression. Bonding can also be delayed if a mom's exhausted and in pain following a prolonged, difficult delivery.

If your baby spends some time in intensive care, you may initially be put off by the amount and complexity of equipment. But bonding with your baby is still important. The hospital staff can help you hold and handle your baby through openings in the isolette (a special nursery bassinet) and will encourage you to spend time watching, touching, and talking with your baby. Soon, your baby will recognize you and respond to your voice and touch.

Nurses will help you learn to bathe and feed your baby. If you're using breast milk you've pumped, the staff, including a lactation consultant, can help you make the transition to breastfeeding before your baby goes home. Some intensive care units also offer rooming-in before you take your baby home to ease the transition.

Is There a Problem?

If you don't feel that you're bonding by the time you take your baby to the first office visit with your child's doctor, discuss your concerns at that appointment. It may be a sign of postpartum depression. Or bonding can be delayed if your baby has had significant, unexpected health issues. It may just be because you feel exhausted and overwhelmed by your child's arrival.

In any event, the sooner a problem is identified, the better. Health care providers are accustomed to dealing with these issues and can help you be better prepared to form a bond with your child.

Also, it often helps to share your feelings about bonding with other new parents. Ask your childbirth educator about parenting classes for parents of newborns.

Bonding is a complex, personal experience that takes time. There's no magic formula and it can't be forced. A baby whose basic needs are being met won't suffer if the bond isn't strong at first. As you become more comfortable with your baby and your new routine becomes more predictable, both you and your partner will likely feel more confident about all of the amazing aspects of raising your little one.

Chapter 74

Working after Birth: Parental Leave Considerations

Chapter Contents

Section 74.1

Maternity Leave in the United States

"Maternity Leave in the United States,"
August 2007. © 2007 Institute for Women's Policy Research
(www.iwpr.org). Reprinted with permission.

Paid Parental Leave Is Still Not Standard, Even among the Best U.S. Employers

Nearly one-quarter (24 percent) of the best employers for working mothers provide four or fewer weeks of paid maternity leave, and half (52 percent) provide six weeks or less, according to an Institute for Women's Policy Research analysis of data provided by Working Mother Media, Inc., publisher of *Working Mother* magazine. Nearly half of the best companies fail to provide any paid leave for paternity or adoption. Each year *Working Mother* selects the 100 family-friendliest companies in the United States by reviewing employer questionnaires describing their "workforce profile, compensation, child care, flexibility, time off and leaves, family-friendly programs and company culture."[1] While more than one-quarter of companies (28 percent) provide nine or more weeks of paid maternity leave, many of the winners' paid parental leave policies fall far short of families' needs. No company provides more than six weeks of paid paternity leave and only 7 of the 100 best companies provide seven weeks or more of paid adoptive leave.

An Institute for Women's Policy Research review of the Working Mother 2006 100 Best Companies finds that 7 percent of the highest-ranked companies offer no paid maternity leave, and another 7 percent provide only one to two weeks, as shown in Table 74.1. Some companies model more adequate standards, however. Goldman, Sachs & Co. offers 16 weeks of paid maternity leave, plus 4 weeks for new fathers and 8 for adoptive parents. Eighteen weeks of paid leave is standard for birth mothers at Pillsbury Winthrop Shaw Pittman LLP. New moms with five years of job tenure at Johnson & Johnson, ranked in the top ten of the 100 winners, receive 26 paid weeks of maternity leave.

Half of the 2006 Working Mother 100 Best Companies do not report any paternity leave, and paid leave is much less available for adoptive

Table 74.1. Working Mother 100 Best Companies, 2006: Percent Offering Paid Maternity Leave for Birth Mothers, by Maximum Leave Length

Number of weeks of paid maternity leave	Percent of companies offering specified number of weeks	Cumulative percent of companies offering some paid maternity leave
more than 12 weeks	8%	8%
11 to 12 weeks	11%	19%
9 to 10 weeks	9%	28%
7 to 8 weeks	20%	48%
5 to 6 weeks	28%	76%
3 to 4 weeks	10%	86%
1 to 2 weeks	7%	93%
0 weeks*	7%	

Note: Years on the job influence the amount of paid maternity leave an individual worker may be entitled to in many establishments. This table shows the longest possible amount of paid leave.

*Zero weeks includes companies for which no data are provided on paid maternity leave.

Source: Institute for Women's Policy Research analysis of Working Mother Media, Inc.'s employment survey for the 2006 Working Mother 100 Best Companies, as presented at http://www.workingmother.com/web?service=vpage/77 (copyright 2007; retrieved 7/12/2007).

parents than for birth mothers (Table 74.2). Thirty-five percent of the "100 Best" companies provide only one to two weeks of paternity leave, 8 percent provide three to four paid weeks, and 7 percent provide up to six paid weeks for new fathers. Of the 54 companies that reported paid leave policies for adoptive parents, 17 provide one to two weeks, 13 companies offer three to four weeks, and 16 provide five weeks or more for adoptive parents to bond with their new child.

Paid Maternity Leave Results in Better Health

Outcomes for Mothers and Children

Research establishes that mothers and children benefit from paid maternity leave.

- Women with any combination of paid vacation or sick time tend to take more time off after childbirth, resulting in positive health effects for both women and children.[2]

- Women workers who have some form of paid leave take on average 10.5 weeks off after childbirth, while women without any paid leave take 6.6 weeks.[3]

- The majority of new mothers report one or more physical side effects five weeks after childbirth, and those who had a cesarean section had significantly more health impacts.[4]

- Newborns have decreased access to follow-up care, lower rates of immunization, and decreased breast-feeding by four and one-half weeks on average as a result of early returns to work.[5]

Paid Maternity Leave Is Not Required by Any Federal Law

While no federal law requires paid maternity leave, two laws give workers important rights related to pregnancy, parenthood, and taking care of seriously ill family members. The Pregnancy Discrimination Act of 1978 (PDA) requires that employers treat pregnant workers the

Table 74.2. Working Mother 100 Best Companies, 2006: Percent Offering Paid Leave for Fathers and Adoptive Parents, by Maximum Leave Length

Number of weeks of paid paternity leave	Percent of companies offering paid paternity leave	Percent of companies offering paid adoptive leave
more than 12 weeks	0%	1%
11 to 12 weeks	0%	3%
9 to 10 weeks	0%	0%
7 to 8 weeks	0%	3%
5 to 6 weeks	7%	9%
3 to 4 weeks	8%	13%
1 to 2 weeks	35%	17%
0 weeks*	50%	46%

Note: Years on the job influence the amount of paid leave an individual worker may be entitled to in many establishments. This table shows the longest possible amount of paid leave.

*Zero weeks includes companies for which no data are provided.

Source: Institute for Women's Policy Research analysis of Working Mother Media, Inc.'s employment survey for the 2006 Working Mother 100 Best Companies, as presented at http://www.workingmother.com/web?service=vpage/77 (copyright 2007; retrieved 7/12/2007).

same as other employees with temporary medical disabilities in all conditions of employment, such as pay and fringe benefits, including paid sick days, health insurance coverage, and temporary disability insurance.[6] It also forbids employers from discriminating against pregnant women or forcing them to take pregnancy leave. The law does not require employers to provide paid leave, but if they provide it for some medical conditions, they must include pregnancy. (The PDA applies to firms that are subject to the 1964 Civil Rights Act—those with 15 or more workers.)

The federal Family and Medical Leave Act of 1993 (FMLA) protects workers' job security during leave taken for the employee's own disability or illness (including pregnancy and childbirth); the care of the employee's newly born, adopted, or fostered child; or to care for an immediate family member (spouse, child, or parent) with a serious health condition. The FMLA applies to employees who work 20 or more weeks in a year and have worked at least 12 months for their current employer and who work for a firm employing at least 50 workers. This federal policy ensures that eligible employees receive:

- up to 12 weeks of unpaid leave annually (leave may be taken all at once or intermittently, and for part or all of a day);

- continued health insurance benefits (if ordinarily provided by the employer); and

- a guarantee of return to the same, or an equivalent, job.

Very Few U.S. Workers Have Paid Family Leave

Expanding from the "100 Best" companies to the entire private sector workforce, an even more inadequate picture emerges of access to paid family leave in the United States. The U.S. Department of Labor (DOL) tracks the kinds of leave offered by employers. According to the most recent DOL data, family leave is nearly absent in U.S. workplaces.[7] Only 8 percent of workers have paid family leave to care for newborns and other family members. Managerial and professional workers and those in larger establishments have a distinct advantage over service and blue-collar workers and those employed in smaller firms. Full-time workers are nearly twice as likely as part-timers to have paid family leave. Workers in the Pacific Northwest and New England are also more likely to have paid family leave. Only 5 percent of the lowest-earning workers (earning less than $15 per home) have paid family leave. Even the federal government, which is typically thought of as a model employer, fails to give its employees paid parental leave. Instead, federal employees who become parents must use paid vacation or sick days or unpaid time off.[8]

State-Level Initiatives Improve on the FMLA

Several states have enacted policies to provide workers with family leave above the Family and Medical Leave Act requirements. These policies provide eligible workers in covered establishments with pay and/or more time to care for a newly born or adopted child or to care for an ill parent, child or spouse.

- Temporary Disability Insurance (TDI) is offered to all workers in California, Hawaii, New Jersey, New York, Rhode Island, and Puerto Rico, by state mandate. These programs provide temporary income to workers with non-work related, short-term disabilities, including pregnancy and childbirth. Funded by employee or employer contributions, or both, TDI ranges in coverage from 26 to 52 weeks.[9]

- The State of California gives workers in all firm sizes the right to six weeks of partially paid family leave to care for a newborn, an adoptive child, or an ill family member. The payment amounts to 55% of wages, to a maximum of $728 per week.[10] This provision was enacted in 2002 by expanding the state's TDI program.

- Washington State's 2007 Family Leave Insurance Law (S 5659) instructed a task force to form a Leave Insurance program to begin October 1, 2009. The program will provide $250 per week for up to five weeks to a full-time worker (pro-rated for part-time workers) to care for a newborn or newly adopted child.[11]

- Some states have elected to mandate family leave policies for firms smaller than the federal FMLA guideline of 50 employees or more. The family and medical leave policy of the District of Columbia covers employees of all firm sizes. Maine covers establishment with 15 or more employees, and Minnesota covers those with 21 or more, though the entitled length of leave is less than the FMLA 12-week period. Oregon covers firms with 25 or more employees and requires more than the 12-week federal minimum.[12]

Congress Is Considering New Proposals to Support Working Parents

Two bills have been introduced in the 110th Congress to provide paid time off for new parents and other workers. The proposed Family Leave Insurance Act (S 1681) would offer up to eight weeks of paid leave to new parents or those caring for seriously ill family members. It is co-sponsored by Senators Chris Dodd (CT) and Ted Stevens (AK).

Eligibility criteria mirror the FMLA. Representatives Carolyn Maloney (NY), Steny Hoyer (MD), and Tom Davis (VA) are co-sponsors of the proposed Federal Employees Paid Parental Leave Act (HR 3158), which would give federal employees up to eight weeks of paid parental leave. These bills, if passed, would provide U.S. workers with much more paid family leave than they currently have, on average, improving families' economic security and health outcomes for mothers and children.

Resources

1. Information collected by Working Mother Media, Inc. from employers and edited by Working Mother Media, Inc. 2007. <http://www.workingmother.com/web?service=vpage/77> (downloaded July 12, 2007).

2. Patricia McGovern, Bryan Dowd, Dwenda Gjerdingen, Ira Moscovice, Laura Kochevar, and Sarah Murphy, 2000. "The Determinants of Time Off Work After Childbirth." *Journal of Health Politics, Policy and Law* 25 (June 2000): 528–564.

3. Ibid.

4. Patricia McGovern, Bryan Dowd, Dwenda Gjerdingen, Cynthia R. Gross, Sally Kenney, Laurie Ukestad, David McCaffrey, and Ulf Lundberg, 2006. "Postpartum Health of Employed Mothers 5 Weeks After Childbirth." *Annals of Family Medicine.* 4 (March/April 2006): 159–167.

5. Lawrence M. Berger, Jennifer Hill, and Jane Waldfogel, 2005. "Maternity Leave, Early Maternal Employment and Child Health and Development in the U.S.," *The Economic Journal,* 115 (February 2005): F29–F47.

6. Roberta M. Spalter-Roth, Claudia Withers, and Sheila R. Gibbs, *Improving Employment Opportunities for Women Workers: An Assessment of The Ten Year Economic and Legal Impact of the Pregnancy Discrimination Act of 1978,* Publication #A108, Washington, DC: Institute for Women's Policy Research, 1990.

7. According to the Bureau of Labor Statistics, the National Compensation Survey considers paid family leave a paid leave given to an employee to care for a family member. The leave may be available to care for a newborn child, an adopted child, a sick child, or a sick adult relative. Paid family leave is granted

in addition to any sick leave, annual leave, vacation, personal leave, or short-term disability leave that is available to the employee. Unpaid family leave is unpaid leave given to an employee to care for a family member. The leave may be for caring for a newborn child, an adopted child, a sick child, or a sick adult relative (personal communication, August 30, 2007).

8. United States Office of Personnel Management. 2001. *Report to Congress on Paid Parental Leave,* http://www.opm.gov/oca/Leave/HTML/ParentalReport.htm (August 29, 2007).

9. Vicky Lovell and Hedieh Rahmanou. Paid Family and Medical Leave: *Essential Support for Working Women and Men,* Publication #A124. Washington, DC: Institute for Women's Policy Research, 2000.

10. Employment Standards Administration. *Federal vs. State Family and Medical Leave Laws.* Washington, DC: Department of Labor. <http://www.dol.gov/esa/programs/whd/state/fmla/index.htm> (downloaded August 3, 2007).

11. Ibid.

12. Ibid.

Section 74.2

Family and Medical Leave Act

Excerpted from "Fact Sheet #28: The Family and Medical Leave Act of 1993," by the Employment Standards Administration, Wage and Hour Division, part of the U.S. Department of Labor (www.dol.gov), revised January 2009.

The U.S. Department of Labor's Employment Standards Administration, Wage and Hour Division, administers and enforces the Family and Medical Leave Act (FMLA) for all private, state and local government employee and some federal employees. Most federal and certain congressional employees are also covered by the law and are subject to the jurisdiction of the U.S. Office of Personnel Management or the Congress.

The FMLA became effective on August 5, 1993 for most employers and entitles eligible employees to take up to 12 weeks of unpaid, job-protected leave in a 12-month period for specified family and medical reasons. Amendments to the FMLA by the National Defense Authorization Act for FY 2008 (NDAA), Public Law 110-181, expanded the FMLA to allow eligible employees to take up to 12 weeks of job-protected leave in the applicable 12-month period for any "qualifying exigency" arising out of the fact that a covered military member is on active duty, or has been notified of an impending call or order to active duty, in support of a contingency operation. The NDAA also amended the FMLA to allow eligible employees to take up to 26 weeks of job-protected leave in a "single 12-month period" to care for a covered service member with a serious injury or illness.

Employer Coverage

FMLA applies to all public agencies, including state, local and federal employers, local education agencies (schools), and private-sector employers who employed 50 or more employees in 20 or more workweeks in the current or preceding calendar year, including joint employers and successors of covered employers.

Employee Eligibility

To be eligible for FMLA benefits, an employee must:

- work for a covered employer;
- have worked for the employer for a total of 12 months;
- have worked at least 1,250 hours over the previous 12 months; and
- work at a location in the United States or in any territory or possession of the United States where at least 50 employees are employed by the employer within 75 miles.

While the 12 months of employment need not be consecutive, employment periods prior to a break in service of seven years or more need not be counted unless the break is occasioned by the employee's fulfillment of his or her National Guard or Reserve military obligation (as protected under the Uniformed Services Employment and Reemployment Rights Act [USERRA]), or a written agreement, including a collective bargaining agreement, exists concerning the employer's intention to rehire the employee after the break in service.

Leave Entitlement

A covered employer must grant an eligible employee up to a total of 12 workweeks of unpaid leave during any 12-month period for one or more of the following reasons:

- for the birth and care of a newborn child of the employee;
- for placement with the employee of a son or daughter for adoption or foster care;
- to care for a spouse, son, daughter, or parent with a serious health condition;
- to take medical leave when the employee is unable to work because of a serious health condition; or
- for qualifying exigencies arising out of the fact that the employee's spouse, son, daughter, or parent is on active duty or call to active duty status as a member of the National Guard or Reserves in support of a contingency operation.

A covered employer also must grant an eligible employee who is a spouse, son, daughter, parent, or next of kin of a current member of the Armed Forces, including a member of the National Guard or Reserves, with a serious injury or illness up to a total of 26 workweeks of unpaid leave during a "single 12-month period" to care for the service member.

Spouses employed by the same employer are limited in the amount of family leave they may take for the birth and care of a newborn child, placement of a child for adoption or foster care, or to care for a parent who has a serious health condition to a combined total of 12 weeks (or 26 weeks if leave to care for a covered service member with a serious injury or illness is also used). Leave for birth and care, or placement for adoption or foster care, must conclude within 12 months of the birth or placement.

Under some circumstances, employees may take FMLA leave intermittently—taking leave in separate blocks of time for a single qualifying reason—or on a reduced leave schedule—reducing the employee's usual weekly or daily work schedule. When leave is needed for planned medical treatment, the employee must make a reasonable effort to schedule treatment so as not to unduly disrupt the employer's operation. If FMLA leave is for birth and care, or placement for adoption or foster care, use of intermittent leave is subject to the employer's approval.

Under certain conditions, employees or employers may choose to "substitute" (run concurrently) accrued paid leave (such as sick or vacation leave) to cover some or all of the FMLA leave. An employee's ability to substitute accrued paid leave is determined by the terms and conditions of the employer's normal leave policy.

"Serious health condition" means an illness, injury, impairment, or physical or mental condition that involves either:

- inpatient care (i.e., an overnight stay) in a hospital, hospice, or residential medical-care facility, including any period of incapacity (i.e., inability to work, attend school, or perform other regular daily activities) or subsequent treatment in connection with such inpatient care; or

- continuing treatment by a health care provider, which includes:

  1. a period of incapacity lasting more than three consecutive, full calendar days, and any subsequent treatment or period of incapacity relating to the same condition, that also includes:

     - treatment two or more times by or under the supervision of a health care provider (i.e., in-person visits, the first within 7 days and both within 30 days of the first day of incapacity); or

     - one treatment by a health care provider (i.c., an in-person visit within 7 days of the first day of incapacity) with a continuing regimen of treatment (e.g., prescription medication, physical therapy); or

  2. any period of incapacity related to pregnancy or for prenatal care. A visit to the health care provider is not necessary for each absence; or

  3. any period of incapacity or treatment for a chronic serious health condition which continues over an extended period of time, requires periodic visits (at least twice a year) to a health care provider, and may involve occasional episodes of incapacity. A visit to a health care provider is not necessary for each absence; or

  4. a period of incapacity that is permanent or long-term due to a condition for which treatment may not be effective. Only supervision by a health care provider is required, rather than active treatment; or

5. any absences to receive multiple treatments for restorative surgery or for a condition that would likely result in a period of incapacity of more than three days if not treated.

Maintenance of Health Benefits

A covered employer is required to maintain group health insurance coverage for an employee on FMLA leave whenever such insurance was provided before the leave was taken and on the same terms as if the employee had continued to work. If applicable, arrangements will need to be made for employees to pay their share of health insurance premiums while on leave. In some instances, the employer may recover premiums it paid to maintain health coverage for an employee who fails to return to work from FMLA leave.

Job Restoration

Upon return from FMLA leave, an employee must be restored to the employee's original job, or to an equivalent job with equivalent pay, benefits, and other terms and conditions of employment. An employee's use of FMLA leave cannot result in the loss of any employment benefit that the employee earned or was entitled to before using FMLA leave, nor be counted against the employee under a "no fault" attendance policy. If a bonus or other payment, however, is based on the achievement of a specified goal such as hours worked, products sold, or perfect attendance, and the employee has not met the goal due to FMLA leave, payment may be denied unless it is paid to an employee on equivalent leave status for a reason that does not qualify as FMLA leave.

An employee has no greater right to restoration or to other benefits and conditions of employment than if the employee had been continuously employed.

Part Eight

Additional Help
and Information

Chapter 75

Glossary of Terms Related to Pregnancy and Birth

amniocentesis: A test performed between 15 and 20 weeks of pregnancy that can indicate chromosomal abnormalities such as Down syndrome, or genetic disorders such as Tay Sachs disease, sickle cell disease, cystic fibrosis, and others. It also can detect the baby's sex and risk of spina bifida (a condition in which the brain or spine do not develop properly).

amniotic fluid: Clear, slightly yellowish liquid that surrounds the unborn baby (fetus) during pregnancy. It is contained in the amniotic sac.

amniotic sac: A sac is formed within the uterus that encloses the fetus. This sac bursts normally during the birthing process, releasing the amniotic fluid. A popular term for the amniotic sac with the amniotic fluid is the bag of waters.

anemia: When the amount of red blood cells or hemoglobin (the substance in the blood that carries oxygen to organs) becomes reduced, causing fatigue that can be severe.

birth center: A special place for women to give birth. They have all the required equipment for birthing, but are specially designed for a woman, her partner, and family. Birth centers may be free standing (separate from a hospital) or located within a hospital.

This glossary contains terms excerpted from glossaries and documents produced by the National Institute of Child Health and Human Development, Substance Abuse and Mental Health Services Administration, Office of Women's Health, and U.S. Food and Drug Administration.

carpal tunnel syndrome: A group of problems that includes swelling, pain, tingling, and loss of strength in the wrist and hand. Women deal with strong hormonal changes during pregnancy that make them more likely to suffer from carpal tunnel syndrome.

cervix: The lower, narrow part of the uterus (womb). The cervix forms a canal that opens into the vagina, which leads to the outside of the body.

cesarean section (C-section): Procedure where the baby is delivered through an abdominal incision. Also called cesarean delivery or cesarean birth.

colostrum: Thick, yellowish fluid secreted from breast during pregnancy and the first few days after childbirth before the onset of mature breast milk. Also called "first milk," it provides nutrients and protection against infectious diseases.

doula: An expert support person who helps give physical support during labor and birth. A doula offers advice on how to breathe, relax, and move. She also gives emotional support and comfort. Doulas and midwives often work together during a woman's labor.

eclampsia: A more severe form of preeclampsia that can cause seizures and coma in the mother.

ectopic pregnancy: A pregnancy that is not in the uterus. It happens when a fertilized egg settles and grows in a place other than the inner lining of the uterus. Most happen in the fallopian tube, but can happen in the ovary, cervix, or abdominal cavity.

embryo: A period during pregnancy where the baby has rapid growth, and the main external features begin to take form.

epidural: When a needle is inserted into the epidural space at the end of the spine to numb the lower body and reduce pain. This allows a woman to have more energy and strength for the end stage of labor, when it is time to push the baby out of the birth canal.

episiotomy: A procedure where an incision is made in the perineum (area between the vagina and the anus) to make the vaginal opening larger in order to prevent the area from tearing during delivery.

estrogen: A group of female hormones that are responsible for the development of breasts and other secondary sex characteristics in women. Estrogen is produced by the ovaries and other body tissues. Estrogen, along with progesterone, is important in preparing a woman's body for pregnancy.

Family and Medical Leave Act (FMLA): A federal regulation that allows eligible employees to take up to 12 work weeks of unpaid leave during any 12-month period for the serious health condition of the employee, parent, spouse or child, or for pregnancy or care of a newborn child, or for adoption or foster care of a child.

fetal alcohol spectrum disorders (FASD): A term used to describe the full range of harmful effects that can occur when a fetus is exposed to alcohol.

fetus: A developing being, usually from 3 months after conception until birth for humans. Prior to that time, the developing being is typically referred to as an embryo.

gestational diabetes: Diabetes that occurs during pregnancy.

group B strep (GBS): A type of bacteria often found in the vagina and rectum of healthy women. One in 4 women has it. GBS usually is not harmful to the mother, but can be deadly to the baby if passed during childbirth.

hemorrhoids: Veins around the anus or lower rectum that are swollen and inflamed.

hormone: Substance produced by one tissue and conveyed by the bloodstream to another to effect a function of the body, such as growth or metabolism.

human chorionic gonadotropin (hCG): A hormone that is made when a fertilized egg implants in the uterus. hCG is only found in the body during pregnancy. The amount of hCG rapidly builds up in a woman's body with each passing day she is pregnant. Pregnancy tests work by detecting hCG in either the urine or blood.

hyperemesis gravidarum: Severe, persistent nausea and vomiting during pregnancy; more extreme than morning sickness.

infertility: A condition in which a couple has problems conceiving, or getting pregnant, after 1 year of regular sexual intercourse without using any birth control methods. If a woman keeps having miscarriages, it's also called infertility. Infertility can be caused by a problem with the man or the woman, or both.

lactation: Breastfeeding, or the secretion of breast milk.

low birth weight: Having a weight at birth that is less than 2500 grams, or 5 pounds, 8 ounces.

mastitis: A condition that occurs mostly in breastfeeding women, causing a hard spot on the breast that can be sore or uncomfortable. It is caused by infection from bacteria that enters the breast through a break or crack in the skin on the nipple or by a plugged milk duct.

menstrual cycle: A recurring cycle in which the lining of the uterus thickens in preparation for pregnancy and then is shed if pregnancy does not occur.

mifepristone: Used, together with another medication called miso-prostol, to end an early pregnancy (within 49 days of the start of a woman's last menstrual period).

miscarriage: An unplanned loss of a pregnancy. Also called a spon-taneous abortion.

neural tube defect: A major birth defect caused by abnormal development of the neural tube, or the structure in an embryo which develops into the brain and spinal cord. Neural tube defects are among the most common birth defects that cause infant death and serious disability. The most common neural tube defects are anencephaly, spina bifida, and encephalocele.

nurse-midwife: A nurse who has undergone special training and has received certification on birthing (labor and delivery). Nurse-midwives can perform most of the same tasks as physicians and have emergency physician backup when they deliver a baby.

OB or OB/GYN (obstetrician/gynecologist): A medical doctor who is an expert in prenatal care, labor, and in delivering babies.

ovaries: The ovaries (part of the reproductive system) produce a woman's eggs. Each month, through the process called ovulation, the ovaries release eggs into the fallopian tubes, where they travel to the uterus, or womb. If an egg is fertilized by a man's sperm, a woman becomes pregnant and the egg grows and develops inside the uterus. If the egg is not fertilized, the egg and the lining of the uterus are shed during a woman's monthly menstrual period.

ovulation: The release of a single egg from a follicle that developed in the ovary. It usually occurs regularly, around day 14 of a 28-day menstrual cycle.

oxytocin: A hormone that increases during pregnancy and acts on the breast to help produce the milk-ejection reflex. Oxytocin also causes uterine contractions.

604

perinatal depression: Depression that occurs during pregnancy or within a year after delivery.

peripartum depression: Depression after pregnancy.

placenta previa: When the placenta covers part or entire opening of cervix inside of the uterus.

placenta: During pregnancy, a temporary organ joining the mother and fetus. The placenta transfers oxygen and nutrients from the mother to the fetus, and permits the release of carbon dioxide and waste products from the fetus. The placenta is expelled during the birth process with the fetal membranes.

placental abruption: When the placenta separates from the uterine wall before delivery, which can mean the fetus doesn't get enough oxygen.

postpartum depression: A serious condition that requires treatment from a health care provider. With this condition, feelings of the baby blues (feeling sad, anxious, afraid, or confused after having a baby) do not go away or get worse.

preconception health: A woman's health before she becomes pregnant. It involves knowing how health conditions and risk factors could affect a woman or her unborn baby if she becomes pregnant.

preeclampsia: Also known as toxemia, it is a syndrome occurring in a pregnant woman after her 20th week of pregnancy that causes high blood pressure and problems with the kidneys and other organs.

preterm birth: Also called premature birth, it is a birth that occurs before the 37th week of pregnancy.

preterm labor: Labor that occurs before 37 completed weeks of pregnancy.

progesterone: A female hormone produced by the ovaries. Progesterone, along with estrogen, prepares the uterus (womb) for a possible pregnancy each month and supports the fertilized egg if conception occurs. Progesterone also helps prepare the breasts for milk production and breastfeeding.

progestin: A hormone that works by causing changes in the uterus. When taken with the hormone estrogen, progestin works to prevent thickening of the lining of the uterus.

prolactin: A hormone that increases during pregnancy and breast-feeding. It stimulates the human breast to produce milk. Prolactin also helps inhibit ovulation.

Rh factor: A protein found on most people's red blood cells. If you do not have the protein, you are Rh negative. Most pregnant women who are Rh negative need treatment to protect the fetus from getting a blood disease that can lead to anemia.

semen: The fluid (which contains sperm) a male releases from his penis when he becomes sexually aroused or has an orgasm.

stillbirth: When a fetus dies during birth, or when the fetus dies during the late stages of pregnancy when it would have been otherwise expected to survive.

toxoplasmosis: An infection caused by the parasite named *Toxoplasma gondii* that can invade tissues and damage the brain, especially in a fetus and in a newborn baby.

trimester: Pregnancy is divided into three time periods, or trimesters, that are each about three months in duration—the first, second, and third trimesters.

ultrasound: A painless, harmless test that uses sound waves to produce images of the organs and structures of the body on a screen. Also called sonography.

umbilical cord: Connected to the placenta and provides the transfer of nutrients and waste between the woman and the fetus.

uterine contractions: During the birthing process, a woman's uterus tightens, or contracts. Contractions can be strong and regular (meaning that they can happen every 5 minutes, every 3 minutes, and so on) during labor until the baby is delivered. Women can have contractions before labor starts; these are not regular and do not progress, or increase in intensity or duration.

uterus: A woman's womb, or the hollow, pear-shaped organ located in a woman's lower abdomen between the bladder and the rectum.

vagina: The muscular canal that extends from the cervix to the outside of the body. Its walls are lined with mucus membranes and tiny glands that make vaginal secretions.

Chapter 76

Directory of Organizations That Provide Help and Information about Pregnancy and Birth

Government Agencies That Provide Information about Pregnancy

Agency for Healthcare Research and Quality
Office of Communications and Knowledge Transfer
540 Gaither Road, Second Floor
Rockville, MD 20850
Phone: 301-427-1364
Fax: 301-427-1873
Website: www.ahrq.gov

Center for the Evaluation of Risks to Human Reproduction
P.O. Box 12233
Research Triangle Park, NC 27709
Phone: 919-541-3455
Fax: 919-316-4511
Website: cerhr.niehs.nih.gov
E-mail: shelby@niehs.nih.gov

Centers for Disease Control and Prevention
1600 Clifton Road
Atlanta, GA 30333
Toll-Free: 800-CDC-INFO (232-4636)
Phone: 404-639-3311
Website: www.cdc.gov
E-mail: cdcinfo@cdc.gov

Healthfinder®
National Health Information Center
P.O. Box 1133
Washington, DC 20013-1133
Toll-Free: 800-336-4797
Phone: 301-565-4167
Fax: 301-984-4256
Website: www.healthfinder.gov
E-mail: healthfinder@nhic.org

Resources in this chapter were compiled from several sources deemed reliable; all contact information was verified and updated in May 2009.

National Cancer Institute
Cancer Information Service
6116 Executive Boulevard
Room 3036A
Bethesda, MD 20892-8322
Toll-Free: 800-4-CANCER
(422-6237)
TTY Toll-Free: 800-332-8615
Website: www.cancer.gov
E-mail:
cancergovstaff@mail.nih.gov

National Center for Complementary and Alternative Medicine
National Institutes of Health
9000 Rockville Pike
Bethesda, MD 20892
Toll-Free: 888-644-6226
TTY: 866-464-3615
Fax: 866-464-3616
Website: nccam.nih.gov
E-mail: info@nccam.nih.gov

National Heart, Lung and Blood Institute
P.O. Box 30105
Bethesda, MD 20824-0105
Phone: 301 592 8573
Fax: 301-592-8563
Website: www.nhlbi.nih.gov
E-mail: nhlbiinfo@nhlbi.nih.gov

National Human Genome Research Institute
National Institutes of Health
Building 31, Room 4B09
31 Center Drive, MSC 2152
9000 Rockville Pike
Bethesda, MD 20892-2152
Phone: 301-402-0911
Fax: 301-402-4831
Website: www.genome.gov

National Institute of Arthritis and Musculoskeletal and Skin Diseases
National Institutes of Health
1 AMS Circle
Bethesda, MD 20892-3675
Toll Free: 877-22-NIAMS
(226-4267)
TTY: 301–565–2966
Phone: 301-495-4484
Fax: 301-718-6366
Website: www.niams.nih.gov
E-mail:
NIAMSinfo@mail.nih.gov

National Institute of Child Health and Human Development
P.O. Box 3006
Rockville, MD 20847
Toll-Free: 800-370-2943
TTY: 888-320-6942
Fax: 866-760-5947
Website: www.nichd.nih.gov
E-mail: NICHDInformation
ResourceCenter@mail.nih.gov

National Institute of Diabetes, Digestive and Kidney Diseases
Building 31, Rm. 9A06
31 Center Drive, MSC 2560
Bethesda, MD 20892-2560
Phone: 301-496-3583
Website: www.niddk.nih.gov

National Institute of Environmental Health Sciences
P.O. Box 12233
Research Triangle Park, NC 27709-2233
Phone: 919-541-3345
Fax: 919-541-4395
Website: www.niehs.nih.gov

National Institute of Mental Health
National Institutes of Health, DHIIS
6001 Executive Boulevard
Room 8184, MSC 9663
Bethesda, MD 20892-9663
Toll-Free: 866-615-NIMH (615-6464)
Phone: 301-443-4513
TTY: 301-443-8431
Toll-Free TTY: 866-415-8051
Fax: 301-443-4279
Website: www.nimh.nih.gov
E-mail: nimhinfo@nih.gov

National Institute of Neurological Disorders and Stroke
NIH Neurological Institute
P.O. Box 5801
Bethesda, MD 20824
Toll-Free: 800-352-9424
Phone: 301-496-5751
TTY: 301-468-5981
Website: www.ninds.nih.gov
E-mail: braininfo@ninds.nih.gov

National Institutes of Health
9000 Rockville Pike
Bethesda, MD 20892
Phone: 301-496-4000
TTY: 301-402-9612
Website: www.nih.gov
E-mail: NIHinfo@od.nih.gov

National Women's Health Information Center
8270 Willow Oaks Corporate Drive
Fairfax, VA 22031
Toll-Free: 800-994-9662
TDD: 888-220-5446
Website: www.4women.gov

Office of Minority Health
P.O. Box 37337
Washington, DC 20013-7337
Toll-Free: 800-444-6472
Fax: 301-251-2160
Website: www.omhrc.gov
E-mail: info@omhrc.gov

U.S. Department of Health and Human Services
200 Independent Avenue, SW
Washington, DC 20201
Toll-Free: 877-696-6775
Phone: 202-619-0257
Website: www.hhs.gov

U.S. Food and Drug Administration
10903 New Hampshire Avenue
Silver Spring, MD 20903
Toll-Free: 888-463-6332
Website: www.fda.gov

U.S. National Library of Medicine
8600 Rockville Pike
Bethesda, MD 20894
Toll-Free: 888-346-3656
Phone: 301-594-5983
TDD: 800-735-2258
Website: www.nlm.nih.gov
E-mail: custserv@nlm.nih.gov

Private Agencies That Provide Information about Pregnancy

American Academy of Family Physicians
11400 Tomahawk Creek Parkway
Leawood, KS 66211-2680
Toll-Free: 800-274-2237
Fax: 913-906-6075
Website: www.aafp.org

American Academy of Pediatrics
141 Northwest Point Boulevard
Elk Grove Village, IL 60007
Phone: 847-434-4000
Fax: 847-434-8000
Website: www.aap.org
E-mail: kidsdocs@aap.org

American Association of Birth Centers
3123 Gottschall Road
Perkiomenville, PA 18074
Toll-Free: 866-54-BIRTH
(542-4784)
Phone: 215-234-8068
Fax: 215-234-8829
Website: www.birthcenters.org

American College of Allergy, Asthma and Immunology
85 West Algonquin Road
Suite 550
Arlington Heights, IL 60005
Website: www.acaai.org
E-mail: mail@acaai.org

American College of Obstetricians and Gynecologists
409 12th Street, SW
P.O. Box 96920
Washington, DC 20090-6920
Phone: 202-638-5577
Website: www.acog.org

American College of Nurse-Midwives
8403 Colesville Road
Suite 1550
Silver Spring, MD 20910
Phone: 240-485-1800
Fax: 240-485-1818
Website: www.midwife.org
E-mail: info@acnm.org

American College of Surgeons
633 N. Saint Clair Street
Chicago, IL 60611-3211
Toll-Free: 800-621-4111
Phone: 312-202-5000
Fax: 312-202-5001
Website: www.facs.org
E-mail: postmaster@facs.org

American Diabetes Association
1701 North Beauregard Street
Alexandria, VA 22311
Toll-Free: 800-DIABETES
(342-2383)
Website: www.diabetes.org
E-mail: AskADA@diabetes.org

American Fertility Association
305 Madison Avenue
Suite 449
New York, NY 10165
Toll-Free: 888-917-3777
Website: www.theafa.org
E-mail: Info@TheAFA.org

American Institute of Ultrasound in Medicine
14750 Sweitzer Lane
Suite 100
Laurel, MD 20707
Toll-Free: 800-638-5352
Phone: 301-498-4100
Fax: 301-498-4450
Website: www.aium.org

American Medical Association/Medem
100 Pine Street, 3rd Floor
San Francisco, CA 94111
Toll-Free: 877-926-3336
Phone: 415-644-3800
Fax: 415-644-3950
Website: www.medem.com
E-mail: info@medem.com

American Pregnancy Association
1425 Greenway Drive
Irving, TX 75038
Phone: 972-550-0140
Fax: 972-550-0800
Website:
www.americanpregnancy.org
E-mail: questions
@americanpregnancy.org

American Society for Reproductive Medicine
1209 Montgomery Highway
Birmingham, AL 35216-2809
Phone: 205-978-5000
Fax: 205-978-5005
Website: www.asrm.org
E-mail: asrm@asrm.org

American Society of Anesthesiologists
520 N. Northwest Highway
Park Ridge, IL 60068-2573
Phone: 847-825-5586
Fax: 847-825-1692
Website: www.asahq.org
E-mail: mail@asahq.org

Association of Maternal and Child Health Programs
2030 M Street, NW
Suite 350
Washington, DC 20036
Phone: 202-775-0436
Fax: 202-775-0061
Website: www.amchp.org

Association of Women's Health, Obstetric and Neonatal Nurses
2000 L Street, NW
Suite 740
Washington, DC 20036
Toll-Free: 800-673-8499
Phone: 202-261-2400
Fax: 202-728-0575
Website: www.awhonn.org
E-mail:
customerservice@awhonn.org

Center for Research on Reproduction and Women's Health
1355 Biomedical Research
Building II/III
University of Pennsylvania
Health System
421 Curie Boulevard
Philadelphia, PA 19104-6160
Phone: 215-898-0147
Fax: 215-573-5408
Website: www.med.upenn.edu/
crrwh

Childbirth and Postpartum Professional Association
P.O. Box 491448
Lawrenceville, GA 30049
Website: www.cappa.net
E-mail: info@cappa.net

Childbirth Connection
281 Park Avenue South
5th Floor
New York, NY 10010
Phone: 212-777-5000
Fax: 212-777-9320
Website:
www.childbirthconnection.org

Cleveland Clinic
9500 Euclid Avenue
Cleveland, OH 44195
Toll-Free: 800-223-2273
Phone: 216-444-2200
TTY: 216-444-0261
Website:
www.clevelandclinic.org

DONA International
P.O. Box 626
Jasper, IN 47547
Toll-Free: 888-788-DONA
(788-3662)
Fax: 812-634-1491
Website: www.dona.org
E-mail: info@DONA.org

Guttmacher Institute
1301 Connecticut Avenue NW,
Suite 700
Washington, DC 20036
Phone: 202-296-4012
Toll Free: 877-823-0262
Fax: 202-223-5756
Website: www.guttmacher.org

Hyperemesis Education & Research Foundation
932 Edwards Ferry Road, #23
Leesburg, VA 20176
Fax: 703-935-2369
Website: www.hyperemesis.org
E-mail: info@helpHER.org

Institute for Women's Policy Research
1707 L Street, NW, Suite 750
Washington, DC 20036
Website: www.iwpr.org
E-mail: iwpr@iwpr.org

International Childbirth Education Association
1500 Sunday Drive, Suite 102
Raleigh, NC 27607
Toll-Free: 800-624-4934
Phone: 919-863-9487
Fax: 919-787-4916
Website: www.icea.org
E-mail: info@icea.org

International Council on Infertility Information Dissemination
P.O. Box 6836
Arlington, VA 22206
Phone: 703-379-9178
Fax: 703-379-1593
Website: www.inciid.org
E-mail: INCIIDinfo@inciid.org

La Leche League
P.O. Box 4079
Schaumburg, IL 60168-4079
Phone: 847-519-7730
Toll-Free: 800-LALECHE
(525-3243)
Fax: 847-969-0460
TTY: 847-592-7570
Website: www.llli.org

Lamaze International
2025 M Street, NW, Suite 800
Washington, DC 20036-3309
Toll-Free: 800-368-4404
Fax: 202-367-2128
Website: www.lamaze.org

March of Dimes
1275 Mamaroneck Avenue
White Plains, NY 10605
Phone: 914-997-4488
Website: www.marchofdimes.com

Midwives Alliance of North America
611 Pennsylvania Avenue, SE
#1700
Washington, DC 20003-4303
Toll-Free: 888-923-MANA
(923-6262)
Website: www.mana.org
E-mail: info@mana.org

Motherisk Program
Phone: 416-813-6780
Website: www.motherisk.org

*National Campaign to
Prevent Teen and
Unplanned Pregnancy*
1776 Massachusetts Avenue,
NW, Suite 200
Washington, DC 20036
Phone: 202-478-8500
Fax: 202-478-8588
Website:
www.thenationalcampaign.org

*Nemours Foundation
Center for Children's
Health Media*
1600 Rockland Road
Wilmington, DE 19803
Phone: 302-651-4000
Fax: 302-651-4055
Website: www.kidshealth.org
E-mail: info@kidshealth.org

*Organization of Teratology
Information Specialists*
University of Arizona
Drachman Hall
P.O. Box 210202
1295 N. Martin, Room B308
Tucson, AZ 85721-0202
Toll-Free: 866-626-OTIS
(626-6847)
Phone: 520-626-3547
Website: www.otispregnancy.org

*Planned Parenthood
Federation of America*
434 West 33rd Street
New York, NY 10001
Toll-Free: 800-230-7526
Phone: 212-541-7800
Fax: 212-245-1845
Website:
www.plannedparenthood.org

Preeclampsia Foundation
5353 Wayzata Boulevard
Suite 207
Minneapolis, MN 55416
Toll-Free: 800-665-9341
Phone: 952-252-3573
Fax: 952-252-8096
Website: www.preeclampsia.org
E-mail: info@preeclampsia.org

*RESOLVE: The National
Infertility Association*
1760 Old Meadow Road
Suite 500
McLean, VA 22102
Phone: 703-556-7172
Fax: 703-506-3266
Website: www.resolve.org

*Sidelines National Support
Network*
P. O. Box 1808
Laguna Beach, CA 92652
Toll-Free: 888-447-4754
Fax: 949-497-5598
Website: www.sidelines.org
E-mail: sidelines@sidelines.org

Information on Public Health Assistance for Low-Income Pregnant Women

American Public Human Services Association
1133 Nineteenth Street, NW
Suite 400
Washington, DC 20036
Phone: 202-682-0100
Fax: 202-289-6555
Website: www.aphsa.org

Center for Health Care Strategies, Inc.
200 American Metro Boulevard
Suite 119
Hamilton, NJ 08619
Phone: 609-528-8400
Fax: 609-586-3679
Website: www.chcs.org
E-mail: mail@chcs.org

Centers for Medicare and Medicaid Services
7500 Security Boulevard
Baltimore, MD 21244-1850
Toll-Free: 800-633-4227
Website: www.medicare.gov

Early Head Start
Administration for Children and Families
370 L'Enfant Promenade, SW
Washington, DC 20447
Website: www.ehsnrc.org

Institute for Health Policy Solutions
1444 Eye Street NW
Suite 900
Washington, DC 20005
Phone: 202-789-1491
Fax: 202-789-1879
Website: www.ihps.org
E-mail: ajavier@ihps.org

National Advocates for Pregnant Women
15 West 36th Street
Suite 901
New York, NY 10018-7910
Phone: 212-255-9252
Fax: 212-255-9253
Website: www.advocatesfor
pregnantwomen.org
E-mail: info @advocatesfor
pregnantwomen.org

National Association of Public Hospitals and Health Systems
1301 Pennsylvania Avenue, NW
Suite 950
Washington, DC 20004
Phone: 202-585-0100
Fax: 202-585-0101
Website: www.naph.org
E-mail: info@naph.org

National Coalition on Health Care
1120 G Street, NW
Suite 810
Washington, DC 20005
Phone: 202-638-7151
Website: www.nchc.org
E-mail: info@nchc.org

National Rural Health Association
521 E. 63rd Street
Kansas City, MO 64110-3329
Phone: 816-756-3140
Fax: 816-756-3144
Website:
www.ruralhealthweb.org

Planned Parenthood Federation of America
434 West 33rd Street
New York, NY 10001
Phone: 212-541-7800
Fax: 212-245-1845
Website:
www.plannedparenthood.org

Robert Wood Johnson Foundation
P.O. Box 2316
Route 1 and College Road East
Princeton, NJ 08543
Toll-Free: 877-843-RWJF
(843-7953)
Website: www.rwjf.org

State Children's Health Insurance Program (SCHIP)
National Conference of State Legislatures
444 North Capitol Street, NW
Suite 515
Washington, DC 20001
Phone: 202-624-5400
Fax: 202-737-1069
Website: www.ncsl.org/programs/health/chiphome.htm

Urban Institute
2100 M Street, NW
Washington, DC 20037
Phone: 202-833-7200
Website: www.urban.org

Women, Infants, and Children
Website: www.fns.usda.gov/wic
E-mail: wichq-web@fns.usda.gov

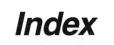

Index

Index

Health Reference Series

Complete Catalog

List price $93 per volume. School and library price $84 per volume.

Adolescent Health Sourcebook, 2nd Edition

Basic Consumer Health Information about the Physical, Mental, and Emotional Growth and Development of Adolescents, Including Medical Care, Nutritional and Physical Activity Requirements, Puberty, Sexual Activity, Acne, Tanning, Body Piercing, Common Physical Illnesses and Disorders, Eating Disorders, Attention Deficit Hyperactivity Disorder, Depression, Bullying, Hazing, and Adolescent Injuries Related to Sports, Driving, and Work

Along with Substance Abuse Information about Nicotine, Alcohol, and Drug Use, a Glossary, and Directory of Additional Resources

Edited by Joyce Brennfleck Shannon. 655 pages. 2007. 978-0-7808-0943-7.

"A particularly good resource for both parents and teens. The concise presentation of the material in brief and well-organized chapters creates an easy volume to browse."
—*School Library Journal*, Jun '07

"I don't believe there are any other books written in such easy to understand language that encompass such a breadth of topics. This is a complete revision of the book and is an excellent resource for parents and teens."
—*Doody's Review Service*, 2007

Adult Health Concerns Sourcebook

Basic Consumer Health Information about Medical and Mental Concerns of Adults, Including Facts about Choosing Healthcare Providers, Navigating Insurance Options, Maintaining Wellness, Preventing Cancer, Heart Disease, Stroke, Diabetes, and Osteoporosis, and Understanding Aging-Related Health Concerns, Including Menopause, Cognitive Changes, and Changes in the Coronary and Vascular Systems

Along with Tips on Caring for Aging Parents and Dealing with Health-Related Work and Travel Issues, a Glossary, and a Directory of Resources for Additional Help and Information

Edited by Sandra J. Judd. 648 pages. 2008. 978-0-7808-0999-4.

"Provides a thorough list of topics that are important to adult health and for caregivers."
—*CHOICE*, Nov '08

"Written in easy-to-understand language . . . the content is well-organized and is intended to aid adults in making health care-related decisions."
—*AORN Journal*, Dec '08

AIDS Sourcebook, 4th Edition

Basic Consumer Health Information about Human Immunodeficiency Virus (HIV) and Acquired Immunodeficiency Syndrome (AIDS), Featuring Updated Statistics and Facts about Risks, Prevention, Screening, Diagnosis, Treatments, Side Effects, and Complications, and Including a Section about the Impact of HIV/AIDS on the Health of Women, Children, and Adolescents

Along with Tips on Managing Life with AIDS, Reports on Current Research Initiatives and Clinical Trials, a Glossary of Related Terms, and Resource Directories for Further Help and Information

Edited by Ivy L. Alexander. 680 pages. 2008. 978-0-7808-0997-0.

SEE ALSO Contagious Diseases Sourcebook, 2nd Edition

Alcoholism Sourcebook, 2nd Edition

Basic Consumer Health Information about Alcohol Use, Abuse, and Dependence, Featuring Facts about the Physical, Mental, and Social Health Effects of Alcohol Addiction, Including Alcoholic Liver Disease, Pancreatic Disease, Cardiovascular Disease, Neurological Disorders, and the Effects of Drinking during Pregnancy

Along with Information about Alcohol Treatment, Medications, and Recovery Programs, in Addition to Tips for Reducing the Prevalence of Underage Drinking, Statistics about Alcohol Use, a Glossary of Related Terms, and Directories of Resources for More Help and Information

Edited by Amy L. Sutton. 625 pages. 2007. 978-0-7808-0942-0.

"A comprehensive look at the adverse effects of alcohol on people of all ages . . . It serves to whet the reader's appetite to continue learning using other resources. It is practical, easy to read, and enlightening, and is the first book a lay person should consult to learn about alcoholism."
—*Doody's Review Service, 2007*

"Should be a basic acquisition for any serious public or college-level library including health reference titles for general-interest readers."
—*California Bookwatch, Feb '07*

SEE ALSO *Drug Abuse Sourcebook, 2nd Edition*

Allergies Sourcebook, 3rd Edition

Basic Consumer Health Information about Allergic Disorders, Such as Anaphylaxis, Hives, Eczema, Rhinitis, Sinusitis, and Conjunctivitis, and Their Triggers, Including Pollen, Mold, Dust Mites, Animal Dander, Insects, Chemicals, Food, Food Additives, and Medications

Along with Advice about the Diagnosis and Treatment of Allergy Symptoms, a Glossary of Related Terms, a Directory of Resources for Help and Information, and Suggestions for Additional Reading

Edited by Amy L. Sutton. 588 pages. 2007. 978-0-7808-0950-5.

SEE ALSO *Asthma Sourcebook, 2nd Edition*

Alzheimer Disease Sourcebook, 4th Edition

Basic Consumer Health Information about Alzheimer Disease, Other Dementias, and Related Disorders, Including Multi-Infarct Dementia, Dementia with Lewy Bodies, Frontotemporal Dementia (Pick Disease), Wernicke-Korsakoff Syndrome (Alcohol-Related Dementia), AIDS Dementia Complex, Huntington Disease, Creutzfeldt-Jacob Disease, and Delirium

Along with Information about Coping with Memory Loss and Forgetfulness, Maintaining

Skills, and Long-Term Planning for People with Dementia, and Suggestions Addressing Common Caregiver Concerns, Updated Information about Current Research Efforts, a Glossary of Related Terms, and Directories of Sources for Additional Help and Information

Edited by Karen Bellenir. 603 pages. 2008. 978-0-7808-1001-3.

"An invaluable resource for persons who have received a diagnosis, for caregivers, and for family members dealing with this insidious disease. It is recommended for public, community college, and ready-reference sections in academic libraries."
—*ARBAonline, Jul '08*

SEE ALSO *Brain Disorders Sourcebook, 2nd Edition*

Arthritis Sourcebook, 2nd Edition

Basic Consumer Health Information about Osteoarthritis, Rheumatoid Arthritis, Other Rheumatic Disorders, Infectious Forms of Arthritis, and Diseases with Symptoms Linked to Arthritis, Featuring Facts about Diagnosis, Pain Management, and Surgical Therapies

Along with Coping Strategies, Research Updates, a Glossary, and Resources for Additional Help and Information

Edited by Amy L. Sutton. 567 pages. 2004. 978-0-7808-0667-2.

"This easy-to-read volume is recommended for consumer health collections within public or academic libraries."
—*E-Streams, May '05*

"As expected, this updated edition continues the excellent reputation of this series in providing sound, usable health information. . . . Highly recommended."
—*American Reference Books Annual, 2005*

Asthma Sourcebook, 2nd Edition

Basic Consumer Health Information about the Causes, Symptoms, Diagnosis, and Treatment of Asthma in Infants, Children, Teenagers, and Adults, Including Facts about Different Types of Asthma, Common Co-Occurring Conditions, Asthma Management Plans, Triggers, Medications, and Medication Delivery Devices

Along with Asthma Statistics, Research Updates, a Glossary, a Directory of Asthma Related Resources, and More

Edited by Karen Bellenir. 581 pages. 2006. 978-0-7808-0866-9.

Attention Deficit Disorder Sourcebook

Basic Consumer Health Information about Attention Deficit/Hyperactivity Disorder in Children and Adults, Including Facts about Causes, Symptoms, Diagnostic Criteria, and Treatment Options Such as Medications, Behavior Therapy, Coaching, and Homeopathy

Along with Reports on Current Research Initiatives, Legal Issues, and Government Regulations, and Featuring a Glossary of Related Terms, Internet Resources, and a List of Additional Reading Material

Edited by Dawn D. Matthews. 447 pages. 2002. 978-0-7808-0624-5.

"Recommended reference source."
—Booklist, Jan '03

SEE ALSO Learning Disabilities Sourcebook, 3rd Edition

Autism and Pervasive Developmental Disorders Sourcebook

Basic Consumer Health Information about Autism Spectrum and Pervasive Developmental Disorders, Such as Classical Autism, Asperger Syndrome, Rett Syndrome, and Childhood Disintegrative Disorder, Including Information about Related Genetic Disorders and Medical Problems and Facts about Causes, Screening Methods, Diagnostic Criteria, Treatments and Interventions, and Family and Education Issues

Along with a Glossary of Related Terms, Tips for Evaluating the Validity of Health Claims, and a Directory of Resources for Additional Help and Information

Edited by Sandra J. Judd. 603 pages. 2007. 978-0-7808-0953-6.

"Recommended for public libraries"
—SciTech Book News, Mar '08

SEE ALSO Learning Disabilities Sourcebook, 3rd Edition

Back and Neck Disorders Sourcebook, 2nd Edition

Basic Consumer Health Information about Spinal Pain, Spinal Cord Injuries, and Related Disorders, Such as Degenerative Disk Disease, Osteoarthritis, Scoliosis, Sciatica, Spina Bifida, and Spinal Stenosis, and Featuring Facts about Maintaining Spinal Health, Self-Care, Pain Management, Rehabilitative Care, Chiropractic Care, Spinal Surgeries, and Complementary Therapies

Along with Suggestions for Preventing Back and Neck Pain, a Glossary of Related Terms, and a Directory of Resources

Edited by Amy L. Sutton. 607 pages. 2004. 978-0-7808-0738-9.

"Recommended. ...An easy to use, comprehensive medical reference book."
—E-Streams, Sep '05

"For anyone who has back or neck problems, this book is ideal. Its easy-to-understand language and variety of topics makes this sourcebook a worthwhile read. The price...is reasonable for the amount of information contained in the book"
—Occupational Therapy in Health Care, 2007

Blood and Circulatory Disorders Sourcebook, 2nd Edition

Basic Consumer Health Information about the Blood and Circulatory System and Related Disorders, Such as Anemia and Other Hemoglobin Diseases, Cancer of the Blood and Associated Bone Marrow Disorders, Clotting and Bleeding Problems, and Conditions That Affect the Veins, Blood Vessels, and Arteries, Including Facts about the Donation and Transplantation of Bone Marrow, Stem Cells, and Blood and Tips for Keeping the Blood and Circulatory System Healthy

Along with a Glossary of Related Terms and Resources for Additional Help and Information

Edited by Amy L. Sutton. 634 pages. 2005. 978-0-7808-0746-4.

"Highly recommended pick for basic consumer health reference holdings at all levels."
—The Bookwatch, Aug '05

Brain Disorders Sourcebook, 2nd Edition

Basic Consumer Health Information about Acquired and Traumatic Brain Injuries, Infections of the Brain, Epilepsy and Seizure Disorders, Cerebral Palsy, and Degenerative Neurological Disorders, Including Amyotrophic Lateral Sclerosis (ALS), Dementias, Multiple Sclerosis, and More

Along with Information on the Brain's Structure and Function, Treatment and Rehabilitation Options, Reports on Current Research Initiatives, a Glossary of Terms Related to Brain Disorders and Injuries, and a Directory of Sources for Further Help and Information

Edited by Sandra J. Judd. 600 pages. 2005. 978-0-7808-0744-0.

"This easy-to-read volume provides up-to-date health information... Recommended for consumer health collections within public or academic libraries."

—E-Streams, Feb '06

SEE ALSO Alzheimer Disease Sourcebook, 4th Edition

Breast Cancer Sourcebook, 3rd Edition

Basic Consumer Health Information about Breast Health and Breast Cancer, Including Facts about Environmental, Genetic, and Other Risk Factors, Prevention Efforts, Screening and Diagnostic Methods, Surgical Treatment Options and Other Care Choices, Complementary and Alternative Therapies, and Post-Treatment Concerns

Along with Statistical Data, News about Research Advances, a Glossary of Related Terms, and Directories of Resources for Additional Information and Support

Edited by Karen Bellenir. 606 pages. 2009. 978-0-7808-1030-3.

SEE ALSO Cancer Sourcebook for Women, 3rd Edition, Women's Health Concerns Sourcebook, 3rd Edition

Breastfeeding Sourcebook

Basic Consumer Health Information about the Benefits of Breastmilk, Preparing to Breastfeed, Breastfeeding as a Baby Grows, Nutrition, and More, Including Information on Special Situations and Concerns Such as Mastitis, Illness, Medications, Allergies, Multiple Births, Prematurity, Special Needs, and Adoption

Along with a Glossary and Resources for Additional Help and Information

Edited by Jenni Lynn Colson. 367 pages. 2002. 978-0-7808-0332-9.

SEE ALSO Pregnancy and Birth Sourcebook, 2nd Edition

Burns Sourcebook

Basic Consumer Health Information about Various Types of Burns and Scalds, Including Flame, Heat, Cold, Electrical, Chemical, and Sun Burns

Along with Information on Short-Term and Long-Term Treatments, Tissue Reconstruction, Plastic Surgery, Prevention Suggestions, and First Aid

Edited by Allan R. Cook. 604 pages. 1999. 978-0-7808-0204-9.

"This is an exceptional addition to the series and is highly recommended for all consumer health collections, hospital libraries, and academic medical centers."

—E-Streams, Mar '00

"This key reference guide is an invaluable addition to all health care and public libraries in confronting this ongoing health issue."

—American Reference Books Annual, 2000

SEE ALSO Dermatological Disorders Sourcebook, 2nd Edition

Cancer Sourcebook, 5th Edition

Basic Consumer Health Information about Major Forms and Stages of Cancer, Featuring Facts about Head and Neck Cancers, Lung Cancers, Gastrointestinal Cancers, Genitourinary Cancers, Lymphomas, Blood Cell Cancers, Endocrine Cancers, Skin Cancers, Bone Cancers, Metastatic Cancers, and More

Along with Facts about Cancer Treatments, Cancer Risks and Prevention, a Glossary of Related Terms, Statistical Data, and a Directory of Resources for Additional Information

Edited by Karen Bellenir. 1105 pages. 2007. 978-0-7808-0947-5.

"The 5th, updated edition of *Cancer Source-book* should be in every public and health lending library collection... An unparalleled discussion essential for any health collections considering an all-in-one basic general reference."

—*California Bookwatch, Aug '07*

SEE ALSO *Breast Cancer Sourcebook, 3rd Edition, Cancer Sourcebook for Women, 3rd Edition, Cancer Survivorship Sourcebook, Leukemia Sourcebook*

Cancer Sourcebook for Women, 3rd Edition

Basic Consumer Health Information about Leading Causes of Cancer in Women, Featuring Facts about Gynecologic Cancers and Related Concerns, Such as Breast Cancer, Cervical Cancer, Endometrial Cancer, Uterine Sarcoma, Vaginal Cancer, Vulvar Cancer, and Common Non-Cancerous Gynecologic Conditions, in Addition to Facts about Lung Cancer, Colorectal Cancer, and Thyroid Cancer in Women

Along with Information about Cancer Risk Factors, Screening and Prevention, Treatment Options, and Tips on Coping with Life after Cancer Treatment, a Glossary of Cancer Terms, and a Directory of Resources for Additional Help and Information

Edited by Amy L. Sutton. 687 pages. 2006. 978-0-7808-0867-6.

"This excellent book provides the general public with information compiled in a way that will help them to gain the knowledge they need. 4 Stars!"

—*Doody's Review Service, Dec '06*

"An indispensable reference for health consumers and cancer patients. Recommended for public libraries and academic libraries with a medical department."

—*E-Streams, Sep '08*

Cancer Survivorship Sourcebook

Basic Consumer Health Information about the Physical, Educational, Emotional, Social, and Financial Needs of Cancer Patients from Diagnosis, through Cancer Treatment, and Beyond, Including Facts about Researching Specific Types of Cancer and Learning about Clinical Trials and Treatment Options, and

Featuring Tips for Coping with the Side Effects of Cancer Treatments and Adjusting to Life after Cancer Treatment Concludes

Along with Suggestions for Caregivers, Friends, and Family Members of Cancer Patients, a Glossary of Cancer Care Terms, and Directories of Related Resources

Edited by Karen Bellenir. 633 pages. 2007. 978-0-7808-0985-7.

"Well organized and comprehensive in coverage, the book speaks to issues encountered both during and after cancer treatment. Recommended for consumer health and public libraries."

—*Library Journal, Aug 1 '07*

"*Cancer Survivorship Sourcebook* will be useful to anyone who has a friend or loved one with a cancer diagnosis."

—*American Reference Books Annual, 2008*

SEE ALSO *Cancer Sourcebook, 5th Edition*

Cardiovascular Diseases and Disorders Sourcebook, 3rd Edition

Basic Consumer Health Information about Heart and Vascular Diseases and Disorders, Such as Angina, Heart Attacks, Arrhythmias, Cardiomyopathy, Valve Disease, Atherosclerosis, and Aneurysms, with Information about Managing Cardiovascular Risk Factors and Maintaining Heart Health, Medications and Procedures Used to Treat Cardiovascular Disorders, and Concerns of Special Significance to Women

Along with Reports on Current Research Initiatives, a Glossary of Related Medical Terms, and a Directory of Sources for Further Help and Information

Edited by Sandra J. Judd. 687 pages. 2005. 978-0-7808-0739-6.

"This updated sourcebook is still the best first stop for comprehensive introductory information on cardiovascular diseases."

—*American Reference Books Annual, 2006*

"Recommended for public libraries and libraries supporting health care professionals."

—*E-Streams, Sep '05*

Caregiving Sourcebook

Basic Consumer Health Information for Caregivers, Including a Profile of Caregivers, Caregiving Responsibilities and Concerns, Tips for Specific Conditions, Care Environments, and the Effects of Caregiving

Along with Facts about Legal Issues, Financial Information, and Future Planning, a Glossary, and a Listing of Additional Resources

Edited by Joyce Brennfleck Shannon. 583 pages. 2001. 978-0-7808-0331-2.

"Essential for most collections."
—*Library Journal, Apr 1 '02*

"An ideal addition to the reference collection of any public library. Health sciences information professionals may also want to acquire the *Caregiving Sourcebook* for their hospital or academic library for use as a ready reference tool by health care workers interested in aging and caregiving."
—*E-Streams, Jan '02*

Child Abuse Sourcebook, 2nd Edition

Basic Consumer Health Information about the Physical, Sexual, and Emotional Abuse of Children, Neglect, Münchhausen Syndrome by Proxy (MSBP), and Shaken Baby Syndrome, and Featuring Facts about Withholding Medical Care, Corporal Punishment, Child Maltreatment in Youth Sports, and Parental Substance Abuse

Along with Information about Child Protective Services, Foster Care, Adoption, Parenting Challenges, Abuse Prevention Programs, and Intervention, Treatment, and Recovery Guidelines, a Glossary of Related Terms, and Resources for Additional Help and Information

Edited by Joyce Brennfleck Shannon. 600 pages. 2009. 978-0-7808-1037-2.

SEE ALSO *Domestic Violence Sourcebook, 3rd Edition*

Childhood Diseases and Disorders Sourcebook, 2nd Edition

Basic Consumer Health Information about the Physical, Mental, and Developmental

Health of Pre-Adolescent Children, Including Facts about Infectious Diseases, Asthma, Allergies, Diabetes, and Other Acute and Chronic Conditions Affecting the Gastrointestinal Tract, Ears, Nose, Throat, Liver, Kidneys, Heart, Blood, Brain, Muscles, Bones, and Skin

Along with Reports on Recommended Childhood Vaccinations, Wellness Guidelines, a Glossary of Related Medical Terms, and a List of Resources for Parents

Edited by Sandra J. Judd. 694 pages. 2009. 978-0-7808-1031-0.

SEE ALSO *Healthy Children Sourcebook*

Colds, Flu and Other Common Ailments Sourcebook

Basic Consumer Health Information about Common Ailments and Injuries, Including Colds, Coughs, the Flu, Sinus Problems, Headaches, Fever, Nausea and Vomiting, Menstrual Cramps, Diarrhea, Constipation, Hemorrhoids, Back Pain, Dandruff, Dry and Itchy Skin, Cuts, Scrapes, Sprains, Bruises, and More

Along with Information about Prevention, Self-Care, Choosing a Doctor, Over-the-Counter Medications, Folk Remedies, and Alternative Therapies, and Including a Glossary of Important Terms and a Directory of Resources for Further Help and Information

Edited by Chad T. Kimball. 622 pages. 2001. 978-0-7808-0435-7.

"A good starting point for research on common illnesses. It will be a useful addition to public and consumer health library collections."
—*American Reference Books Annual, 2002*

"Will prove valuable to any library seeking to maintain a current, comprehensive reference collection of health resources. . . Excellent reference."
—*The Bookwatch, Aug '01*

Communication Disorders Sourcebook

Basic Information about Deafness and Hearing Loss, Speech and Language Disorders, Voice Disorders, Balance and Vestibular Disorders, and Disorders of Smell, Taste, and Touch

Edited by Linda M. Ross. 533 pages. 1996. 978-0-7808-0077-9.

Complementary and Alternative Medicine Sourcebook, 3rd Edition

Basic Consumer Health Information about Complementary and Alternative Medical Therapies, Including Acupuncture, Ayurveda, Traditional Chinese Medicine, Herbal Medicine, Homeopathy, Naturopathy, Biofeedback, Hypnotherapy, Yoga, Art Therapy, Aromatherapy, Clinical Nutrition, Vitamin and Mineral Supplements, Chiropractic, Massage, Reflexology, Crystal Therapy, Therapeutic Touch, and More

Along with Facts about Alternative and Complementary Treatments for Specific Conditions Such as Cancer, Diabetes, Osteoarthritis, Chronic Pain, Menopause, Gastrointestinal Disorders, Headaches, and Mental Illness, a Glossary, and a Resource List for Additional Help and Information

Edited by Sandra J. Judd. 630 pages. 2006. 978-0-7808-0864-5.

Congenital Disorders Sourcebook, 2nd Edition

Basic Consumer Health Information about Nonhereditary Birth Defects and Disorders Related to Prematurity, Gestational Injuries, Congenital Infections, and Birth Complications, Including Heart Defects, Hydrocephalus, Spina Bifida, Cleft Lip and Palate, Cerebral Palsy, and More

Along with Facts about the Prevention of Birth Defects, Fetal Surgery and Other Treatment Options, Research Initiatives, a Glossary of Related Terms, and Resources for Additional Information and Support

Edited by Sandra J. Judd. 619 pages. 2007. 978-0-7808-0945-1.

SEE ALSO *Pregnancy and Birth Sourcebook, 2nd Edition*

Contagious Diseases Sourcebook, 2nd Edition

Basic Consumer Health Information about Diseases Spread from Person to Person through Direct Physical Contact, Airborne Transmissions, Sexual Contact, or Contact with Blood or Other Body Fluids, Including Pneumococcal, Staphylococcal, and Streptococcal Diseases, Colds, Influenza, Lice, Measles, Mumps, Tuberculosis, and Others

Along with Facts about Self-Care and Over-the-Counter Medications, Antibiotics and Drug Resistance, Disease Prevention, Vaccines, and Bioterrorism, a Glossary, and a Directory of Resources for More Information

Edited by Joyce Brennfleck Shannon. 600 pages. 2009. 978-0-7808-1075-4.

SEE ALSO *AIDS Sourcebook, 4th Edition, Hepatitis Sourcebook*

Cosmetic and Reconstructive Surgery Sourcebook, 2nd Edition

Basic Consumer Information about Plastic Surgery and Non-Surgical Appearance-Enhancing Procedures, Including Facts about Botulinum Toxin, Collagen Replacement, Dermabrasion,

Chemical Peels, Eyelid Surgery, Nose Reshaping, Lip Augmentation, Liposuction, Breast Enlargement and Reduction, Tummy Tucking, and Other Skin, Hair, Facial, and Body Shaping Procedures

Along with Information about Reconstructive Procedures for Congenital Disorders, Disfiguring Diseases, Burns, and Traumatic Injuries, a Glossary of Related Terms, and a Directory of Additional Resources

Edited by Karen Bellenir. 483 pages. 2007. 978-0-7808-0951-2.

"A practical guide for health care consumers and health care workers. . . . This easy-to-read reference guide would be useful for novice and veteran health care consumers, surgical technology students, nursing students, and perioperative nurses new to plastic and reconstructive surgery. It also may be helpful for medical-surgical nurses as a guide for patient teaching in their practices."

—AORN Journal, Aug '08

SEE ALSO Surgery Sourcebook, 2nd Edition

Death and Dying Sourcebook, 2nd Edition

Basic Consumer Health Information about End-of-Life Care and Related Perspectives and Ethical Issues, Including End-of-Life Symptoms and Treatments, Pain Management, Quality-of-Life Concerns, the Use of Life Support, Patients' Rights and Privacy Issues, Advance Directives, Physician-Assisted Suicide, Caregiving, Organ and Tissue Donation, Autopsies, Funeral Arrangements, and Grief

Along with Statistical Data, Information about the Leading Causes of Death, a Glossary, and Directories of Support Groups and Other Resources

Edited by Joyce Brennfleck Shannon. 626 pages. 2006. 978-0-7808-0871-3.

Dental Care and Oral Health Sourcebook, 3rd Edition

Basic Consumer Health Information about Dental Care and Oral Health Throughout the Lifespan, Including Facts about Cavities, Bad Breath, Cold and Canker Sores, Dry Mouth,

Toothaches, Gum Disease, Malocclusion, Temporomandibular Joint and Muscle Disorders, Oral Cancers, and Dental Emergencies

Along with Information about Mouth Hygiene, Crowns, Bridges, Implants, and Fillings, Surgical, Orthodontic, and Cosmetic Dental Procedures, Pain Management, Health Conditions that Impact Oral Care, a Glossary of Related Terms, and a Directory of Additional Resources

Edited by Amy L. Sutton. 619 pages. 2008. 978-0-7808-1032-7.

Depression Sourcebook, 2nd Edition

Basic Consumer Health Information about Unipolar Depression, Bipolar Disorder, Dysthymia, Seasonal Affective Disorder, Postpartum Depression, and Other Depressive Disorders, Including Facts about Populations at Special Risk, Coexisting Medical Conditions, Symptoms, Treatment Options, and Suicide Prevention

Along with Statistical Data, a Glossary of Related Terms, and a Directory of Resources for Additional Help and Information

Edited by Sandra J. Judd. 646 pages. 2008. 978-0-7808-1003-7.

"Recommended for public libraries."
—ARBAonline, Nov '08

SEE ALSO Mental Health Disorders Sourcebook, 4th Edition

Dermatological Disorders Sourcebook, 2nd Edition

Basic Consumer Health Information about Conditions and Disorders Affecting the Skin, Hair, and Nails, Such as Acne, Rosacea, Rashes, Dermatitis, Pigmentation Disorders, Birthmarks, Skin Cancer, Skin Injuries, Psoriasis, Scleroderma, and Hair Loss, Including Facts about Medications and Treatments for Dermatological Disorders and Tips for Maintaining Healthy Skin, Hair, and Nails

Along with Information about How Aging Affects the Skin, a Glossary of Related Terms, and a Directory of Resources for Additional Help and Information

Edited by Amy L. Sutton. 617 pages. 2006. 978-0-7808-0795-2.

Diabetes Sourcebook, 4th Edition

Basic Consumer Health Information about Type 1 and Type 2 Diabetes Mellitus, Gestational Diabetes, Monogenic Forms of Diabetes, and Insulin Resistance, with Guidelines for Lifestyle Modifications and the Medical Management of Diabetes, Including Facts about Insulin, Insulin Delivery Devices, Oral Diabetes Medications, Self-Monitoring of Blood Glucose, Meal Planning, Physical Activity Recommendations, Foot Care, and Treatment Options for People with Kidney Failure

Along with a Section about Diabetes Complications and Co-Occurring Conditions, a Glossary of Related Terms, and Directories of Resources for Additional Help and Information

Edited by Karen Bellenir. 627 pages. 2008. 978-0-7808-1005-1.

SEE ALSO *Endocrine and Metabolic Disorders Sourcebook, 2nd Edition*

Diet and Nutrition Sourcebook, 3rd Edition

Basic Consumer Health Information about Dietary Guidelines and the Food Guidance System, Recommended Daily Nutrient Intakes, Serving Proportions, Weight Control, Vitamins and Supplements, Nutrition Issues for Different Life Stages and Lifestyles, and the Needs of People with Specific Medical Concerns, Including Cancer, Celiac Disease, Diabetes, Eating Disorders, Food Allergies, and Cardiovascular Disease

Along with Facts about Federal Nutrition Support Programs, a Glossary of Nutrition and Dietary Terms, and Directories of Additional Resources for More Information about Nutrition

Edited by Joyce Brennfleck Shannon. 605 pages. 2006. 978-0-7808-0800-3.

SEE ALSO *Digestive Diseases and Disorders Sourcebook, Eating Disorders Sourcebook, 2nd Edition, Gastrointestinal Diseases and Disorders Sourcebook, 2nd Edition, Vegetarian Sourcebook*

Digestive Diseases and Disorders Sourcebook

Basic Consumer Health Information about Diseases and Disorders that Impact the Upper and Lower Digestive System, Including Celiac Disease, Constipation, Crohn's Disease, Cyclic Vomiting Syndrome, Diarrhea, Diverticulosis and Diverticulitis, Gallstones, Heartburn, Hemorrhoids, Hernias, Indigestion (Dyspepsia), Irritable Bowel Syndrome, Lactose Intolerance, Ulcers, and More

Along with Information about Medications and Other Treatments, Tips for Maintaining a Healthy Digestive Tract, a Glossary, and Directory of Digestive Diseases Organizations

Edited by Karen Bellenir. 323 pages. 2000. 978-0-7808-0327-5.

SEE ALSO *Diet and Nutrition Sourcebook, 3rd Edition, Gastrointestinal Diseases and Disorders Sourcebook, 2nd Edition*

Disabilities Sourcebook

Basic Consumer Health Information about Physical and Psychiatric Disabilities, Including Descriptions of Major Causes of Disability, Assistive and Adaptive Aids, Workplace Issues, and Accessibility Concerns

Along with Information about the Americans with Disabilities Act, a Glossary, and Resources for Additional Help and Information

Edited by Dawn D. Matthews. 602 pages. 2000. 978-0-7808-0389-3.

"A must for libraries with a consumer health section."
—American Reference Books Annual, 2002

"A much needed addition to the Omnigraphics Health Reference Series. A current reference work to provide people with disabilities, their families, caregivers or those who work with them, a broad range of information in one volume, has not been available until now. . . . It is recommended for all public and academic library reference collections."
—E-Streams, May '01

"An excellent source book in easy-to-read format covering many current topics; highly recommended for all libraries."
—CHOICE, Jan '01

Disease Management Sourcebook

Basic Consumer Health Information about Coping with Chronic and Serious Illnesses, Navigating the Health Care System, Communicating with Health Care Providers, Assessing Health Care Quality, and Making Informed Health Care Decisions, Including Facts about Second Opinions, Hospitalization, Surgery, and Medications

Along with a Section about Children with Chronic Conditions, Information about Legal, Financial, and Insurance Issues, a Glossary of Related Terms, and Directories of Additional Resources

Edited by Joyce Brennfleck Shannon. 621 pages. 2008. 978-0-7808-1002-0.

"Consumers need to know how to manage their health care the same way they manage anything else in their lives. The text is very readable and is written for the layperson and consumer. The cost is not prohibitive. This book should be in all collections of health care libraries and public libraries."
—ARBAonline, Jul '08

"The information is very current, and the selection of font and layout make the book easy to read. A hardback that will stand up to much usage, this is an excellent resource for consumers. . . . Recommended. General readers."
—CHOICE, Nov '08

"Intended for lay readers, this resource clarifies the many confusing and overwhelming details associated with chronic disease care. Meticulous and clearly explained, the book even includes diagrams intended to ease comprehension of over-the-counter medication labels. An essential guide to navigating the health-care rapids."
—Library Journal, Aug '08

Domestic Violence Sourcebook, 3rd Edition

Basic Consumer Health Information about Warning Signs, Risk Factors, and Health Consequences of Intimate Partner Violence, Sexual Violence and Rape, Stalking, Human Trafficking, Child Maltreatment, Teen Dating Violence, and Elder Abuse

Along with Facts about Victims and Perpetrators, Strategies for Violence Prevention, and Emergency Interventions, Safety Plans, and Financial and Legal Tips for Victims, a Glossary of Related Terms, and Directories of Resources for Additional Information and Support

Edited by Joyce Brennfleck Shannon. 600 pages. 2009. 978-0-7808-1038-9.

SEE ALSO Child Abuse Sourcebook, 2nd Edition

Drug Abuse Sourcebook, 2nd Edition

Basic Consumer Health Information about Illicit Substances of Abuse and the Misuse of Prescription and Over-the-Counter Medications, Including Depressants, Hallucinogens, Inhalants, Marijuana, Stimulants, and Anabolic Steroids

Along with Facts about Related Health Risks, Treatment Programs, Prevention Programs, a Glossary of Abuse and Addiction Terms, a Glossary of Drug-Related Street Terms, and a Directory of Resources for More Information

Edited by Catherine Ginther. 581 pages. 2004. 978-0-7808-0740-2.

"Commendable for organizing useful, normally scattered government and association-produced data into a logical sequence."
—American Reference Books Annual, 2006

"An excellent library reference."
—*The Bookwatch, May '05*

SEE ALSO *Alcoholism Sourcebook, 2nd Edition*

Ear, Nose, and Throat Disorders Sourcebook, 2nd Edition

Basic Consumer Health Information about Disorders of the Ears, Hearing Loss, Vestibular Disorders, Nasal and Sinus Problems, Throat and Vocal Cord Disorders, and Otolaryngologic Cancers, Including Facts about Ear Infections and Injuries, Genetic and Congenital Deafness, Sensorineural Hearing Disorders, Tinnitus, Vertigo, Ménière Disease, Rhinitis, Sinusitis, Snoring, Sore Throats, Hoarseness, and More

Along with Reports on Current Research Initiatives, a Glossary of Related Medical Terms, and a Directory of Sources for Further Help and Information

Edited by Sandra J. Judd. 631 pages. 2007. 978-0-7808-0872-0.

"A resource book for the general public that provides comprehensive coverage of basic up-to-date medical information about the causes, symptoms, diagnosis, and treatment of diseases and disorders that affect the ears, nose, sinuses, throat, and voice. . . . The majority of information is presented in question and answer format, much like questions a patient might ask of a health care provider. An extensive index facilitates the reader's ability to easily access information on any specific topic."
—*Journal of Dental Hygiene, Oct '07*

"A handy compilation of information on common and some not so common ailments of the ears, nose, and throat."
—*Doody's Review Service, 2007*

Eating Disorders Sourcebook, 2nd Edition

Basic Consumer Health Information about Anorexia Nervosa, Bulimia, Binge Eating, Compulsive Exercise, Female Athlete Triad, and Other Eating Disorders, Including Facts about Body Image and Other Cultural and Age-Related Risk Factors, Prevention Efforts, Adverse Health Effects, Treatment Options, and the Recovery Process

Along with Guidelines for Healthy Weight Control, a Glossary, and Directories of Additional Resources

Edited by Joyce Brennfleck Shannon. 557 pages. 2007. 978-0-7808-0948-2.

"Recommended for the reference collection of large public libraries."
—*American Reference Books Annual, 2008*

"A basic health reference any health or general library needs."
—*Internet Bookwatch, Jun '07*

SEE ALSO *Diet and Nutrition Sourcebook, 3rd Edition, Mental Health Disorders Sourcebook, 4th Edition*

Emergency Medical Services Sourcebook

Basic Consumer Health Information about Preventing, Preparing for, and Managing Emergency Situations, When and Who to Call for Help, What to Expect in the Emergency Room, the Emergency Medical Team, Patient Issues, and Current Topics in Emergency Medicine

Along with Statistical Data, a Glossary, and Sources of Additional Help and Information

Edited by Jenni Lynn Colson. 472 pages. 2002. 978-0-7808-0420-3.

"Handy and convenient for home, public, school, and college libraries. Recommended."
—*CHOICE, Apr '03*

"This reference can provide the consumer with answers to most questions about emergency care in the United States, or it will direct them to a resource where the answer can be found."
—*American Reference Books Annual, 2003*

SEE ALSO *Injury and Trauma Sourcebook*

Endocrine and Metabolic Disorders Sourcebook, 2nd Edition

Basic Consumer Health Information about Hormonal and Metabolic Disorders that Affect the Body's Growth, Development, and Functioning, Including Disorders of the Pancreas, Ovaries and Testes, and Pituitary, Thyroid, Parathyroid, and Adrenal Glands, with Facts

657

about Growth Disorders, Addison Disease, Cushing Syndrome, Conn Syndrome, Diabetic Disorders, Multiple Endocrine Neoplasia, Inborn Errors of Metabolism, and More

Along with Information about Endocrine Functioning, Diagnostic and Screening Tests, a Glossary of Related Terms, and Directories of Additional Resources

Edited by Joyce Brennfleck Shannon. 597 pages. 2007. 978-0-7808-0952-9.

SEE ALSO Diabetes Sourcebook, 4th Edition

Environmental Health Sourcebook, 2nd Edition

Basic Consumer Health Information about the Environment and Its Effect on Human Health, Including the Effects of Air Pollution, Water Pollution, Hazardous Chemicals, Food Hazards, Radiation Hazards, Biological Agents, Household Hazards, Such as Radon, Asbestos, Carbon Monoxide, and Mold, and Information about Associated Diseases and Disorders, Including Cancer, Allergies, Respiratory Problems, and Skin Disorders

Along with Information about Environmental Concerns for Specific Populations, a Glossary of Related Terms, and Resources for Further Help and Information

Edited by Dawn D. Matthews. 650 pages. 2003. 978-0-7808-0632-0.

"Recommended for teenage and adult students and readers, and for public and academic libraries, as well as any library focusing on consumer health."
—E-Streams, May '04

"This recently updated edition continues the level of quality and the reputation of the numerous other volumes in Omnigraphics' Health Reference Series."
—American Reference Books Annual, 2004

Ethnic Diseases Sourcebook

Basic Consumer Health Information for Ethnic and Racial Minority Groups in the United States, Including General Health Indicators and Behaviors, Ethnic Diseases, Genetic Testing, the Impact of Chronic Diseases, Women's Health, Mental Health Issues, and Preventive Health Care Services

Along with a Glossary and a Listing of Additional Resources

Edited by Joyce Brennfleck Shannon. 648 pages. 2001. 978-0-7808-0336-7.

"Not many books have been written on this topic to date, and the Ethnic Diseases Sourcebook is a strong addition to the list. It will be an important introductory resource for health consumers, students, health care personnel, and social scientists. It is recommended for public, academic, and large hospital libraries."
—American Reference Books Annual, 2002

"Will prove valuable to any library seeking to maintain a current, comprehensive reference collection of health resources. . . . An excellent source of health information about genetic disorders which affect particular ethnic and racial minorities in the U.S."
—The Bookwatch, Aug '01

Eye Care Sourcebook, 3rd Edition

Basic Consumer Health Information about Eye Care and Eye Disorders, Including Facts about the Diagnosis, Prevention, and Treatment of Refractive Disorders, Cataracts, Glaucoma, Macular Degeneration, and Problems Affecting the Cornea, Retina, and Lacrimal Glands

Along with Advice about Preventing Eye Injuries and Tips for Living with Low Vision or Blindness, a Glossary of Related Terms, and Directories of Resources for More Help and Information

Edited by Amy L. Sutton. 646 pages. 2008. 978-0-7808-1000-6.

Family Planning Sourcebook

Basic Consumer Health Information about Planning for Pregnancy and Contraception, Including Traditional Methods, Barrier Methods, Hormonal Methods, Permanent Methods, Future Methods, Emergency Contraception, and Birth Control Choices for Women at Each Stage of Life

Along with Statistics, a Glossary, and Sources of Additional Information

Edited by Amy Marcaccio Keyzer. 503 pages. 2001. 978-0-7808-0379-4.

"Recommended for public, health, and undergraduate libraries as part of the circulating collection."
—E-Streams, Mar '02

"Will prove valuable to any library seeking to maintain a current, comprehensive reference collection of health resources. . . . Excellent reference."

—*The Bookwatch, Aug '01*

SEE ALSO *Pregnancy and Birth Sourcebook, 2nd Edition*

Fitness and Exercise Sourcebook, 3rd Edition

Basic Consumer Health Information about the Physical and Mental Benefits of Fitness, Including Cardiorespiratory Endurance, Muscular Strength, Muscular Endurance, and Flexibility, with Facts about Sports Nutrition and Exercise-Related Injuries and Tips about Physical Activity and Exercises for People of All Ages and for People with Health Concerns

Along with Advice on Selecting and Using Exercise Equipment, Maintaining Exercise Motivation, a Glossary of Related Terms, and a Directory of Resources for More Help and Information

Edited by Amy L. Sutton. 635 pages. 2007. 978-0-7808-0946-8.

"Updates the consumer information on the physical and mental benefits of physical activity throughout the lifespan offered in earlier editions. . . . Recommended. All readers; all levels."

—*CHOICE, Oct '07*

"An exceptionally well-rounded coverage perfect for any concerned about developing and understanding a fitness program."

—*California Bookwatch, Jun '07*

SEE ALSO *Sports Injuries Sourcebook, 3rd Edition*

Food Safety Sourcebook

Basic Consumer Health Information about the Safe Handling of Meat, Poultry, Seafood, Eggs, Fruit Juices, and Other Food Items, and Facts about Pesticides, Drinking Water, Food Safety Overseas, and the Onset, Duration, and Symptoms of Foodborne Illnesses, Including Types of Pathogenic Bacteria, Parasitic Protozoa, Worms, Viruses, and Natural Toxins

Along with the Role of the Consumer, the Food Handler, and the Government in Food Safety; a Glossary, and Resources for Additional Help and Information

Edited by Dawn D. Matthews. 327 pages. 1999. 978-0-7808-0326-8.

"Recommended reference source."

—*Booklist, May '00*

"This book takes the complex issues of food safety and foodborne pathogens and presents them in an easily understood manner. [It does] an excellent job of covering a large and often confusing topic."

— *American Reference Books Annual, 2000*

Forensic Medicine Sourcebook

Basic Consumer Information for the Layperson about Forensic Medicine, Including Crime Scene Investigation, Evidence Collection and Analysis, Expert Testimony, Computer-Aided Criminal Identification, Digital Imaging in the Courtroom, DNA Profiling, Accident Reconstruction, Autopsies, Ballistics, Drugs and Explosives Detection, Latent Fingerprints, Product Tampering, and Questioned Document Examination

Along with Statistical Data, a Glossary of Forensics Terminology, and Listings of Sources for Further Help and Information

Edited by Annemarie S. Muth. 574 pages. 1999. 978-0-7808-0232-2.

"Given the expected widespread interest in its content and its easy to read style, this book is recommended for most public and all college and university libraries."

—*E-Streams, Feb '01*

"A wealth of information, useful statistics, references are up-to-date and extremely complete. This wonderful collection of data will help students who are interested in a career in any type of forensic field. It is a great resource for attorneys who need information about types of expert witnesses needed in a particular case. It also offers useful information for fiction and nonfiction writers whose work involves a crime. A fascinating compilation. All levels."

—*CHOICE, Jan '00*

"There are several items that make this book attractive to consumers who are seeking certain forensic data. . . . This is a useful current

source for those seeking general forensic medical answers."
—*American Reference Books Annual, 2000*

Gastrointestinal Diseases and Disorders Sourcebook, 2nd Edition

Basic Consumer Health Information about the Upper and Lower Gastrointestinal (GI) Tract, Including the Esophagus, Stomach, Intestines, Rectum, Liver, and Pancreas, with Facts about Gastroesophageal Reflux Disease, Gastritis, Hernias, Ulcers, Celiac Disease, Diverticulitis, Irritable Bowel Syndrome, Hemorrhoids, Gastrointestinal Cancers, and Other Diseases and Disorders Related to the Digestive Process

Along with Information about Commonly Used Diagnostic and Surgical Procedures, Statistics, Reports on Current Research Initiatives and Clinical Trials, a Glossary, and Resources for Additional Help and Information

Edited by Sandra J. Judd. 654 pages. 2006. 978-0-7808-0798-3.

"The text is designed for the general reader seeking information on prevention, disease warning signs, diagnostic and therapeutic questions. . . . It is an excellent resource for the general reader to conveniently locate credible, coordinated and indexed information. . . . The sourcebook will prove very helpful for patients, caregivers and should be available in every physician waiting room."
—*Doody's Review Service, 2006*

SEE ALSO *Diet and Nutrition Sourcebook, 3rd Edition, Digestive Diseases and Disorders Sourcebook*

Genetic Disorders Sourcebook, 4th Edition

Basic Consumer Health Information about Hereditary Diseases and Disorders, Including Facts about the Human Genome, Genetic Inheritance Patterns, Disorders Associated with Specific Genes, Such as Sickle Cell Disease, Hemophilia, and Cystic Fibrosis, Chromosome Disorders, Such as Down Syndrome, Fragile X Syndrome, and Turner Syndrome, and Complex Diseases and Disorders Resulting from the Interaction of Environmental and Genetic Factors, Such as Allergies, Cancer, and Obesity

Along with Facts about Genetic Testing, Suggestions for Parents of Children with Special Needs, Reports on Current Research Initiatives, a Glossary of Genetic Terminology, and Resources for Additional Help and Information

Edited by Sandra J. Judd. 600 pages. 2009. 978-0-7808-1076-1.

Head Trauma Sourcebook

Basic Information for the Layperson about Open-Head and Closed-Head Injuries, Treatment Advances, Recovery, and Rehabilitation

Along with Reports on Current Research Initiatives

Edited by Karen Bellenir. 414 pages. 1997. 978-0-7808-0208-7.

Headache Sourcebook

Basic Consumer Health Information about Migraine, Tension, Cluster, Rebound and Other Types of Headaches, with Facts about the Cause and Prevention of Headaches, the Effects of Stress and the Environment, Headaches during Pregnancy and Menopause, and Childhood Headaches

Along with a Glossary and Other Resources for Additional Help and Information

Edited by Dawn D. Matthews. 342 pages. 2002. 978-0-7808-0337-4.

"Highly recommended for academic and medical reference collections."
—*Library Bookwatch, Sep '02*

SEE ALSO *Pain Sourcebook, 3rd Edition*

Healthy Aging Sourcebook

Basic Consumer Health Information about Maintaining Health through the Aging Process, Including Advice on Nutrition, Exercise, and Sleep, Help in Making Decisions about Midlife Issues and Retirement, and Guidance Concerning Practical and Informed Choices in Health Consumerism

Along with Data Concerning the Theories of Aging, Different Experiences in Aging by Minority Groups, and Facts about Aging Now and Aging in the Future; and Featuring a Glossary, a Guide to Consumer Help, Additional Suggested Reading, and Practical Resource Directory

Edited by Jenifer Swanson. 537 pages. 1999.
978-0-7808-0390-9.

"Recommended reference source."
—*Booklist, Feb '00*

SEE ALSO *Physical and Mental Issues in Aging Sourcebook*

Healthy Children Sourcebook

Basic Consumer Health Information about the Physical and Mental Development of Children between the Ages of 3 and 12, Including Routine Health Care, Preventative Health Services, Safety and First Aid, Healthy Sleep, Dental Care, Nutrition, and Fitness, and Featuring Parenting Tips on Such Topics as Bedwetting, Choosing Day Care, Monitoring TV and Other Media, and Establishing a Foundation for Substance Abuse Prevention

Along with a Glossary of Commonly Used Pediatric Terms and Resources for Additional Help and Information.

Edited by Chad T. Kimball. 624 pages. 2003.
978-0-7808-0247-6.

"Should be required reading for parents and teachers."
—*E-Streams, Jun '04*

"It is hard to imagine that any other single resource exists that would provide such a comprehensive guide of timely information on health promotion and disease prevention for children aged 3 to 12."
—*American Reference Books Annual, 2004*

"This easy-to-read volume is a tremendous resource."
—*AORN Journal, May '05*

SEE ALSO *Childhood Diseases and Disorders Sourcebook, 2nd Edition*

Healthy Heart Sourcebook for Women

Basic Consumer Health Information about Cardiac Issues Specific to Women, Including Facts about Major Risk Factors and Prevention, Treatment and Control Strategies, and Important Dietary Issues

Along with a Special Section Regarding the Pros and Cons of Hormone Replacement Therapy and Its Impact on Heart Health, and Additional Help, Including Recipes, a Glossary, and a Directory of Resources

Edited by Dawn D. Matthews. 321 pages.
2000. 978-0-7808-0329-9.

"A good reference source and recommended for all public, academic, medical, and hospital libraries."
—*Medical Reference Services Quarterly, Summer '01*

"Contains very important information about coronary artery disease that all women should know. The information is current and presented in an easy-to-read format. The book will make a good addition to any library."
—*American Medical Writers Association Journal, Summer '00*

SEE ALSO *Cardiovascular Diseases and Disorders Sourcebook, 3rd Edition, Women's Health Concerns Sourcebook, 3rd Edition*

Hepatitis Sourcebook

Basic Consumer Health Information about Hepatitis A, Hepatitis B, Hepatitis C, and Other Forms of Hepatitis, Including Autoimmune Hepatitis, Alcoholic Hepatitis, Nonalcoholic Steatohepatitis, and Toxic Hepatitis, with Facts about Risk Factors, Screening Methods, Diagnostic Tests, and Treatment Options

Along with Information on Liver Health, Tips for People Living with Chronic Hepatitis, Reports on Current Research Initiatives, a Glossary of Terms Related to Hepatitis, and a Directory of Sources for Further Help and Information

Edited by Sandra J. Judd. 570 pages. 2006. 978-0-7808-0749-5.

"The breadth of information found in this one book would not be readily found in another source. Highly recommended."
—*American Reference Books Annual, 2006*

SEE ALSO *Contagious Diseases Sourcebook*

Household Safety Sourcebook

Basic Consumer Health Information about Household Safety, Including Information about Poisons, Chemicals, Fire, and Water Hazards in the Home

Along with Advice about the Safe Use of Home Maintenance Equipment, Choosing Toys and Nursery Furniture, Holiday and Recreation Safety, a Glossary, and Resources for Further Help and Information

Edited by Dawn D. Matthews. 587 pages. 2002. 978-0-7808-0338-1.

"As a sourcebook on household safety this book meets its mark. It is encyclopedic in scope and covers a wide range of safety issues that are commonly seen in the home."
—*E-Streams, Jul '02*

Hypertension Sourcebook

Basic Consumer Health Information about the Causes, Diagnosis, and Treatment of High Blood Pressure, with Facts about Consequences, Complications, and Co-Occurring Disorders, Such as Coronary Heart Disease, Diabetes, Stroke, Kidney Disease, and Hypertensive Retinopathy, and Issues in Blood Pressure Control, Including Dietary Choices, Stress Management, and Medications

Along with Reports on Current Research Initiatives and Clinical Trials, a Glossary, and Resources for Additional Help and Information

Edited by Dawn D. Matthews and Karen Bellenir. 588 pages. 2004. 978-0-7808-0674-0.

"Academic, public, and medical libraries will want to add the *Hypertension Sourcebook* to their collections."
—*E-Streams, Aug '05*

"The strength of this source is the wide range of information given about hypertension."
—*American Reference Books Annual, 2005*

SEE ALSO *Stroke Sourcebook, 2nd Edition*

Immune System Disorders Sourcebook, 2nd Edition

Basic Consumer Health Information about Disorders of the Immune System, Including Immune System Function and Response, Diagnosis of Immune Disorders, Information about Inherited Immune Disease, Acquired Immune Disease, and Autoimmune Diseases, Including Primary Immune Deficiency, Acquired Immunodeficiency Syndrome (AIDS), Lupus, Multiple Sclerosis, Type 1 Diabetes, Rheumatoid Arthritis, and Graves' Disease

Along with Treatments, Tips for Coping with Immune Disorders, a Glossary, and a Directory of Additional Resources

Edited by Joyce Brennfleck Shannon. 643 pages. 2005. 978-0-7808-0748-8.

"Highly recommended for academic and public libraries."
—*American Reference Books Annual, 2006*

"The updated second edition is a 'must' for any consumer health library seeking a solid resource covering the treatments, symptoms, and options for immune disorder sufferers. . . . An excellent guide."
—*MBR Bookwatch, Jan '06*

SEE ALSO *AIDS Sourcebook, 4th Edition, Arthritis Sourcebook, 2nd Edition*

Infant and Toddler Health Sourcebook

Basic Consumer Health Information about the Physical and Mental Development of Newborns, Infants, and Toddlers, Including Neonatal Concerns, Nutrition Recommendations, Immunization Schedules, Common Pediatric Disorders, Assessments and Milestones, Safety Tips, and Advice for Parents and Other Caregivers

Along with a Glossary of Terms and Resource Listings for Additional Help

Edited by Jenifer Swanson. 570 pages. 2000. 978-0-7808-0246-9.

"As a reference for the general public, this would be useful in any library."
—*E-Streams, May '01*

"Recommended reference source."
—*Booklist, Feb '01*

Infectious Diseases Sourcebook

Basic Consumer Health Information about Non-Contagious Bacterial, Viral, Prion, Fungal, and Parasitic Diseases Spread by Food and Water, Insects and Animals, or Environmental Contact, Including Botulism, E. Coli, Encephalitis, Legionnaires' Disease, Lyme Disease, Malaria, Plague, Rabies, Salmonella, Tetanus, and Others, and Facts about Newly Emerging Diseases, Such as Hantavirus, Mad Cow Disease, Monkeypox, and West Nile Virus

Along with Information about Preventing Disease Transmission, the Threat of Bioterrorism, and Current Research Initiatives, with a Glossary and Directory of Resources for More Information

Edited by Karen Bellenir. 610 pages. 2004. 978-0-7808-0675-7.

"This reference continues the excellent tradition of the *Health Reference Series* in consolidating a wealth of information on a selected topic into a format that is easy to use and accessible to the general public."
—*American Reference Books Annual, 2005*

"Recommended for public and academic libraries."
—*E-Streams, Jan '05*

Injury and Trauma Sourcebook

Basic Consumer Health Information about the Impact of Injury, the Diagnosis and Treatment of Common and Traumatic Injuries, Emergency Care, and Specific Injuries Related to Home, Community, Workplace, Transportation, and Recreation

Along with Guidelines for Injury Prevention, a Glossary, and a Directory of Additional Resources

Edited by Joyce Brennfleck Shannon. 675 pages. 2002. 978-0-7808-0421-0.

"Practitioners should be aware of guides such as this in order to facilitate their use by patients and their families."
—*Doody's Health Sciences Book Review Journal, Sep-Oct '02*

"Recommended reference source."
—*Booklist, Sep '02*

"Highly recommended for academic and medical reference collections."
—*Library Bookwatch, Sep '02*

SEE ALSO *Emergency Medical Services Sourcebook, Sports Injuries Sourcebook, 3rd Edition*

Learning Disabilities Sourcebook, 3rd Edition

Basic Consumer Health Information about Dyslexia, Auditory and Visual Processing Disorders, Communication Disorders, Dyscalculia, Dysgraphia, and Other Conditions That Impede Learning, Including Attention Deficit/ Hyperactivity Disorder, Autism Spectrum Disorders, Hearing and Visual Impairments, Chromosome-Based Disorders, and Brain Injury

Along with Facts about Brain Function, Assessment, Therapy and Remediation, Accommodations, Assistive Technology, Legal Protections, and Tips about Family Life, School Transitions, and Employment Strategies, a Glossary of Related Terms, and Directories of Additional Resources

Edited by Joyce Brennfleck Shannon. 613 pages. 2009. 978-0-7808-1039-6.

SEE ALSO *Attention Deficit Disorder Sourcebook, Autism and Pervasive Developmental Disorders Sourcebook*

Leukemia Sourcebook

Basic Consumer Health Information about Adult and Childhood Leukemias, Including Acute Lymphocytic Leukemia (ALL), Chronic Lymphocytic Leukemia (CLL), Acute Myelogenous Leukemia (AML), Chronic Myelogenous Leukemia (CML), and Hairy Cell Leukemia, and Treatments Such as Chemotherapy, Radiation Therapy, Peripheral Blood Stem Cell and Marrow Transplantation, and Immunotherapy

Along with Tips for Life During and After Treatment, a Glossary, and Directories of Additional Resources

Edited by Joyce Brennfleck Shannon. 564 pages. 2003. 978-0-7808-0627-6.

"Unlike other medical books for the layperson, . . . the language does not talk down to the reader. . . . This volume is highly recommended for all libraries."
—*American Reference Books Annual, 2004*

"A fine title which ranges from diagnosis to alternative treatments, staging, and tips for life during and after diagnosis."
—*The Bookwatch, Dec '03*

SEE ALSO *Cancer Sourcebook, 5th Edition*

Liver Disorders Sourcebook

Basic Consumer Health Information about the Liver and How It Works; Liver Diseases, Including Cancer, Cirrhosis, Hepatitis, and Toxic and Drug Related Diseases; Tips for Maintaining a Healthy Liver; Laboratory Tests, Radiology Tests, and Facts about Liver Transplantation

Along with a Section on Support Groups, a Glossary, and Resource Listings

Edited by Joyce Brennfleck Shannon. 580 pages. 2000. 978-0-7808-0383-1.

"This title is recommended for health sciences and public libraries with consumer health collections."
—*E-Streams, Oct '00*

"Recommended reference source."
—*Booklist, Jun '00*

SEE ALSO *Gastrointestinal Diseases and Disorders Sourcebook, 2nd Edition, Hepatitis Sourcebook*

Lung Disorders Sourcebook

Basic Consumer Health Information about Emphysema, Pneumonia, Tuberculosis, Asthma, Cystic Fibrosis, and Other Lung Disorders, Including Facts about Diagnostic Procedures, Treatment Strategies, Disease Prevention Efforts, and Such Risk Factors as Smoking, Air Pollution, and Exposure to Asbestos, Radon, and Other Agents

Along with a Glossary and Resources for Additional Help and Information

Edited by Dawn D. Matthews. 657 pages. 2002. 978-0-7808-0339-8.

"Highly recommended for academic and medical reference collections."
—*Library Bookwatch, Sep '02*

SEE ALSO *Respiratory Disorders Sourcebook, 2nd Edition*

Medical Tests Sourcebook, 3rd Edition

Basic Consumer Health Information about X-Rays, Blood Tests, Stool and Urine Tests, Biopsies, Mammography, Endoscopic Procedures, Ultrasound Exams, Computed Tomography, Magnetic Resonance Imaging (MRI), Nuclear Medicine, Genetic Testing, Home-Use Tests, and More

Along with Facts about Preventive Care and Screening Test Guidelines, Screening and Assessment Tests Associated with Such Specific Concerns as Cancer, Heart Disease, Allergies, Diabetes, Thyroid Disfunction, and Infertility, a Glossary of Related Terms, and a Directory of Resources for Additional Help and Information

Edited by Karen Bellenir. 627 pages. 2008. 978-0-7808-1040-2

"This volume has a wide scope that makes it useful . . . Can be a valuable reference guide."
—*ARBAonline, Nov '08*

Men's Health Concerns Sourcebook, 3rd Edition

Basic Consumer Health Information about Wellness in Men and Gender-Related Differences in Health, With Facts about Heart Disease, Cancer, Traumatic Injury, and Other Leading Causes of Death in Men, Reproductive Concerns, Sexual Dysfunction, Disorders of the Prostate, Penis, and Testes, Sex-Linked Genetic Disorders, and Other Medical and Mental Concerns of Men

Along with Statistical Data, a Glossary of Related Terms, and a Directory of Resources for Additional Information

Edited by Sandra J. Judd. 600 pages. 2009. 978-0-7808-1033-4.

SEE ALSO *Prostate and Urological Disorders Sourcebook*

Mental Health Disorders Sourcebook, 4th Edition

Basic Consumer Health Information about the Causes and Symptoms of Mental Health Problems, Including Depression, Bipolar Disorder, Anxiety Disorders, Posttraumatic Stress Disorder, Obsessive-Compulsive Disorder, Eating Disorders, Addictions, and Personality and Psychotic Disorders

Along with Information about Medications and Treatments, Mental Health Concerns in Children, Adolescents, and Adults, Tips on Living with Mental Health Disorders, a Glossary of Related Terms, and a Directory of Resources for Additional Help and Information

Edited by Amy L. Sutton. 600 pages. 2009. 978-0-7808-1041-9.

SEE ALSO *Depression Sourcebook, 2nd Edition, Stress-Related Disorders Sourcebook, 2nd Edition*

Mental Retardation Sourcebook

Basic Consumer Health Information about Mental Retardation and Its Causes, Including

Down Syndrome, Fetal Alcohol Syndrome, Fragile X Syndrome, Genetic Conditions, Injury, and Environmental Sources

Along with Preventive Strategies, Parenting Issues, Educational Implications, Health Care Needs, Employment and Economic Matters, Legal Issues, a Glossary, and a Resource Listing for Additional Help and Information

Edited by Joyce Brennfleck Shannon. 627 pages. 2000. 978-0-7808-0377-0.

"Public libraries will find the book useful for reference and as a beginning research point for students, parents, and caregivers."
—American Reference Books Annual, 2001

"The strength of this work is that it compiles many basic fact sheets and addresses for further information in one volume. It is intended and suitable for the general public."
—E-Streams, Nov '00

"An invaluable overview."
—Reviewer's Bookwatch, Jul '00

Movement Disorders Sourcebook, 2nd Edition

Basic Consumer Health Information about the Symptoms and Causes of Movement Disorders, Including Parkinson Disease, Amyotrophic Lateral Sclerosis, Cerebral Palsy, Muscular Dystrophy, Multiple Sclerosis, Myasthenia, Myoclonus, Spina Bifida, Dystonia, Essential Tremor, Choreatic Disorders, Huntington Disease, Tourette Syndrome, and Other Disorders That Cause Slowed, Absent, or Excessive Movements

Along with Information about Surgical and Nonsurgical Interventions, Physical Therapies, Strategies for Independent Living, a Glossary of Related Terms, and a Directory of Resources for Additional Help and Information

Edited by Amy L. Sutton. 600 pages. 2009. 978-0-7808-1034-1.

SEE ALSO Multiple Sclerosis Sourcebook, Muscular Dystrophy Sourcebook

Multiple Sclerosis Sourcebook

Basic Consumer Health Information about Multiple Sclerosis (MS) and Its Effects on Mobility, Vision, Bladder Function, Speech,

Swallowing, and Cognition, Including Facts about Risk Factors, Causes, Diagnostic Procedures, Pain Management, Drug Treatments, and Physical and Occupational Therapies

Along with Guidelines for Nutrition and Exercise, Tips on Choosing Assistive Equipment, Information about Disability, Work, Financial, and Legal Issues, a Glossary of Related Terms, and a Directory of Additional Resources

Edited by Joyce Brennfleck Shannon. 553 pages. 2007. 978-0-7808-0998-7.

SEE ALSO Movement Disorders Sourcebook, 2nd Edition

Muscular Dystrophy Sourcebook

Basic Consumer Health Information about Congenital, Childhood-Onset, and Adult-Onset Forms of Muscular Dystrophy, Such as Duchenne, Becker, Emery-Dreifuss, Distal, Limb-Girdle, Facioscapulohumeral (FSHD), Myotonic, and Ophthalmoplegic Muscular Dystrophies, Including Facts about Diagnostic Tests, Medical and Physical Therapies, Management of Co-Occurring Conditions, and Parenting Guidelines

Along with Practical Tips for Home Care, a Glossary, and Directories of Additional Resources

Edited by Joyce Brennfleck Shannon. 552 pages. 2004. 978-0-7808-0676-4.

"This book is highly recommended for public and academic libraries as well as health care offices that support the information needs of patients and their families."
—E-Streams, Apr '05

"Excellent reference."
—The Bookwatch, Jan '05

SEE ALSO Movement Disorders Sourcebook, 2nd Edition

Obesity Sourcebook

Basic Consumer Health Information about Diseases and Other Problems Associated with Obesity, and Including Facts about Risk Factors, Prevention Issues, and Management Approaches

Along with Statistical and Demographic Data, Information about Special Populations,

Research Updates, a Glossary, and Source Listings for Further Help and Information

Edited by Wilma Caldwell and Chad T. Kimball. 360 pages. 2001. 978-0-7808-0333-6.

"The book synthesizes the reliable medical literature on obesity into one easy-to-read and useful resource for the general public."
—American Reference Books Annual, 2002

"Well suited for the health reference collection of a public library or an academic health science library that serves the general population."
—E-Streams, Sep '01

Osteoporosis Sourcebook

Basic Consumer Health Information about Primary and Secondary Osteoporosis and Juvenile Osteoporosis and Related Conditions, Including Fibrous Dysplasia, Gaucher Disease, Hyperthyroidism, Hypophosphatasia, Myeloma, Osteopetrosis, Osteogenesis Imperfecta, and Paget's Disease

Along with Information about Risk Factors, Treatments, Traditional and Non-Traditional Pain Management, a Glossary of Related Terms, and a Directory of Resources

Edited by Allan R. Cook. 568 pages. 2001. 978-0-7808-0239-1.

"This resource is recommended as a great reference source for public, health, and academic libraries, and is another triumph for the editors of Omnigraphics."
—American Reference Books Annual, 2002

"Will prove valuable to any library seeking to maintain a current, comprehensive reference collection of health resources. . . . From prevention to treatment and associated conditions, this provides an excellent survey."
—The Bookwatch, Aug '01

SEE ALSO Healthy Aging Sourcebook, Women's Health Concerns Sourcebook, 3rd Edition

Pain Sourcebook, 3rd Edition

Basic Consumer Health Information about Acute and Chronic Pain, Including Nerve Pain, Bone Pain, Muscle Pain, Cancer Pain, and Disorders Characterized by Pain, Such as Arthritis, Temporomandibular Muscle and Joint (TMJ) Disorder, Carpal Tunnel Syndrome,

Headaches, Heartburn, Sciatica, and Shingles, and Facts about Diagnostic Tests and Treatment Options for Pain, Including Over-the-Counter and Prescription Drugs, Physical Rehabilitation, Injection and Infusion Therapies, Implantable Technologies, and Complementary Medicine

Along with Tips for Living with Pain, a Glossary of Related Terms, and a Directory of Additional Resources

Edited by Joyce Brennfleck Shannon. 644 pages. 2008. 978-0-7808-1006-8.

"Excellent for ready-reference users and can be used for beginning students in health fields . . . appropriate for the consumer health collection in both public and academic libraries."
—ARBAonline, Nov '08

Pediatric Cancer Sourcebook

Basic Consumer Health Information about Leukemias, Brain Tumors, Sarcomas, Lymphomas, and Other Cancers in Infants, Children, and Adolescents, Including Descriptions of Cancers, Treatments, and Coping Strategies

Along with Suggestions for Parents, Caregivers, and Concerned Relatives, a Glossary of Cancer Terms, and Resource Listings

Edited by Edward J. Prucha. 575 pages. 1999. 978-0-7808-0245-2.

"An excellent source of information. Recommended for public, hospital, and health science libraries with consumer health collections."
—E-Streams, Jun '00

"A valuable addition to all libraries specializing in health services and many public libraries."
—American Reference Books Annual, 2000

SEE ALSO Childhood Diseases and Disorders Sourcebook, 2nd Edition, Healthy Children Sourcebook

Physical and Mental Issues in Aging Sourcebook

Basic Consumer Health Information on Physical and Mental Disorders Associated with the Aging Process, Including Concerns about Cardiovascular Disease, Pulmonary Disease, Oral Health, Digestive Disorders, Musculoskeletal and Skin Disorders, Metabolic

Changes, Sexual and Reproductive Issues, and Changes in Vision, Hearing, and Other Senses

Along with Data about Longevity and Causes of Death, Information on Acute and Chronic Pain, Descriptions of Mental Concerns, a Glossary of Terms, and Resource Listings for Additional Help

Edited by Jenifer Swanson. 660 pages. 1999. 978-0-7808-0233-9.

"This is a treasure of health information for the layperson."
—CHOICE Health Sciences Supplement, May '00

"Recommended for public libraries."
—American Reference Books Annual, 2000

SEE ALSO Healthy Aging Sourcebook

Podiatry Sourcebook, 2nd Edition

Basic Consumer Health Information about Disorders, Diseases, and Deformities that Affect the Foot and Ankle, Including Sprains, Corns, Calluses, Bunions, Plantar Warts, Plantar Fasciitis, Neuromas, Clubfoot, Flat Feet, Achilles Tendonitis, and Much More

Along with Information about Selecting a Foot Care Specialist, Foot Fitness, Shoes and Socks, Diagnostic Tests and Corrective Procedures, Financial Assistance for Corrective Devices, a Glossary of Related Terms, and a Directory of Resources for Additional Help and Information

Edited by Ivy L. Alexander. 516 pages. 2007. 978-0-7808-0944-4.

"An excellent resource. . . . Although there have been various types of 'foot books' published in the past, none are as comprehensive as this one. 5 Stars (out of 5)!"
—Doody's Review Service, 2007

"Perfect for both health libraries and general-interest lending collections."
—Internet Bookwatch, Jul '07

Pregnancy and Birth Sourcebook, 3rd Edition

Basic Consumer Health Information about Pregnancy and Fetal Development, Including Facts about Fertility and Conception, Physical

and Emotional Changes during Pregnancy, Prenatal Care and Diagnostic Tests, High-Risk Pregnancies and Complications, Labor, Delivery, and the Postpartum Period

Along with Tips on Maintaining Health and Wellness during Pregnancy and Caring for Newborn Infants, a Glossary of Related Terms, and Directories of Resources for Additional Help and Information

Edited by Amy L. Sutton. 600 pages. 2009. 978-0-7808-1074-7.

SEE ALSO Breastfeeding Sourcebook, Congenital Disorders Sourcebook, 2nd Edition, Family Planning Sourcebook, Women's Health Concerns Sourcebook, 3rd Edition

Prostate and Urological Disorders Sourcebook

Basic Consumer Health Information about Urogenital and Sexual Disorders in Men, Including Prostate and Other Andrological Cancers, Prostatitis, Benign Prostatic Hyperplasia, Testicular and Penile Trauma, Cryptorchidism, Peyronie Disease, Erectile Dysfunction, and Male Factor Infertility, and Facts about Commonly Used Tests and Procedures, Such as Prostatectomy, Vasectomy, Vasectomy Reversal, Penile Implants, and Semen Analysis

Along with a Glossary of Andrological Terms and a Directory of Resources for Additional Information

Edited by Karen Bellenir. 604 pages. 2006. 978-0-7808-0797-6.

"Certain to be a popular pick among library reference holdings. . . . No prior knowledge is assumed for any of the conditions or terms herein, making it a most accessible general-interest reference."
—California Bookwatch, Apr '06

SEE ALSO Men's Health Concerns Sourcebook, 3rd Edition, Urinary Tract and Kidney Diseases and Disorders Sourcebook, 2nd Edition

Prostate Cancer Sourcebook

Basic Consumer Health Information about Prostate Cancer, Including Information about the Associated Risk Factors, Detection, Diagnosis, and Treatment of Prostate Cancer

Along with Information on Non-Malignant Prostate Conditions, and Featuring a Section

Listing Support and Treatment Centers and a Glossary of Related Terms

Edited by Dawn D. Matthews. 340 pages. 2001. 978-0-7808-0324-4.

"Recommended reference source."
—Booklist, Jan '02

"A valuable resource for health care consumers seeking information on the subject. . . . All text is written in a clear, easy-to-understand language that avoids technical jargon. Any library that collects consumer health resources would strengthen their collection with the addition of the *Prostate Cancer Sourcebook*."
—American Reference Books Annual, 2002

SEE ALSO Cancer Sourcebook, 5th Edition, Men's Health Concerns Sourcebook, 3rd Edition

Rehabilitation Sourcebook

Basic Consumer Health Information about Rehabilitation for People Recovering from Heart Surgery, Spinal Cord Injury, Stroke, Orthopedic Impairments, Amputation, Pulmonary Impairments, Traumatic Injury, and More, Including Physical Therapy, Occupational Therapy, Speech/Language Therapy, Massage Therapy, Dance Therapy, Art Therapy, and Recreational Therapy

Along with Information on Assistive and Adaptive Devices, a Glossary, and Resources for Additional Help and Information

Edited by Dawn D. Matthews. 519 pages. 2000. 978-0-7808-0236-0.

"This is an excellent resource for public library reference and health collections."
—American Reference Books Annual, 2001

"Recommended reference source."
—Booklist, May '00

Respiratory Disorders Sourcebook, 2nd Edition

Basic Consumer Health Information about Infectious, Inflammatory, and Chronic Conditions Affecting the Lungs and Respiratory System, Including Pneumonia, Bronchitis, Influenza, Tuberculosis, Sarcoidosis, Asthma, Cystic Fibrosis, Chronic Obstructive Pulmonary Disease, Lung Abscesses, Pulmonary Embolism, Occupational Lung Diseases, and Other Bacterial, Viral, and Fungal Infections

Along with Facts about the Structure and Function of the Lungs and Airways, Methods of Diagnosing Respiratory Disorders, and Treatment and Rehabilitation Options, a Glossary of Related Terms, and a Directory of Resources for Additional Help and Information

Edited by Sandra L. Judd. 638 pages. 2008. 978-0-7808-1007-5.

"A great addition for public and school libraries because it provides concise health information . . . readers can start with this reference source and get satisfactory answers before proceeding to other medical reference tools for more in depth information . . . A good guide for health education on lung disorders."
—ARBAonline, Nov '08

SEE ALSO Lung Disorders Sourcebook

Sexually Transmitted Diseases Sourcebook, 4th Edition

Basic Consumer Health Information about Chlamydial Infections, Gonorrhea, Hepatitis, Herpes, HIV/AIDS, Human Papillomavirus, Pubic Lice, Scabies, Syphilis, Trichomoniasis, Vaginal Infections, and Other Sexually Transmitted Diseases, Including Facts about Risk Factors, Symptoms, Diagnosis, Treatment, and the Prevention of Sexually Transmitted Infections

Along with Updates on Current Research Initiatives, a Glossary of Related Terms, and Resources for Additional Help and Information

Edited by Laura Larsen. 600 pages. 2009. 978-0-7808-1073-0.

SEE ALSO AIDS Sourcebook, 4th Edition, Contagious Diseases Sourcebook, 2nd Edition, Men's Health Concerns Sourcebook, 3rd Edition, Women's Health Concerns Sourcebook, 3rd Edition

Sleep Disorders Sourcebook, 2nd Edition

Basic Consumer Health Information about Sleep and Sleep Disorders, Including Insomnia, Sleep Apnea, Restless Legs Syndrome, Narcolepsy, Parasomnias, and Other Health Problems That Affect Sleep, Plus Facts about Diagnostic Procedures, Treatment Strategies,

Sleep Medications, and Tips for Improving Sleep Quality

Along with a Glossary of Related Terms and Resources for Additional Help and Information

Edited by Amy L. Sutton. 567 pages. 2005. 978-0-7808-0743-3.

"This book will be useful for just about everybody, especially the 40 million Americans with sleep disorders."
—*American Reference Books Annual, 2006*

"A welcome addition to public libraries and consumer health libraries."
—*Medical Reference Services Quarterly, Summer '06*

Smoking Concerns Sourcebook

Basic Consumer Health Information about Nicotine Addiction and Smoking Cessation, Featuring Facts about the Health Effects of Tobacco Use, Including Lung and Other Cancers, Heart Disease, Stroke, and Respiratory Disorders, Such as Emphysema and Chronic Bronchitis

Along with Information about Smoking Prevention Programs, Suggestions for Achieving and Maintaining a Smoke-Free Lifestyle, Statistics about Tobacco Use, Reports on Current Research Initiatives, a Glossary of Related Terms, and Directories of Resources for Additional Help and Information

Edited by Karen Bellenir. 595 pages. 2004. 978-0-7808-0323-7.

"Provides everything needed for the student or general reader seeking practical details on the effects of tobacco use."
—*The Bookwatch, Mar '05*

"Public libraries and consumer health care libraries will find this work useful."
—*American Reference Books Annual, 2005*

SEE ALSO *Respiratory Disorders Sourcebook, 2nd Edition*

Sports Injuries Sourcebook, 3rd Edition

Basic Consumer Health Information about Sprains and Strains, Fractures, Growth Plate Injuries, Overtraining Injuries, and Injuries to the Head, Face, Shoulders, Elbows, Hands, Spinal Column, Knees, Ankles, and Feet, and with Facts about Heat-Related Illness, Steroids and Sport Supplements, Protective Equipment, Diagnostic Procedures, Treatment Options, and Rehabilitation

Along with a Glossary of Related Terms and a Directory of Resources for Additional Help and Information

Edited by Sandra J. Judd. 623 pages. 2007. 978-0-7808-0949-9.

SEE ALSO *Fitness and Exercise Sourcebook, 3rd Edition*

Stress-Related Disorders Sourcebook, 2nd Edition

Basic Consumer Health Information about Stress and Stress-Related Disorders, Including Types of Stress, Sources of Acute and Chronic Stress, the Impact of Stress on the Body's Systems, and Mental and Emotional Health Problems Associated with Stress, Such as Depression, Anxiety Disorders, Substance Abuse, Posttraumatic Stress Disorder, and Suicide

Along with Advice about Getting Help for Stress-Related Disorders, Information about Stress Management Techniques, a Glossary of Stress-Related Terms, and a Directory of Resources for Additional Help and Information

Edited by Amy L. Sutton. 608 pages. 2007. 978-0-7808-0996-3

"Accessible to the lay reader. Highly recommended for medical and psychiatric collections."
—*Library Journal, Mar '08*

"Well-written for a general readership, the 2nd Edition of *Stress-Related Disorders Sourcebook* is a useful addition to the health reference literature."
—*American Reference Books Annual, 2008*

SEE ALSO *Mental Health Disorders Sourcebook, 4th Edition*

Stroke Sourcebook, 2nd Edition

Basic Consumer Health Information about Stroke, Including Ischemic, Hemorrhagic, and Mini Strokes, as Well as Risk Factors, Prevention Guidelines, Diagnostic Tests, Medications and

Surgical Treatments, and Complications of Stroke

Along with Rehabilitation Techniques and Innovations, Tips on Staying Healthy and Maintaining Independence after Stroke, a Glossary of Related Terms, and a Directory of Resources for Stroke Survivors and Their Families

Edited by Amy L. Sutton. 626 pages. 2008. 978-0-7808-1035-8.

"An encyclopedic handbook on stroke that is written in a language the layperson can understand. . . . This is one of the most helpful, readable books on stroke. This volume is highly recommended and should be in every medical, hospital and public library; in addition, every family practitioner should have a copy in his or her office."
—ARBAonline Dec '08

SEE ALSO *Hypertension Sourcebook*

Surgery Sourcebook, 2nd Edition

Basic Consumer Health Information about Common Inpatient and Outpatient Surgeries, Including Critical Care and Trauma, Gastrointestinal, Gynecologic and Obstetric, Cardiac and Vascular, Neurologic, Ophthalmologic, Orthopedic, Reconstructive and Cosmetic, and Other Major and Minor Surgeries

Along with Information about Anesthesia and Pain Relief Options, Risks and Complications, Postoperative Recovery Concerns, and Innovative Surgical Techniques and Tools, a Glossary of Related Terms, and a Directory of Additional Resources

Edited by Amy L. Sutton. 645 pages. 2008. 978-0-7808-1004-4.

"Large public libraries and medical libraries would benefit from this material in their reference collections."
—ARBAonline Aug '08

SEE ALSO *Cosmetic and Reconstructive Surgery Sourcebook, 2nd Edition*

Thyroid Disorders Sourcebook

Basic Consumer Health Information about Disorders of the Thyroid and Parathyroid Glands, Including Hypothyroidism, Hyperthyroidism,

Graves Disease, Hashimoto Thyroiditis, Thyroid Cancer, and Parathyroid Disorders, Featuring Facts about Symptoms, Risk Factors, Tests, and Treatments

Along with Information about the Effects of Thyroid Imbalance on Other Body Systems, Environmental Factors That Affect the Thyroid Gland, a Glossary, and a Directory of Additional Resources

Edited by Joyce Brennfleck Shannon. 573 pages. 2005. 978-0-7808-0745-7.

"Recommended for consumer health collections."
—American Reference Books Annual, 2006

"Highly recommended pick for basic consumer health reference holdings at all levels."
—The Bookwatch, Aug '05

SEE ALSO *Endocrine and Metabolic Disorders Sourcebook, 2nd Edition*

Transplantation Sourcebook

Basic Consumer Health Information about Organ and Tissue Transplantation, Including Physical and Financial Preparations, Procedures and Issues Relating to Specific Solid Organ and Tissue Transplants, Rehabilitation, Pediatric Transplant Information, the Future of Transplantation, and Organ and Tissue Donation

Along with a Glossary and Listings of Additional Resources

Edited by Joyce Brennfleck Shannon. 610 pages. 2002. 978-0-7808-0322-0.

"Recommended for libraries with an interest in offering consumer health information."
—E-Streams, Jul '02

"This is a unique and valuable resource for patients facing transplantation and their families."
—Doody's Review Service, Jun '02

Traveler's Health Sourcebook

Basic Consumer Health Information for Travelers, Including Physical and Medical Preparations, Transportation Health and Safety, Essential Information about Food and Water, Sun Exposure, Insect and Snake Bites, Camping and Wilderness Medicine, and Travel with Physical or Medical Disabilities

Along with International Travel Tips, Vaccination Recommendations, Geographical Health Issues, Disease Risks, a Glossary, and a Listing of Additional Resources

Edited by Joyce Brennfleck Shannon. 619 pages. 2000. 978-0-7808-0384-8.

"Recommended reference source."
—Booklist, Feb '01

"This book is recommended for any public library, any travel collection, and especially any collection for the physically disabled."
—American Reference Books Annual, 2001

SEE ALSO *Worldwide Health Sourcebook*

Urinary Tract and Kidney Diseases and Disorders Sourcebook, 2nd Edition

Basic Consumer Health Information about the Urinary System, Including the Bladder, Urethra, Ureters, and Kidneys, with Facts about Urinary Tract Infections, Incontinence, Congenital Disorders, Kidney Stones, Cancers of the Urinary Tract and Kidneys, Kidney Failure, Dialysis, and Kidney Transplantation

Along with Statistical and Demographic Information, Reports on Current Research in Kidney and Urologic Health, a Summary of Commonly Used Diagnostic Tests, a Glossary of Related Terms, and a Directory of Resources for Additional Help and Information

Edited by Ivy L. Alexander. 621 pages. 2005. 978-0-7808-0750-1.

"A good choice for a consumer health information library or for a medical library needing information to refer to their patients."
—American Reference Books Annual, 2006

SEE ALSO *Prostate and Urological Disorders Sourcebook*

Vegetarian Sourcebook

Basic Consumer Health Information about Vegetarian Diets, Lifestyle, and Philosophy, Including Definitions of Vegetarianism and Veganism, Tips about Adopting Vegetarianism, Creating a Vegetarian Pantry, and Meeting Nutritional Needs of Vegetarians, with Facts Regarding Vegetarianism's Effect on Pregnant and Lactating Women, Children, Athletes, and Senior Citizens

Along with a Glossary of Commonly Used Vegetarian Terms and Resources for Additional Help and Information

Edited by Chad T. Kimball. 337 pages. 2002. 978-0-7808-0439-5.

"Organizes into one concise volume the answers to the most common questions concerning vegetarian diets and lifestyles. This title is recommended for public and secondary school libraries."
—E-Streams, Apr '03

"Invaluable reference for public and school library collections alike."
—Library Bookwatch, Apr '03

"The articles in this volume are easy to read and come from authoritative sources. The book does not necessarily support the vegetarian diet but instead provides the pros and cons of this important decision. . . . Recommended for public libraries and consumer health libraries."
—American Reference Books Annual, 2003

SEE ALSO *Diet and Nutrition Sourcebook, 3rd Edition*

Women's Health Concerns Sourcebook, 3rd Edition

Basic Consumer Health Information about Issues and Trends in Women's Health and Health Conditions of Special Concern to Women, Including Endometriosis, Uterine Fibroids, Menstrual Irregularities, Menopause, Sexual Dysfunction, Infertility, Cancer in Women, and Other Such Chronic Disorders as Lupus, Fibromyalgia, and Thyroid Disease

Along with Statistical Data, Tips for Maintaining Wellness, a Glossary, and a Directory of Resources for Further Help and Information

Edited by Sandra J. Judd. 600 pages. 2009. 978-0-7808-1036-5.

SEE ALSO *Breast Cancer Sourcebook, 3rd Edition, Cancer Sourcebook for Women, 3rd Edition, Healthy Heart Sourcebook for Women, Osteoporosis Sourcebook*

Workplace Health and Safety Sourcebook

Basic Consumer Health Information about Workplace Health and Safety, Including the Effect of Workplace Hazards on the Lungs,

Skin, Heart, Ears, Eyes, Brain, Reproductive Organs, Musculoskeletal System, and Other Organs and Body Parts

Along with Information about Occupational Cancer, Personal Protective Equipment, Toxic and Hazardous Chemicals, Child Labor, Stress, and Workplace Violence

Edited by Chad T. Kimball. 610 pages. 2000. 978-0-7808-0231-5.

"As a reference for the general public, this would be useful in any library."
—*E-Streams, Jun '01*

"Provides helpful information for primary care physicians and other caregivers interested in occupational medicine. . . . General readers; professionals."
—*CHOICE, May '01*

Worldwide Health Sourcebook

Basic Information about Global Health Issues, Including Malnutrition, Reproductive Health, Disease Dispersion and Prevention, Emerging Diseases, Risky Health Behaviors, and the Leading Causes of Death

Along with Global Health Concerns for Children, Women, and the Elderly, Mental Health Issues, Research and Technology Advancements, and Economic, Environmental, and Political Health Implications, a Glossary, and a Resource Listing for Additional Help and Information

Edited by Joyce Brennfleck Shannon. 597 pages. 2001. 978-0-7808-0330-5.

"Named an Outstanding Academic Title."
—*CHOICE, Jan '02*

"Yet another handy but also unique compilation in the extensive *Health Reference Series*, this is a useful work because many of the international publications reprinted or excerpted are not readily available. Highly recommended."
—*CHOICE, Nov '01*

SEE ALSO *Traveler's Health Sourcebook*

Teen Health Series
Complete Catalog
List price $69 per volume. School and library price $62 per volume.

Abuse and Violence Information for Teens
Health Tips about the Causes and Consequences of Abusive and Violent Behavior
Including Facts about the Types of Abuse and Violence, the Warning Signs of Abusive and Violent Behavior, Health Concerns of Victims, and Getting Help and Staying Safe

Edited by Sandra Augustyn Lawton. 411 pages. 2008. 978-0-7808-1008-2.

"A useful resource for schools and organizations providing services to teens and may also be a starting point in research projects."
—*Reference and Research Book News, Aug '08*

"Violence is a serious problem for teens. . . . This resource gives teens the information they need to face potential threats and get help—either for themselves or for their friends."
—*ARBAonline, Aug '08*

Accident and Safety Information for Teens
Health Tips about Medical Emergencies, Traumatic Injuries, and Disaster Preparedness
Including Facts about Motor Vehicle Accidents, Burns, Poisoning, Firearms, Natural Disasters, National Security Threats, and More

Edited by Karen Bellenir. 420 pages. 2008. 978-0-7808-1046-4.

SEE ALSO *Sports Injuries Information for Teens, 2nd Edition*

Alcohol Information for Teens, 2nd Edition
Health Tips about Alcohol and Alcoholism
Including Facts about Alcohol's Effects on the Body, Brain, and Behavior, the Consequences of Underage Drinking, Alcohol Abuse Prevention and Treatment, and Coping with Alcoholic Parents

Edited by Lisa Bakewell. 400 pages. 2009. 978-0-7808-1043-3.

SEE ALSO *Drug Information for Teens, 2nd Edition*

Allergy Information for Teens
Health Tips about Allergic Reactions Such as Anaphylaxis, Respiratory Problems, and Rashes
Including Facts about Identifying and Managing Allergies to Food, Pollen, Mold, Animals, Chemicals, Drugs, and Other Substances

Edited by Karen Bellenir. 410 pages. 2006. 978-0-7808-0799-0.

"This is a comprehensive, readable text on the subject of allergic diseases in teenagers. 5 Stars (out of 5)!"
—*Doody's Review Service, Jun '06*

"This authoritative and useful self-help title is a solid addition to YA collections, whether for personal interest or reports."
—*School Library Journal, Jul '06*

Asthma Information for Teens
Health Tips about Managing Asthma and Related Concerns
Including Facts about Asthma Causes, Triggers, Symptoms, Diagnosis, and Treatment

Edited by Karen Bellenir. 386 pages. 2005. 978-0-7808-0770-9.

"Highly recommended for medical libraries, public school libraries, and public libraries."
—*American Reference Books Annual, 2006*

"Although this volume is nearly 400 pages long, it is so clearly written and well organized that even hesitant readers will be able to find the facts they need, whether for reports or personal information. . . . A succinct but complete resource."
—*School Library Journal, Sep '05*

Body Information for Teens

Health Tips about Maintaining Well-Being for a Lifetime

Including Facts about the Development and Functioning of the Body's Systems, Organs, and Structures and the Health Impact of Lifestyle Choices

Edited by Sandra Augustyn Lawton. 458 pages. 2007. 978-0-7808-0443-2.

Cancer Information for Teens, 2nd Edition

Health Tips about Cancer Awareness, Symptoms, Prevention, Diagnosis, and Treatment

Including Facts about Common Cancers Affecting Teens, Causes, Detection, Coping Strategies, Clinical Trials, Nutrition and Exercise, Cancer in Friends or Family, and More

Edited by Karen Bellenir and Lisa Bakewell. 400 pages. 2009. 978-0-7808-1085-3.

Complementary and Alternative Medicine Information for Teens

Health Tips about Non-Traditional and Non-Western Medical Practices

Including Information about Acupuncture, Chiropractic Medicine, Dietary and Herbal Supplements, Hypnosis, Massage Therapy, Prayer and Spirituality, Reflexology, Yoga, and More

Edited by Sandra Augustyn Lawton. 407 pages. 2007. 978-0-7808-0966-6.

"This volume covers CAM specifically for teenagers but of general use also. It should be a welcome addition to both public and academic libraries."
—*American Reference Books Annual, 2008*

"This volume provides a solid foundation for further investigation of the subject, making it useful for both public and high school libraries."
—*VOYA: Voice of Youth Advocates, Jun '07*

Diabetes Information for Teens

Health Tips about Managing Diabetes and Preventing Related Complications

Including Information about Insulin, Glucose Control, Healthy Eating, Physical Activity, and Learning to Live with Diabetes

Edited by Sandra Augustyn Lawton. 410 pages. 2006. 978-0-7808-0811-9.

"A comprehensive instructional guide for teens. . . . some of the material may also be directed towards parents or teachers. 5 stars (out of 5)!"
—*Doody's Review Service, 2006*

"Students dealing with their own diabetes or that of a friend or family member or those writing reports on the topic will find this a valuable resource."
—*School Library Journal, Aug '06*

"This text is directed to the teen population and would be an excellent library resource for a health class or for the teacher as a reference for class preparation. It can, however, serve a much wider audience. The clinical educator on diabetes may find it valuable to educate the newly diagnosed client regardless of age. It also would be an excellent reference and education tool for a preventive medicine seminar on diabetes."
—*Physical Therapy, Mar '07*

Diet Information for Teens, 2nd Edition

Health Tips about Diet and Nutrition

Including Facts about Dietary Guidelines, Food Groups, Nutrients, Healthy Meals, Snacks, Weight Control, Medical Concerns Related to Diet, and More

Edited by Karen Bellenir. 432 pages. 2006. 978-0-7808-0820-1.

"A very quick and pleasant read in spite of the fact that it is very detailed in the information it gives. . . . A book for anyone concerned about diet and nutrition."
—*American Reference Books Annual, 2007*

SEE ALSO *Eating Disorders Information for Teens, 2nd Edition*

Drug Information for Teens, 2nd Edition

Health Tips about the Physical and Mental Effects of Substance Abuse

Including Information about Marijuana, Inhalants, Club Drugs, Stimulants, Hallucinogens,

Opiates, Prescription and Over-the-Counter Drugs, Herbal Products, Tobacco, Alcohol, and More

Edited by Sandra Augustyn Lawton. 468 pages. 2006. 978-0-7808-0862-1.

"As with earlier installments in Omnigraphics' *Teen Health Series*, *Drug Information for Teens* is designed specifically to meet the needs and interests of middle and high school students. . . . Strongly recommended for both academic and public libraries."
—*American Reference Books Annual, 2007*

"Solid thoughtful advice is given about how to handle peer pressure, drug-related health concerns, and treatment strategies."
—*School Library Journal, Dec '06*

SEE ALSO *Alcohol Information for Teens, 2nd Edition, Tobacco Information for Teens*

Eating Disorders Information for Teens, 2nd Edition
Health Tips about Anorexia, Bulimia, Binge Eating, And Other Eating Disorders
Including Information about Risk Factors, Diagnosis and Treatment, Prevention, Related Health Concerns, and Other Issues

Edited by Sandra Augustyn Lawton. 377 pages. 2009. 978-0-7808-1044-0.

SEE ALSO *Diet Information for Teens, 2nd Edition*

Fitness Information for Teens, 2nd Edition
Health Tips about Exercise, Physical Well-Being, and Health Maintenance
Including Facts about Conditioning, Stretching, Strength Training, Body Shape and Body Image, Sports Nutrition, and Specific Activities for Athletes and Non-Athletes

Edited by Lisa Bakewell. 432 pages. 2009. 978-0-7808-1045-7.

SEE ALSO *Diet Information for Teens, 2nd Edition, Sports Injuries Information for Teens, 2nd Edition*

Learning Disabilities Information for Teens
Health Tips about Academic Skills Disorders and Other Disabilities That Affect Learning
Including Information about Common Signs of Learning Disabilities, School Issues, Learning to Live with a Learning Disability, and Other Related Issues

Edited by Sandra Augustyn Lawton. 400 pages. 2006. 978-0-7808-0796-9.

"This book provides a wealth of information for any reader interested in the signs, causes, and consequences of learning disabilities, as well as related legal rights and educational interventions. . . . Public and academic libraries should want this title for both students and general readers."
—*American Reference Books Annual, 2006*

Mental Health Information for Teens, 2nd Edition
Health Tips about Mental Wellness and Mental Illness
Including Facts about Mental and Emotional Health, Depression and Other Mood Disorders, Anxiety Disorders, Conduct Disorder, Self-Injury, Psychosis, Schizophrenia, and More

Edited by Karen Bellenir. 424 pages. 2006. 978-0-7808-0863-8.

"This excellent overview of the psychological disorders that affect teens provides clear definitions and descriptions, and discusses resources, therapies, coping mechanisms, and medications."
—*School Library Journal Curriculum Connections, Fall '07*

"A well done reference for a specific, often under-represented group."
—*Doody's Review Service, 2006*

SEE ALSO *Stress Information for Teens*

Pregnancy Information for Teens
Health Tips about Teen Pregnancy and Teen Parenting
Including Facts about Prenatal Care, Pregnancy Complications, Labor and Delivery,

Postpartum Care, Pregnancy-Related Lifestyle Concerns, and More

Edited by Sandra Augustyn Lawton. 434 pages. 2007. 978-0-7808-0984-0.

SEE ALSO *Sexual Health Information for Teens, 2nd Edition*

Sexual Health Information for Teens, 2nd Edition
Health Tips about Sexual Development, Reproduction, Contraception, and Sexually Transmitted Infections
Including Facts about Puberty, Sexuality, Birth Control, Chlamydia, Gonorrhea, Herpes, Human Papillomavirus, Syphilis, and More

Edited by Sandra Augustyn Lawton. 430 pages. 2008. 978-0-7808-1010-5.

"This offering represents the most up-to-date information available on an array of topics including abstinence-only sexual education and pregnancy-prevention methods. . . . The range of coverage—from puberty and anatomy to sexually transmitted diseases—is thorough and extensive. Each chapter includes a bibliographic citation, and the three back sections containing additional resources, further reading, and the index are all first-rate. . . . This volume will be well used by students in need of the facts, whether for educational or personal reasons."
—*School Library Journal, Nov '08*

SEE ALSO *Pregnancy Information for Teens*

Skin Health Information for Teens, 2nd Edition
Health Tips about Dermatological Concerns and Skin Cancer Risks
Including Facts about Acne, Warts, Allergies, and Other Conditions and Lifestyle Choices, Such as Tanning, Tattooing, and Piercing, That Affect the Skin, Nails, Scalp, and Hair

Edited by Edited by Kim Wohlenhaus. 400 pages. 2009. 978-0-7808-1042-6.

Sleep Information for Teens
Health Tips about Adolescent Sleep Requirements, Sleep Disorders, and the Effects of Sleep Deprivation

Including Facts about Why People Need Sleep, Sleep Patterns, Circadian Rhythms, Dreaming, Insomnia, Sleep Apnea, Narcolepsy, and More

Edited by Karen Bellenir. 355 pages. 2008. 978-0-7808-1009-9.

SEE ALSO *Body Information for Teens*

Sports Injuries Information for Teens, 2nd Edition
Health Tips about Acute, Traumatic, and Chronic Injuries in Adolescent Athletes
Including Facts about Sprains, Fractures, and Overuse Injuries, Treatment, Rehabilitation, Sport-Specific Safety Guidelines, Fitness Suggestions, and More

Edited by Karen Bellenir. 429 pages. 2008. 978-0-7808-1011-2.

"An engaging selection of informative articles about the prevention and treatment of sports injuries. . . The value of this book is that the articles have been vetted and are often augmented with inserts of useful facts, definitions of technical terms, and quick tips. Sensitive topics like injuries to genitalia are discussed openly and responsibly. This revised edition contains updated articles and defines sport more broadly than the first edition."
—*School Library Journal, Nov '08*

"This work will be useful in the young adult collections of public libraries as well as high school libraries. . . . A useful resource for student research."
—*ARBAonline, Aug '08*

SEE ALSO *Accident and Safety Information for Teens*

Stress Information for Teens
Health Tips about the Mental and Physical Consequences of Stress
Including Information about the Different Kinds of Stress, Symptoms of Stress, Frequent Causes of Stress, Stress Management Techniques, and More

Edited by Sandra Augustyn Lawton. 392 pages. 2008. 978-0-7808-1012-9.

"Understanding what stress is, what causes it, how the body and the mind are impacted by it, and what teens can do are the general categories addressed here. . . . The chapters are brief but informative, and the list of community-help organizations is exhaustive. Report writers will find information quickly and easily, as will those who have personal concerns. The print is clear and the format is readable, making this an accessible resource for struggling readers and researchers."

—*School Library Journal, Dec '08*

"The articles selected will specifically appeal to young adults and are designed to answer their most common questions."

—*ARBAonline, Aug '08*

SEE ALSO *Mental Health Information for Teens, 2nd Edition*

Suicide Information for Teens

Health Tips about Suicide Causes and Prevention
Including Facts about Depression, Risk Factors, Getting Help, Survivor Support, and More

Edited by Joyce Brennfleck Shannon. 368 pages. 2005. 978-0-7808-0737-2.

"Highly Recommended for libraries serving teenagers as well as those who work with them."

—*E-Streams, Apr '06*

SEE ALSO *Mental Health Information for Teens, 2nd Edition*

Tobacco Information for Teens

Health Tips about the Hazards of Using Cigarettes, Smokeless Tobacco, and Other Nicotine Products
Including Facts about Nicotine Addiction, Immediate and Long-Term Health Effects of Tobacco Use, Related Cancers, Smoking Cessation, Tobacco Use Prevention, and Tobacco Use Statistics

Edited by Karen Bellenir. 440 pages. 2007. 978-0-7808-0976-5.

"A comprehensive resource. Each chapter is written to stand alone, so students can dip in and use the information in each section for reports or to answer personal questions without having to read the entire book. . . . The book is packed full of statistics, with sources to help students look up more."

—*School Library Journal, Sep '07*

"Pulls together a wide variety of authoritative sources to provide a comprehensive overview of tobacco use for this age group. . . . This reasonably priced reference title should be considered a necessary purchase for all public libraries and school media centers, along with academic libraries supporting teacher education."

—*American Reference Books Annual, 2008*

SEE ALSO *Drug Information for Teens, 2nd Edition*

Health Reference Series